Cardiac Emergency Care

DATE DUE

NOV 1 2 1994	
MAR 2 8 1995	
AUG 2 4 1995	
MAR - 5 1996	
MAR 3 0 1996	
APR - 5 1999	
SEP 2 7 2001	
OCT 2 5 2001	
NOV 8 2001	

Cardiac Emergency Care

Edited by

Edward K. Chung, M.D.

Professor of Medicine
Thomas Jefferson University Hospital
Philadelphia, PA

Fourth Edition

Lea & Febiger • Philadelphia • London • 1991

Lea & Febiger
200 Chester Field Parkway
Malvern, Pennsylvania   19355-9725
U.S.A.
(215) 251-2230

Library of Congress Cataloging-in-Publication Data

Cardiac emergency care / edited by Edward K. Chung. – 4th ed.
   p. cm.
   Includes bibliographical references and index.
   ISBN 0-8121-1421-3
   1. Heart–Diseases. 2. Medical emergencies. 3. Coronary care
units. I. Chung, Edward K.
   [DNLM: 1. Coronary Care Units. 2. Emergencies. 3. Heart
Diseases. WG 205 C267]
   RC682.C367   1991
   616.1'2025–dc20
   DNLM/DLC
   for Library of Congress
                                                        91-6362
                                                           CIP

PRINTED IN THE UNITED STATES OF AMERICA

Print number: 5   4   3   2   1

Reprints of chapters may be purchased from Lea & Febiger in quantities of 100 or more.

To My Wife, Lisa
and
Our Children,
Linda and Christopher

PREFACE

Since the third edition of this book was published in 1985, considerable changes have occurred in the therapeutic aspects of various cardiac emergencies. This is particularly true in the management of acute myocardial infarction and other related problems, as reflected in "Acute Coronary Care" (Chapter 5), "Thrombolytic Therapy In Acute Myocardial Infarction" (Chapter 6), and "Coronary Angioplasty" (Chapter 7). These chapters have been expanded significantly and updated.

In addition, "Wolff-Parkinson-White Syndrome" (Chapter 9), "Cardiac Electrophysiologic Studies" (Chapter 22), and "Antiarrhythmic Drug Therapy" (Chapter 12) have been expanded markedly. New information, such as that on automatic implantable cardioverter-defibrillator (AICD), anti-tachycardia pacing, and treatment of life-threatening digitalis intoxication using digoxin-specific Fab antibody fragments have been added because every physician should be familiar with these new therapeutic modalities. The whole text has been revised considerably, although the basic aims and design of the book are essentially unchanged. The unique feature of the book is its practical approach.

The secretarial and editorial duties have been carried out cheerfully by Mrs. Maureen Gamble, personal secretary to the author. Her able assistance and efforts have been most valuable in the completion of this book. The endless cooperation of the staff of Lea & Febiger—and particularly of Mr. R. Kenneth Bussy, Executive Editor—is greatly appreciated.

Lastly, I owe deep gratitude and appreciation to my father, Professor Il-Chun Chung, M.D., who has always provided guidance and inspiration for me.

Philadelphia, Pennsylvania   Edward K. Chung, M.D.

CONTRIBUTORS

Marvin A. Bowers, III, M.D.
   Chief Resident
   Department of Cardiothoracic Surgery
   Thomas Jefferson University Hospital
   Philadelphia, PA
Chung Whee Choue, M.D.
   Research Fellow,
   Division of Cardiology
   Montefiore Hospital
   New York, NY
Edward K. Chung, M.D., F.A.C.P., F.A.C.C.
   Professor of Medicine
   Thomas Jefferson University Hospital
   Philadelphia, PA
Richard N. Edie, M.D., F.A.C.S.
   Professor of Surgery
   Director, Division of Cardiothoracic Surgery
   Thomas Jefferson University Hospital
   Philadelphia, PA
Edward D. Frolich, M.D., F.A.C.P., F.A.C.C.
   Vice President for Academic Affairs
   Alton Ochsner Medical Foundation
   New Orleans, LA
Soo G. Kim, M.D., F.A.C.C.
   Montefiore Hospital
   Associate Professor of Medicine
   Albert Einstein College of Medicine
   New York, NY
Jae Ki Ko, M.D.
   Assistant Professor of Medicine
   Chon Buk National University Hospital
   Chonju City, Korea

Cheryl C. Kurer, M.D.
    Assistant Physician
    The Children's Hospital
    Assistant Professor of Pediatrics
    University of Pennsylvania School of Medicine
    Philadelphia, PA
Hong Soon Lee, M.D.
    Staff Member
    Department of Medicine
    The National Medical Center
    Seoul, Korea
Charles E. Rackley, M.D., F.A.C.C.
    Professor of Medicine
    Georgetown University
    School of Medicine
    Washington, DC
Michael P. Savage, M.D.
    Clinical Assistant Professor of Medicine
    Thomas Jefferson University Hospital
    Philadelphia, PA
Se Woong Seo, M.D.
    Assistant Professor of Medicine
    Soon Chun Hyang University
    College of Medicine
    Seoul, Korea
Yi Shi, M.D.
    Research Associate
    Division of Cardiology
    Thomas Jefferson University Hospital
    Philadelphia, PA
Martha I. Spence, R.N., M.N., C.C.R.N.
    Instructor, University of Miami School of Nursing
    Patient Educator Instructor
    Staff Nurse
    Baptist Hospital
    Miami, Florida
Henry R. Wagner, M.D., F.A.C.C.
    Senior Cardiologist and Director of Outpatient Clinics
    Children's Hospital of Philadelphia
    Professor of Pediatrics
    University of Pennsylvania School of Medicine
    Philadelphia, PA
Andrew Zalewski, M.D.
    Clinical Associate Professor of Medicine
    Thomas Jefferson University Hospital
    Philadelphia, PA

CONTENTS

1

CORONARY ARTERY SPASM

Hong Soon Lee and Edward K. Chung

In the past decade, a considerable change in the understanding of the pathophysiology of coronary artery disease (CAD) has occurred. Particularly, coronary artery spasm has been recognized as a unique clinical entity in the production of myocardial ischemia. Coronary artery spasm was initially suggested by Sir William Osler, Keefer and Resnick. In the 1950s, however, the concept was abandoned as coronary angiography failed to demonstrate the evidence of coronary artery spasm in the development of myocardial ischemia. In 1959, Prinzmetal and his coworkers described the syndrome of variant angina pectoris and interest in coronary artery spasm was revived. They presented 32 cases of this distinct clinical syndrome; contrary to classical angina pectoris, chest pain occurred at rest without exertion, and was associated with the S-T segment elevation.

It is well established that variant angina is often brought on by spasm alone, but the spasm may be superimposed on an atherosclerotic stenotic lesion in the major coronary artery. In addition, various studies confirmed that anginal attacks can be induced by exercise in certain patients with variant angina pectoris.

Since the 1970s many researchers have tried to elucidate the mechanism of coronary artery spasm. Recently, the discovery of endothelium-derived relaxing factor (EDRF) has provided considerable light on this pursuit. Yet much of the mechanism remains to be uncovered.

Coronary artery spasm is now believed to play an important role in the genesis of a variety of CAD including variant angina, unstable angina, post-infarct angina, myocardial infarction (MI), post-percutaneous transluminal coronary angioplasty (PTCA) occlusion, post-operative cardiovascular collapse, and even exertional angina pectoris.

Thus, it is essential to understand coronary artery spasm in every respect for proper diagnosis and management of all patients with CAD.

This chapter will include detailed descriptions of the pathophysiology, diagnosis, and management of this unique cardiac disorder—coronary artery spasm.

I. DEFINITION
1. Coronary artery spasm refers to severe constriction of the epicardial coronary artery; the spasm is transient and reversible in response to stimuli. It may cause only mild constriction in healthy hearts.
2. Coronary artery spasm may occur in both mild and severe atherosclerotic coronary lesions.
3. Coronary artery spasm is the mechanism that leads to a decrease in myocardial blood flow, and the spasm often causes various symptoms of myocardial ischemia.

II. ETIOLOGY AND PATHOPHYSIOLOGY

Although the exact mechanism of coronary artery spasm is not yet fully understood, certain factors are thought to play a role in its pathogenesis. It has been shown that the constriction of the coronary artery per se does not necessarily lead to spasm of the artery. However, coronary artery spasm can result when constriction is compounded by: (1) local hypersensitivity response and/or (2) a series of triggering factors including platelet aggregating effect and platelet activating effect. Suggested mechanisms of coronary artery constriction are as follows.

A. Alpha-Adrenergic Receptor-Mediated Coronary Vasoconstriction

Both alpha- and beta-adrenergic receptors are known to be present in the coronary arteries. Sympathetic amines can directly give rise to vasoconstriction through alpha stimulation. Normally, the activation of alpha and beta receptors contributes to vasodilation. This process is probably endothelium-dependent. In the presence of CAD, such vasodilatory effects are markedly decreased because of endothelial damage. Therefore, sympathetic amines can provoke the constriction of the coronary arteries in patients with CAD.

B. Acetylcholine-Mediated Coronary Vasoconstriction

Acetylcholine, released during parasympathetic activation, is known to stimulate smooth muscles directly, thus contributing to vasoconstriction. At the same time, acetylcholine exerts endothelium-dependent relaxation effects, and normally these effects are prevalent in human coronary arteries. In patients with CAD, however, endothelial damage results in the suppression of such vasodilatory effect. Thus, the parasympathetic release of acetylcholine may cause coronary vasoconstriction in patients with CAD.

C. Serotonin-Mediated Coronary Vasoconstriction

Serotonin has at least 2 different receptors, S_1 and S_2, in the coronary artery system. Coronary artery dilatation appears to be mainly caused by the S_1-mediated endothelium-dependent effect. On the other hand, direct effect of S_2 receptors provokes coronary artery constriction. Although S_1-mediated effect dominates in physiologic conditions, the situation becomes reversed in the presence of CAD. Damaged endothelium triggers the activation of the platelets which, in turn, releases serotonin, leading to coronary artery spasm.

D. Thromboxane-Mediated Coronary Vasoconstriction

Thromboxane, a product of arachidonic acid metabolism, can directly stimulate its receptors on the vascular smooth muscle cells, thereby producing muscle contraction. Also, acetylcholine has a platelet-aggregating effect. Thus, it can induce coronary artery constriction via thromboxane receptors, platelet aggregating effect, and platelet activating effect. Furthermore, damaged endothelium cannot produce prostacyclin.

E. Physicochemical Stimuli-Induced Coronary Vasoconstriction

Hyperoxia decreases serotonin metabolism in the coronary artery. This may induce constriction of the artery. Histamine also can induce coronary vasoconstriction.

The intima of the artery has a defense mechanism against coronary constriction, coronary spasm, and platelet aggregation. Heparan sulfate, plasmin, prostacyclin, and endothelium-derived relaxing factor also can prevent thrombosis and spasm.

III. SYMPTOMS AND SIGNS

1. The majority of patients with coronary artery spasm have significant fixed coronary artery lesions.
2. Less frequently, spasm may occur in mild coronary artery lesions.
3. During episodes of chest pain, total or subtotal occlusion of a major coronary artery may occur.
4. During the coronary artery spasm, three-fourths of the episodes are reported to be symptom-free (silent).
5. The episodes of chest pain in classic exertional angina pectoris are frequently observed in the early morning to the early afternoon. On the other hand, variant angina pectoris has no circadian rhythm, although episodes occur more frequently around midnight and early morning.
6. During anginal attacks, significant cardiac arrhythmias may occur, and may lead to syncope or near-syncope.
7. During the episodes of chest pain, left ventricular dysfunction may occur and alter cardiac output. The skin is frequently diaphoretic, and the pulse may be irregular and weak. Rarely, pulmonary rales may be heard.
8. Coronary artery spasm should be suspected in any patient in whom signs and symptoms of myocardial ischemia de-

velop in the absence of an increased myocardial oxygen demand.

IV. LABORATORY FINDINGS

  A. ECG Findings

    1. S-T Segment Changes

A typical abnormality is the S-T segment elevation during coronary spasm (Fig. 1–1). On rare occasions, the S-T segment depression may occur (Fig. 1–2). In some cases, no S-T segment changes may be seen. For example, during the left circumflex PTCA ballooning, only 40% may show S-T segment depression in leads V_1 and V_2 whereas 30% may show S-T segment elevation in leads II, III, and aVF or V_5 and V_6. Another 30% may show no changes.

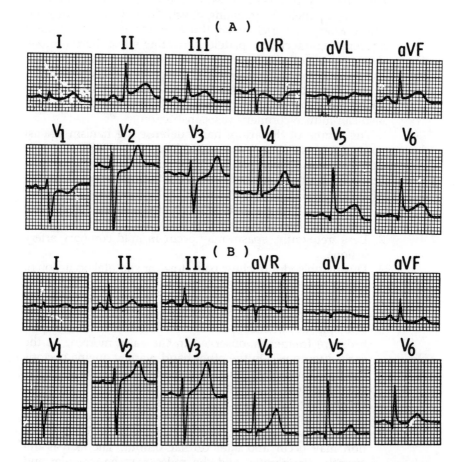

FIG. 1–1. *A,* 12-lead electrocardiogram during chest pain. S-T elevation in leads II, III, aVF, V_5 and V_6, and S-T depression in leads V_{1-3} indicate diaphragmatic posterolateral subepicardial injury. *B,* Following resolution of chest pain, the ECG reverts to normal.

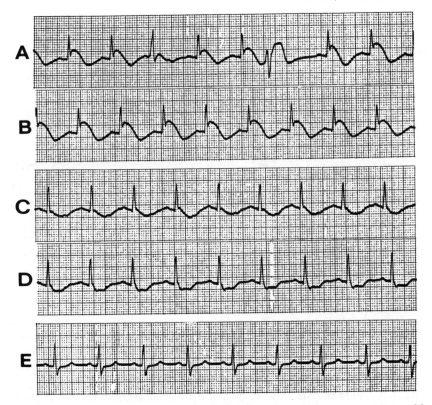

FIG. 1–2. These rhythm strips A to E (lead II) are recorded on a 56-year-old man with coronary artery spasm. The strips A and B, and C and D, are continuous in each given strip. The first 2 strips (A and B), middle 2 strips (C and D), and E are taken only few seconds apart. *A and B,* Sinus rhythm with a ventricular premature contraction and marked S-T segment elevation indicating subepicardial injury. *C and D,* Progressive S-T segment depression indicating gradual worsening of the subendocardial injury. *E,* Normalization of ECG (no S-T segment or T wave change). These ECG changes clearly confirm that coronary artery spasm may cause S-T segment elevation or depression in the same patient depending on the ischemic event that takes place predominantly in the subepicardium or subendocardium.

2. QRS Changes

   Transient Q waves have been reported during the episodes of coronary artery spasm.
3. Cardiac Arrhythmias

   The most frequently documented arrhythmias are ventricular premature contractions (VPCs), that may progress to ventricular tachycardia (VT) or fibrillation (Fig. 1–3). Other reported arrhythmias may include sinoatrial block, sinus arrest, and AV block. Less frequent arrhythmias are atrial premature contractions (APCs), supraventricular tachycardia,

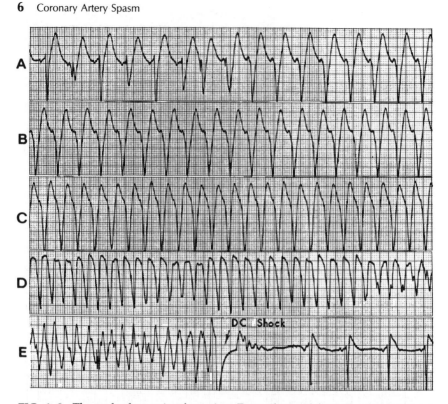

FIG. 1–3. These rhythm strips from A to E are obtained from the same patient (Fig. 1–2). The strips A to D are taken 1 to 2 seconds apart, and the strips D and E are continuous. Note that relatively slow ventricular tachycardia (strip A) progressively speeds up (from A to C), and finally ventricular fibrillation is produced (D and E). DC shock terminates ventricular fibrillation (indicated by arrow), and sinus rhythm is restored.

and atrial fibrillation (AF). During the resolution phase of coronary artery spasm, VPCs and slow ventricular tachycardia (nonparoxysmal VT or idioventricular tachycardia) may be observed.

B. Thallium Study Findings
Single or multiple defects appear in thallium-201 single photon emission computerized rotational tomography (SPECT), and the findings are usually transient and reversible.

C. Coronary Angiographic Findings
  1. Angiography may reveal subtotal or total occlusion of a short or long segment of the coronary artery, which is transient and reversible. The same findings are often induced by various provocative tests (See Diagnosis).
  2. Single or multivessel coronary artery spasm can occur, and can be induced by certain stimuli.

V. DIAGNOSIS
  A. History and Physical Examination
    The diagnosis of coronary artery spasm is based upon the patient's detailed history and physical examination. Attention should be paid to resting anginal pain that is accompanied by increased heart rate or blood pressure, but is promptly reversed by nitroglycerin. It should be noted, however, that coronary artery spasm may be provoked by physical exercise.
  B. Electrocardiogram (ECG)
    A typical ECG finding is the S-T segment elevation, but sometimes S-T segment depression or no change can occur during the episodes of coronary artery spasm (Figs. 1–1 and 1–2). These findings are probably dependent on the location and degree of the spasm. Coronary artery spasm should be differentiated from many other clinical conditions that cause S-T segment elevation (i.e., acute pericarditis, early repolarization pattern, early stage of acute MI, ventricular aneurysm, etc.).
  C. Holter Monitor ECG
    Holter monitor ECG is useful in the diagnosis of symptomatic or silent coronary artery spasm by recognizing transient S-T segment elevation or depression, but one should always be careful about false positive and false negative findings primarily because of various artifacts.
  D. Thallium Test
    Thallium scan is especially useful in diagnosing simultaneous multivessel coronary artery spasm that can be induced by certain drugs or exercise ECG tests. In thallium scan, the S-T segment elevation in the ECG is important to diagnose coronary artery spasm. Unfortunately, however, the S-T segment elevation does not prove that the patient has coronary artery spasm in every case.
  E. Provocative Tests
    When the diagnosis of coronary artery spasm is equivocal because various symptoms are not characteristic or episodes of pain are infrequent, various provocative tests are indicated.
    1. Cold Pressor Test and Exercise (Stress) ECG Test
      Cold pressor tests are carried out as follows. Antianginal therapy is discontinued at least 24 hours before cardiac catheterization. The patient's hand and forearm are immersed in a slurry of ice water for 90 seconds. Serial injections of the study vessel are performed as a control, and then immediately before removal of the forearm from the ice water. These tests can provoke coronary artery spasm by employing alpha-adrenergic stimuli with a local hypersensitivity and/or a triggering mechanism.
    2. Dopamine Test
      Antianginal therapy is discontinued at least 24 hours before the test. Dopamine is infused intravenously at incremental rates of 5, 10, and 15 μg/kg/min for periods of 5 minutes

each. Dopamine is used to provoke alpha-adrenergic stimulation.

3. Acetylcholine Test

Antianginal therapy is discontinued at least 24 hours before the test. Acetylcholine is infused into the coronary artery at incremental doses of 10, 20, 30, 50, 80, and 100 μg for periods of 3 minutes each. Acetylcholine can induce smooth muscle contraction which leads to spasm of the coronary artery.

4. Ergonovine Test

Ergonovine is most commonly used to induce coronary artery constriction and spasm. Ergonovine is not a biogenic amine, but resembles serotonin in its characteristics. The sensitivity of the ergonovine test is around 95%. Studies should be done 24 hours after discontinuation of all antianginal medications. Ergonovine is initially administered 0.05 mg intravenously after a control arteriogram. The onset of the ergonovine effect usually occurs within 3 to 6 minutes after the injection, and the vasoconstrictive effect of ergonovine and the duration of the spasm may last at least 10 to 15 minutes. All coronary arteries should be visualized within 5 minutes, and a second dose (0.1 mg) may be given intravenously, if needed. Total cumulative doses of 0.3 mg can be used for the test. Adverse effects are hypertension, hypotension, severe nausea, vomiting, severe headache, and major arrhythmias (ventricular tachycardia, ventricular fibrillation, complete AV block). Therefore, an artificial pacemaker should be available during the ergonovine test. Presently, intracoronary ergonovine injection is commonly used in place of intravenous injection in order to reduce serious complications.

5. Hyperventilation Test

This test probably induces hyperoxia in the coronary artery and increases the level of serotonin in it.

VI. ROLE OF CORONARY ARTERY SPASM

Coronary artery spasm may predispose to the development of coronary artery atherosclerosis, and the spasm frequently involves atherosclerotic areas of coronary artery (arteries).

A. Exertional Angina Pectoris

1. Exertional angina pectoris is mainly related to oxygen demand. Variability of residual coronary flow reserve is thought to be responsible for myocardial ischemia.

2. Less commonly, S-T segment elevation may be induced by exercise. This finding strongly suggests coronary artery spasm, providing that the patient is not recovering from recent MI.

3. Coronary artery constriction, local hypersensitivity, and triggering effects are probably related to coronary artery spasm in exertional angina pectoris.

B. Unstable Angina Pectoris
   1. Unstable angina refers to angina pectoris of new onset or increased severity or frequency. These findings are reversible and transient.
   2. The S-T segment elevation or depression can occur during the episodes of myocardial ischemia. The S-T segment elevation may be observed at rest, but it may be induced by exercise.
   3. Rest pain has been demonstrated to have reduced blood flow rather than increased oxygen demand, and the pain may be related to coronary artery spasm.
C. Variant Angina Pectoris
   1. Variant angina pectoris is characterized by transient and reversible chest pain occurring at rest associated with S-T segment elevation or depression. However, effort-related chest pain can occur.
   2. Prolonged coronary artery spasm may predispose to the development of atherosclerosis of the coronary artery which can result in severe coronary artery stenosis.
D. Coronary Artery Spasm Induced by Percutaneous Transluminal Coronary Angioplasty (PTCA)
   1. Recently, PTCA-induced coronary artery spasm is found to be very important as the number of PTCA procedures increases.
   2. Acute closure of a balloon-dilated coronary artery during or after PTCA is probably related to severe intimal tear, flap, thrombosis, and coronary artery spasm.
   3. The same factors may be responsible for the restenosis of the balloon-dilated coronary artery.
E. Myocardial Infarction (MI)
   1. Probable underlying mechanisms of thrombosis in the coronary artery are atherosclerotic plaque rupture, ulceration, hemorrhage and/or platelet aggregation, and/or spasm.
   2. The majority of patients who develop acute MI show a severe atherosclerotic narrowing of the infarct-related vessel(s).
   3. Occasionally, insignificant stenosis may be observed on the infarct-related coronary artery.
   4. Rarely, mild luminal irregularity or normal angiogram may follow acute MI.
   5. These findings suggest that transient total occlusion can be caused by coronary artery spasm.
F. Post-Infarction Angina Pectoris
   1. Post-MI angina pectoris refers to the type of angina pectoris that recurs after chest pain (due to acute MI) has subsided. It may occur within 24 hours following the acute MI episode or after discharge.
   2. The main underlying mechanisms are thought to be atherosclerotic plaque, reduction in collateral blood flow, or coronary artery spasm.

VII. MANAGEMENT

In treating coronary artery spasm, the primary objective should be the prevention of myocardial ischemia rather than of recurrent attacks of chest pain because silent ischemia is not uncommon.

Prevention of myocardial ischemic episodes should result in a decrease of malignant ventricular arrhythmias and, probably, a decrease in the incidence of acute MI and sudden death.

It is extremely important to accurately define the underlying CAD, because all patients with coronary artery spasm superimposed upon fixed atherosclerotic obstruction (greater than 75% narrowing) appear to do poorly with medical therapy alone.

A. Drug Therapy

1. Nitroglycerin and Long Acting Nitrate

   a) The basic actions of nitrates are relaxation of vascular smooth muscle, predominantly in the venous system, and, to some extent, in the arterial system as well. In addition, these drugs are capable of dilating the coronary artery stenosis, especially eccentric lesions.

   b) Increased venous capacitance and reduced wall tension and afterload lead to a reduction in cardiac oxygen consumption.

   c) Intravenous, sublingual, long-acting, transdermal patch and ointment forms are available. These undergo considerable first-pass hepatic metabolism.

   d) The usual starting dose of isosorbide dinitrate is 20 mg/day, (3 to 4 times/day p.o.), and the dosage can be increased up to 480 mg/day. Tolerance is reported to develop during treatment.

   e) Side effects of nitroglycerin and long-acting nitrate are common, but generally tolerable. Headache, nausea, vomiting, hypotension, and reflex tachycardia may be encountered.

2. Beta-Blockers

   a) The basic actions of beta-blockers are a negative chronotropic-inotropic effect and a corresponding reduction of cardiac oxygen consumption. The beta-blockers are reported to protect the myocardium during transient coronary artery spasm.

   b) Other potentially beneficial effects are a reduction in catecholamine-induced platelet aggregation and ventricular arrhythmias.

   c) Intravenous and oral forms are available.

   d) The usual starting dose of propranolol is 40 mg/day (3 to 4 times/day p.o.); the dose can be increased up to 480 mg/day (in divided dosage).

   e) Side effects of beta-blockers are hypotension, bradycardia, AV block, congestive heart failure (CHF), and potential exacerbation of pre-existing coronary artery spasm.

   f) Therefore, current wisdom dictates that beta-blockers

should not be used without a vasodilator in patients with coronary artery spasm.

3. Calcium Channel-Blockers

   a) These agents are potent coronary vasodilators but relatively weak direct dilators of stenotic lesions.

   b) Their negative chronotropic-inotropic effects (e.g., verapamil, diltiazem) may be beneficial to reduce cardiac oxygen consumption.

   c) Nifedipine and verapamil also have been reported to have platelet inhibitory effects that may partially explain their antispasmodic action.

   d) The usual dose of verapamil is 80 to 120 mg 3 to 4 times daily; nifedipine is 10 to 30 mg 3 to 4 times daily; and diltiazem is 30 to 40 mg 3 to 4 times daily.

   e) Side effects of calcium channel-blockers are hypotension, bradycardia or tachycardia, AV block, CHF, headache, facial flushing, and leg edema. Calcium channel-blockers may induce coronary steal syndrome in some cases.

B. Surgical Therapy

   1. PTCA and coronary artery bypass graft (CABG) can be used to treat coronary artery spasm when maximal medical therapy fails to eliminate symptoms of recurrent myocardial ischemia.

   2. PTCA and CABG are effective in case of coronary artery obstruction. Although drug therapy significantly reduces coronary artery spasm, it fails to bring sufficient relief of coronary artery obstruction in many cases.

   3. Various complications related to CABG and PTCA may be observed.

VIII. PROGNOSIS

The natural history of variant angina pectoris is frequent exacerbation and remission. Successful reduction of symptoms may reflect appropriate therapy or a fortuitous diminution in the disease progress.

A. Fortunately, the total number of patients with coronary artery spasm is reported to be reduced in recent years. This trend is probably attributed to a ready availability of very effective antianginal drugs, especially calcium channel-blockers.

B. In a series of 100 patients with variant angina who were followed for at least 1 year, nearly 50% remained asymptomatic without treatment, and an additional 30% were symptom-free with proper drug therapy.

C. In patients with pure coronary artery spasm, spontaneous remission has been reported in 39%.

D. It has been reported that patients with less active disease are more likely to undergo spontaneous remission.

E. The incidence of MI is higher in patients with a fixed coronary artery stenosis of 90% or greater.

F. Sudden death, which is probably caused by ventricular ar-

Table 1–1. Commonly Used Calcium Channel-Blockers in the Treatment of Coronary Artery Spasm

Hemodynamic and Electrophysiologic Effects		Nifedipine (Procardia)	Verapamil (Isoptin. Calan)	Diltiazem (Cardizem)
Heart rate	Acute	↑	↑ ↓	NC
	long-term	NC	↓	NC or ↓
Total peripheral resistance	Acute	↓ ↓	↓	↓
	long-term	↓	NC	↓
Inotropic		±	↓ ↓	↓
AV Node	ERP	±	↑ ↑	↑ ↑
	FRP	±	↑ ↑	↑ ↑
Drug interaction c digoxin (increase in serum digoxin)		↑	↑ ↑	↑ ↑
Recommended doses		10–30 mg q 6–8 hrs	80–120 mg q 8 hrs	30–40 mg q 6–8 hrs
Onset of action		15 min (PO) 2–3 min (SL)	15–30 min (PO) 2–3 min (IV)	2 hrs 2–5 min (IV)
Duration of action		3–5 hrs	3–6 hrs	6–8 hrs
Maximum recommended dose		120 mg/24 hrs	480 mg/24 hrs	240 mg/24 hrs
Side effects		Leg edema, flushing, headache, dizziness, hypotension, GI upset, VPCs	Leg edema, muscle cramps, 2 to 3 AV block, hypotension	Headache, dizziness, bradycardia, GI upset, 2 AV block, VPCs
Contraindications		Hypotension, severe depression of LV function	Depressed LV function, AV block, digitalis toxicity	Depressed LV function, AV block, digitalis toxicity

ERP–Effective refractory period: FRP–Functional refractory period: PO–Peroral: SL–Sublingual: IV–Intravenous: q–Every: NC–No change: AV–Atrioventricular: LV–Left ventricle: GI–Gastrointestinal.

rhythmias, may occur in patients with significant fixed coronary artery lesion(s).

G. Long-term prognosis for patients with variant angina pectoris is relatively good. The improvement in prognosis is attributed to the proper use of calcium channel-blockers. Survival rates of 1, 3, 5, and 10 years during follow-up are reported to be 98%, 97%, 97%, and 97%, respectively. Thus, the prognosis seems to be improving in recent years.

H. The effects of antianginal drugs for myocardial ischemia may be evaluated by a Holter monitor ECG judging from S-T segment alterations.

I. Various provocative tests, (e.g., ergonovine test) can be used to evaluate the patient with silent ischemia without any therapy.

IX. CONCLUSION

A. Coronary artery spasm is now recognized as a unique clinical entity which causes various ischemic myocardial syndromes.

B. Coronary artery spasm may be associated with variant angina pectoris, unstable angina pectoris, and even stable angina pectoris. It also may involve dilated vessels after PTCA.

C. Various precipitating factors of coronary artery spasm are not fully defined. However, a local hypersensitivity reaction and triggering mechanism due to a complex interaction between vascular endothelium, smooth muscle, and platelets, may lead to coronary artery spasm.

D. Coronary artery spasm is reported to predispose to the development of atherosclerotic coronary artery lesions.

E. The ECG manifestation of coronary artery spasm is primarily S-T segment elevation, but S-T segment depression may occur on rare occasions. In some cases, no S-T segment alteration may be observed.

F. Various cardiac arrhythmias may be observed in association with the ischemic episodes, and may serve as markers for those patients who are at great risk of developing an acute MI, or even sudden death.

G. Those patients with significant fixed multivessel CAD are less likely to respond to medical therapy alone, and, therefore, PTCA or CABG should be seriously considered under these circumstances.

H. Patients with minimal underlying fixed coronary artery lesions usually respond to medical therapy, and the incidence of various arrhythmias is also reduced with medical therapy.

I. The primary goal of medical therapy is to eliminate all episodes of myocardial ischemia. However, the efficacy of the therapy is difficult to evaluate because of the high incidence of silent myocardial ischemia. Holter monitor ECG is useful to identify S-T segment alteration, especially in patients with silent ischemia.

J. Provocative tests are indicated to confirm the diagnosis of coronary artery spasm when the clinical and ECG findings are equivocal.

K. The total number of patients with coronary artery spasm is significantly reduced in recent years, primarily because of a ready availability of effective calcium channel-blockers.

L. The underlying mechanisms for the production of coronary artery spasm are still not fully understood. Continued efforts should be made to uncover the etiology and pathophysiology of vasospastic CAD.

ACKNOWLEDGMENT

We would like to express our sincere appreciation to Jaeho Lee, M.D., for his valuable assistance in the preparation of this chapter.

SUGGESTED READING

Antman, E., Muller, J., Goldberg, S., et al.: Nifedipine therapy for coronary artery spasm. N. Engl. J. Med. *302*:1269, 1980.

Bassenge, E., and Busse, R.: Endothelial modulation of coronary tone. Prog. Cardiovasc. Dis. *30*:349, 1988.

Berry, C., Zalewski, A., Kovach, R., et al.: Surface electrocardiogram in the detection of transmural myocardial ischemia during coronary artery occlusion. Am. J. Cardiol. *63*:21, 1989.

Chahine, R.A.: Coronary artery spasm. J. Am. Coll. Cardiol. *7*:446, 1986.

Chung, E.K.: Coronary artery spasm. *In* E.K. Chung (ed.): Quick Reference to Cardiovascular Disease. Baltimore, Williams and Wilkins, 1987, p. 21.

Conti, C.R.: Large vessel coronary vasospasm: Diagnosis, natural history and treatment. Am. J. Cardiol. *55*:41B, 1985.

Crea, T., Chierchia, S., Kaski J.C., et al.: Provocation of coronary spasm by dopamine in patients with active variant angina pectoris. Circulation *74*:262, 1986.

Fischell, T.A., Derby, G., Tse, T.M., et al.: Coronary artery vasoconstriction routinely occurs after percutaneous transluminal coronary angioplasty. Circulation *78*:1323, 1988.

Giazier, J.J., Faxon, D.P., Melidossian, C., et al.: The changing face of coronary artery spasm: A decade of experience. Am. Heart J. *116*:572, 1988.

Hacket, D., Larkin, S., Chierchia, S., et al.: Induction of coronary artery spasm by a direct local action of ergonovine. Circulation *75*:577, 1987.

Hugenholtz, P.G., Mitchels, H.R., Serruys, P.W., et al.: Nifedipine in the treatment of unstable angina, coronary spasm and myocardial ischemia. Am. J. Cardiol. *47*:163, 1981.

Johns, J.A., and Gold, H.K.: Management of coronary reocclusion following successful thrombolysis. *In* E.J. Toppol (ed.): Acute Coronary Intervention. New York, Alan R. Liss, Inc., p. 95.

Johnson, S.M., Mauritson, D.R., Willerson, J.T., et al.: A controlled trial of verapamil for Prinzmetal's variant angina. N. Engl. J. Med. *304*:862, 1981.

Lo, Y.S., Lesch, M., and Kaplan, K.: Postinfarction angina. Prog. Cardiovasc. Dis. *30*:111, 1987.

Maseri, A.: Role of coronary artery spasm in symptomatic and silent myocardial ischemia. J. Am. Coll. Cardiol. 9:249, 1987.

Maseri, A.: Clinical syndromes of angina pectoris. Hosp. Pract. (March) 15:65, 1989.

Nabel, E.G., Ganz, P., Gordon, J.B., et al.: Dilation of normal and constriction of atherosclerotic coronary arteries caused by the cold pressor test. Circulation 77:43, 1988.

Nademanee, K., Intrachot, V., Josephson, M.A., et al.: Circadian variation in occurrence of transient overt and silent myocardial ischemia in chronic stable and comparison with Prinzmetal angina in men. Am. J. Cardiol. 60:494, 1987.

Okumura, K., Yasue, H., Horio, Y., et al.: Multivessel coronary spasm in patients with variant angina: A study with intra-coronary injection of acetylcholine. Circulation 77:535, 1988.

Prinzmetal, M., et al.: Angina pectoris 1. A variant form of angina pectoris. Am. J. Med. 27:375, 1959.

Redd, D.C., Roubin, G.S., and Leimgruber, P.P.: The transstenotic pressure gradient trend as a predictor of acute complications after percutaneous transluminal coronary angioplasty. Circulation 76:792, 1987.

Rocco, M.B., and Selwyn, A.P.: Circadian rhythms and ischemic heart disease with particular reference to transient myocardial ischemia. In B.N. Sing (ed.): Silent Myocardial Ischemia and Angina. Elmsford, NY, Pergamon Press, 1988.

Shell, W.E.: Nitroglycerin in the myocardial ischemic syndromes. In B.N. Sing (ed.): Silent Myocardial Ischemia and Angina. Elmsford, NY, Pergamon Press, 1988.

Sing, B.N., Josephson, M.A., and Nademanee, K.N.: Calcium channel blockers in therapeutics. In M.D. Cheitlin, et al. (eds.): Cardiology. Vol 1 (22). Philadelphia, J.B. Lippincott, 1988, p. 1.

Yasue, H., Ogawa, H., and Okumura, K.: Coronary artery spasm in the genesis of myocardial ischemia. Am. J. Cardiol. 63:29E, 1989.

Yasue, H., Takizawa, A., Nagao, M., et al.: Long-term prognosis for patients with variant angina and influential factors. Circulation 78:1, 1988.

Zalewski, A., Goldberg, S., Dervan, J.P., et al.: Myocardial protection during transient coronary artery occlusion in man: Beneficial effects of regional beta-adrenergic blockade. Circulation 73:734, 1986.

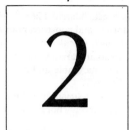

HEART FAILURE AND PULMONARY EDEMA

Se Woong Seo and Edward K. Chung

I. GENERAL CONSIDERATIONS

Heart failure is not a discrete disease entity but a syndrome characterized by the inability of the heart to pump an adequate blood flow to meet the metabolic needs of the body. It is not just cardiac dysfunction, but actually represents a final common pathway of several different causes.

When the cardiac dysfunction develops, compensatory mechanisms are implemented in an attempt to supply adequate blood flow to the body. By the time heart failure is fully developed, the clinical picture is dominated by symptoms and signs caused by those compensatory mechanisms that were previously beneficial. The major clinical manifestations reflect reduced cardiac output and a high diastolic filling pressure that often lead to fluid retention.

Congestive heart failure (CHF) is a common clinical syndrome and, in its advanced stages, a grave prognosis is expected. It is estimated that over 2 million Americans have congestive heart failure, and its prevalence increases with aging. Approximately 400,000 new heart failure cases develop each year in the United States. About 50% of patients with heart failure die within 5 years after the initial diagnosis, and 1 year mortality of severe heart failure approaches 50%.

II. ETIOLOGY

Heart failure can be produced by many different heart diseases. In emergency cardiac care, it is important to identify not only the underlying cause of the heart failure but also the precipitating factors.

A. Underlying Causes
  1. Loss of myocardial mass
     a) Ischemic heart disease
     b) Myocarditis
     c) Cardiomyopathy
     d) Infiltrative disease of the heart.
  2. Increased work load
     a) Pressure overload
        (1) Systemic or pulmonary hypertension
        (2) Aortic or pulmonary stenosis
        (3) Coarctation of aorta
        (4) Obstructive cardiomyopathy
     b) Volume overload
        (1) Valvular regurgitation
        (2) Atrial septal defect (ASD)
        (3) Ventricular septal defect (VSD)
        (4) Patent ductus arteriosus (PDA)
  3. Restriction of ventricular filling
     a) Inflow valvular obstruction
        (1) Mitral stenosis
        (2) Tricuspid stenosis
     b) Decreased myocardial or pericardial compliance
        (1) Constrictive pericarditis
        (2) Restrictive cardiomyopathy
        (3) Cardiac tamponade
        (4) Endomyocardial fibroelastosis
  4. Cardiac rhythm disturbances
  5. Others
     a) Endocrinopathies (e.g., thyrotoxicosis)
     b) Anemia
     c) Paget's disease
     d) Systemic or pulmonary arteriovenous fistula.

B. Precipitating Factors

The underlying causes may exist for a long time with little or no disability. In at least half of the cases, however, the manifestations of clinical heart failure appear when an additional burden is placed on a myocardium that is already excessively strained and has no additional reserve.

There are many precipitating factors which include:
  1. Arrhythmias
  2. Pulmonary infections
  3. Myocardial infarction (MI)
  4. Pulmonary embolism
  5. Anemia

6. Thyrotoxicosis
7. Pregnancy
8. Systemic hypertension
9. Excessive salt intake
10. Discontinuation of medication(s)
11. Emotional crisis.

These additional burdens should be sought in every patient with heart failure. Because the precipitating factors can usually be treated or corrected more effectively than the underlying causes, the prognosis will improve significantly when these precipitating factors can be identified and corrected. Obviously, the prognosis will be grave in patients with far-advanced underlying heart disease.

III. PATHOPHYSIOLOGY

As the heart fails, a decrease in cardiac output rapidly activates several compensatory mechanisms that tend to increase cardiac output back to normal and to maintain blood flow to vital organs.

The initial hemodynamic consequence of heart failure is a decrease in stroke volume. Stretch receptors in the carotid sinus and aorta are activated, causing reflex sympathetic changes in the cardiovascular system. The vasoconstriction caused by increased sympathetic tone increases venous return to the heart, resulting in an increase in end-diastolic volume. This increase in preload leads to an increase in stroke work in accordance with Frank-Starling's law. The arterial vasoconstriction due to increased sympathetic tone maintains systemic blood pressure and results in a redistribution of blood flow to vital organs, such as heart and brain, away from nonvital organs such as skin, kidney, skeletal muscles, and splanchnic organs. Sympathetic stimulation also increases heart rate and contractility, resulting in increased cardiac output.

The increased sympathetic activity and the decreased perfusion pressure in the macula densa due to reduced cardiac output activate the renin-angiotensin-aldosterone system. Dilutional hyponatremia due to antidiuretic hormone or diuretic therapy in heart failure can also activate the renin-angiotensin-aldosterone system. The renin released from the juxtaglomerular apparatus produces angiotensin I from angiotensinogen that was synthesized in the liver. Angiotensin I is converted to angiotensin II by an angiotensin-converting enzyme, which is located throughout the body but mainly in pulmonary capillary endothelial cells. Angiotensin II is a potent vasoconstrictor and contributes, along with the increased sympathetic tone, to the increase in peripheral vascular resistance and to the maintenance of blood pressure. Angiotensin II stimulates secretion of aldosterone, which increases sodium reabsorption in the distal tubule and collecting ducts of the kidney. It also stimulates the brain to provoke thirst and augments myocardial hypertrophy and the release of norepinephrine from the nerve endings. Initially the activation of this system is beneficial in maintaining blood pressure and cardiac output.

As the heart failure progresses, however, the increased peripheral vascular resistance due to increased sympathetic tone and angiotensin II make it more difficult for the heart to eject blood, resulting in decreased cardiac output. The increased venous return and increased ventricular end-diastolic volume and pressure due to increased sympathetic tone and activation of renin-angiotensin-aldosterone system may induce an increase in atrial, pulmonary venous, and pulmonary capillary pressure, resulting in transudation of fluid into the extravascular spaces of the lungs. When the amount of transudate exceeds the capacity of the pulmonary lymphatic drainage system, pulmonary congestion, hepatic congestion, and systemic edema may occur.

The increased heart rate and vasoconstriction from increased sympathetic tone and angiotensin II increase myocardial oxygen consumption and decrease coronary blood flow. This may aggravate the heart failure.

In patients with severe heart failure, the secretion of pituitary antidiuretic hormone, or arginine vasopressin (AVP), is increased. This is a potent vasoconstrictor and may cause systemic vasoconstriction.

The plasma atrial natriuretic factor (ANF) is increased in patients with heart failure. This is synthesized in atrial cells when atrial pressure increases. ANF has natriuretic, diuretic, and vasodilating effects and also inhibits aldosterone production. However, its importance in the pathogenesis of heart failure is not clear.

A chronic compensatory mechanism in heart failure is myocardial hypertrophy. Mechanical ventricular wall stress that results from chronic pressure or volume overload initiates protein synthesis in myocytes, resulting in an increase in the number and/or size of sarcomeres. The myocardial hypertrophy increases cardiac contractility and then raises cardiac output. There are 2 types of myocardial hypertrophy: concentric hypertrophy and eccentric hypertrophy. Concentric hypertrophy is present in patients with pressure overload; the ventricle maintains its normal ellipsoid shape, while wall thickness increases. Eccentric hypertrophy occurs in patients with volume overload, and the heart becomes spherical in shape. In the latter, as the heart failure progresses, the ventricle dilates further, and afterload increases progressively in accordance with the law of Laplace. Myocardial fiber shortening is also decreased as the ventricle dilates. The increased afterload and decreased myocardial fiber shortening induce reduction of cardiac output. In pressure overload, hypertrophy, myocardial contractility, and distensibility decrease, resulting in decreased cardiac output. Decreased coronary blood flow due to decreased cardiac output may induce myocardial ischemia in hypertrophied myocardium that consumes more oxygen than the normal heart. Myocardial ischemia impairs ventricular relaxation and may further decrease cardiac output.

IV. CLASSIFICATION
  A. Low-output and High-output Failure
    1. Low-output Failure.
      Cardiac output is decreased in most forms of heart failure secondary to congenital, valvular, rheumatic, hypertensive, coronary, or cardiomyopathic heart disease.
    2. High-output Failure.
      Cardiac output tends to increase in patients with heart failure secodary to thyrotoxicosis, anemia, beriberi, Paget's disease of bone, arteriovenous fistula, and pregnancy.
  B. Backward and Forward Failure
    These are based on the mechanical reasons for the clinical manifestations in heart failure.
    1. Backward Failure.
      When the heart fails, the end-diastolic volume of the ventricle increases; the pressure and volume of the atrium and venous system behind the failing ventricle become elevated. Retention of fluid due to increased systemic venous pressure results in systemic venous congestion and edema.
    2. Forward Failure.
      The clinical manifestations of heart failure are due to decreased renal perfusion secondary to reduced cardiac output, resulting in activation of the renin-angiotensin-aldosterone system. Activation of this system causes fluid retention.
  C. Right-sided and Left-sided Failure
    In patients with heart failure, fluid localizes behind the cardiac chamber that is affected first.
    1. Right-sided Failure.
      When the right ventricle is affected initially, fluid accumulates in the systemic venous system and produces systemic edema and congestive hepatomegaly.
    2. Left-sided Failure.
      If the left ventricle is affected first, the clinical manifestations are dyspnea and orthopnea due to fluid accumulation in the lungs.
  D. Acute and Chronic Heart Failure
    The clinical manifestations of the heart failure are dependent on:
    1. The rate at which it develops
    2. Whether enough time has elapsed for compensatory mechanisms to become operational and
    3. Whether enough time has elapsed for fluid retention in the interstitial space to occur.
  E. Systolic and Diastolic Heart Failure
    The heart failure can be caused by systolic dysfunction or by abnormalities in diastolic filling. These classifications are often useful in the early stage of heart failure. However, because of ventricular interdependence, the specific lesions that place an

abnormal load on one ventricle may eventually be responsible for failure of the other ventricle.
  F. Functional Classification of New York Heart Association
    1. Class I. No limitation of physical activity. Ordinary physical activity does not cause symptoms.
    2. Class II. Slight limitation of physical activity. Comfortable at rest. Extraordinary physical activity results in fatigue, palpitations, dyspnea or anginal pain.
    3. Class III. Marked limitation of physical activity. Comfortable at rest. Ordinary physical activity causes symptoms.
    4. Class IV. Inability to carry on any physical activity without discomfort. Symptoms may be present even at rest. With any physical activity, discomfort is increased.
      Although there are limitations, this classification is useful in comparing the general state of patients and at different times in the same patient.
V. CLINICAL MANIFESTATIONS
  A. Symptoms
    1. Dyspnea.
      The most common symptom of heart failure is dyspnea—breathlessness, or shortness of breath. Elevated pulmonary venous and capillary pressures cause pulmonary congestion, and then decreased pulmonary compliance. Breathing with noncompliant lungs requires more work, resulting in dyspnea. The shallow, rapid, breathing caused by activation of pulmonary receptors may also contribute to the development of dyspnea. Inadequate blood flow to the respiratory muscles also plays a role in the development of dyspnea. In the early stage, dyspnea is observed only during physical activity; however, as the heart failure becomes severe, it can also be seen at rest.
    2. Orthopnea.
      Orthopnea is defined as dyspnea that develops in the recumbent position. In the recumbent position, fluid moves from the abdomen and lower extremities to the chest, resulting in pulmonary congestion and reduction of pulmonary compliance. This occurs within several minutes of assuming a recumbent position and is relieved immediately by sitting upright with the legs dependent. In severe cases, dyspnea is so extreme that the patients cannot lie down and have to spend the night in a sitting position.
    3. Paroxysmal Nocturnal Dyspnea (PND).
      PND is severe dyspnea that occurs at night and awakens the patient from sleep. Patients may sit on the side of the bed or go to an open window to breathe fresh air. It takes more than 30 minutes in this position for relief to occur.
      Bronchospasm due to congestion of bronchial mucosa is commonly also present and associated with wheezing (cardiac asthma). A combination of nocturnal depression of the

respiratory center, increase in venous return to the lungs, and reduced adrenergic support during the night leads to pulmonary venous congestion and edema so that a sudden attack of severe dyspnea occurs.

4. Acute Pulmonary Edema (See below).
5. Cough.
    Cough usually occurs in chronic heart failure and at night. Edema of the bronchial tree or increased pressure on the bronchial tree by the dilated left atrium may cause cough.
6. Fatigue and Weakness.
    These symptoms are common but nonspecific, and they are related to the decreased blood flow to the skeletal muscles, at least in part.
7. Gastrointestinal Symptoms.
    Anorexia, nausea, abdominal distension and fullness, and abdominal pain are commonly observed. These symptoms may be due to congestion of the liver and the gastrointestinal tract.
8. Cerebral Symptoms.
    Confusion, difficulty in concentration, impairment of memory, headache, and anxiety may occur. These symptoms are usually observed in elderly patients with accompanying cerebral arteriosclerosis, arterial hypoxemia, and decreased cerebral perfusion.
9. Urinary Symptoms.
    Nocturia usually occurs in the early stage of heart failure. In the recumbent position at night, renal blood flow increases and urine formation increases. Oliguria develops in the late stage and relates to the markedly reduced cardiac output.

B. Physical Signs
    1. Cardiac Findings
        Point of maximal cardiac intensity (PMI) is displaced toward the left and often downward due to cardiomegaly. As the left ventricle dilates, the mitral valve leaflets fail to close properly, resulting in mitral regurgitation. If the right ventricle dilates, there may be tricuspid regurgitation as well. As pulmonary arterial pressure increases, the pulmonary component of the second heart sound will be accentuated. There may actually be a decrease in the pulmonary component if pulmonary regurgitation occurs.

        Ventricular gallop rhythm (protodiastolic gallop or S_3 gallop) occurs early in diastole during rapid ventricular filling, due to ventricular wall vibrations by the abrupt deceleration of blood flow. In children and young adults, this is a normal variant. However, after the age of 40 years, it is a reliable sign of heart failure. Left ventricular gallop is best heard at the apex in the left lateral recumbent position, and right ventricular gallop is best heard at the left sternal border in the 4th or 5th interspace in supine position. Atrial gallop is not a specific indicator of heart failure.

In patients with severe heart failure, the intensity of heart sounds may alternate between strong and weak beats (pulsus alternans). This is usually observed in patients with heart failure due to systemic hypertension, aortic stenosis, coronary atherosclerosis, or dilated cardiomyopathy. Pulsus alternans is caused by alternations in fiber length or alternating increase and decrease in the number of contractile units or both. Not uncommonly, pulsus alternans is associated with electrical alternans.

Sinus tachycardia is usually observed due to increased sympathetic tone. Other cardiac arrhythmias, such as atrial flutter or fibrillation, may occur as a complication in the course of advanced heart failure.

2. Rales.

Most rales, caused by transudation of fluid into the alveoli, are heard over the lung bases and are accompanied by some dullness to percussion. Wheezing and rhonchi may also be heard as a consequence of pulmonary congestion, excessive bronchial secretion, or bronchospasm.

3. Cheyne-Stokes Respiration.

This is a periodic breathing characterized by alternate periods of apnea and hyperventilation due to prolonged circulation time between lungs and the respiratory center in the brain. As the phases change from the beginning of apnea to that of hyperventilation, arterial PO_2 decreases from its peak to nadir, and arterial PCO_2 increases from its nadir to peak. During hyperventilation, arterial PO_2 increases from its nadir and PCO_2 decreases from its peak. The changes in arterial blood gases cause the periodic changes in respiration.

4. Abdomino-Jugular Reflex.

Jugular venous distension reflects systemic venous hypertension. Compression of the abdomen may increase venous return, resulting in increased jugular venous pressure and pulsation.

5. Cyanosis.

Decreased blood supply to peripheral tissues and increased oxygen extraction in peripheral tissues cause higher concentration of reduced hemoglobin (more than 5 gm/100 ml), resulting in cyanosis.

6. Peripheral Edema.

This occurs symmetrically and first in the dependent portions of the body. In the late stage, edema becomes massive and generalized (anasarca).

7. Hydrothorax and Ascites.

Pleural effusion from transudation of fluids into the pleural cavities occurs when systemic and pulmonary venous pressures are increased markedly. This is more frequently observed in the right pleural cavity than the left. Increased intra-abdominal venous pressure can cause ascites. Hypoalbuminemia due to malabsorption that combines with late stage heart failure may also contribute to the development of ascites and hydrothorax.

8. Hepatosplenomegaly.

Systemic venous hypertension may result in an enlarged, tender liver and, less commonly, splenomegaly. If there is tricuspid regurgitation, hepatic pulsation is palpable. In chronic heart failure, there may be jaundice caused by impairment of hepatic function and cardiac cirrhosis.

C. Pulmonary Edema

Increase in pulmonary venous and capillary pressures cause increased fluid flux across the alveolar-capillary membrane. Dilatation of pulmonary vessels competes for space with airways in the bronchovascular sheaths, resulting in airway compression. If the fluid' flux exceeds the capacity of pulmonary lymphatic drainage, fluid begins to accumulate in the interstitial space around the large vessels and airways, also leading to airway compression and thickening of alveolar walls. After the fluid fills the interstitial space, it begins to accumulate in the alveolar space, resulting in hypoxemia, hypocapnea, or hypercapnea, in severe cases.

This is the most dramatic symptom of left heart failure. The patient may sit or stand in upright position and is extremely anxious. The skin is cyanotic, cold, and clammy. Respiration is rapid and shallow, the alae nasi are dilated, and retraction of intercostal spaces and supraclavicular fossae is present. The patient coughs and expectorates frothy, watery, or blood-tinged sputum.

On auscultation, bubbling rales, wheezing, and rhonchi are heard over the whole lung field and may obscure the heart sounds and murmurs.

VI. LABORATORY FINDINGS

A. Routine Laboratory Tests.

Tests may show some abnormalities in the function of liver and kidney, but they are not diagnostic of heart failure.

B. Electrocardiogram.

Though there is no specific ECG finding of heart failure itself, an ECG may show right or left ventricular hypertrophy, atrial enlargement, or nonspecific S-T segment and T wave abnormalities according to the underlying heart disease. It may show ischemia or infarction if the underlying heart disease is coronary artery disease (CAD). At end-stage heart failure, there may be low voltage in QRS complexes. Some rhythm disturbances, such as atrial or ventricular premature beats or atrial tachycardia or flutter, may be seen. Atrial fibrillation (AF) is very common in patients with chronic heart failure.

C. Echocardiography

This cannot be used to diagnose heart failure itself. However, it is of great value in detecting the underlying heart disease, such as valvular or congenital heart disease, pericardial effusion, or mass in the cardiac chambers.

D. Radionuclide Angiography

Angiography is helpful in evaluating the cardiac function, but there is no specific radionuclide angiographic finding in patients with heart failure. It is useful in detecting the underlying heart disease, such as myocardial infarction (MI), or pulmonary embolism.

E. Chest X-ray

Cardiac chamber enlargement, pulmonary congestion, and fluid accumulation can be seen on chest films. If the pulmonary venous pressure is above the upper limit of normal (about 13 mm Hg), the pulmonary veins begin to dilate. Fluid begins to move from capillaries into the interstitial space of the lungs when it exceeds the normal plasma oncotic pressure (25 to 30 mm Hg). Chest film shows dilatation and redistribution of pulmonary vasculature. If there is interstitial pulmonary edema, the chest film often shows pulmonary clouding. Fluid accumulation in interlobar septa may be seen as a linear density usually up to 3 cm in length and 0.2 cm in width (Kerley's B line). This is usually seen in the base of the lungs, and it develops when the mean pulmonary arterial pressure exceeds 18 mm Hg. As the pulmonary venous pressure increases further, pulmonary edema may produce characteristic butterfly-shaped hazy density on chest film. The heart makes the body of the butterfly, and edema makes the wings. Free pleural fluid causes blunting of the costophrenic angles and is best seen on lateral film. In most cases it occurs bilaterally, but, when unilateral, it occurs more frequently in the right chest. The localized fluid accumulation in the interlobar spaces may produce mass or pseudo-tumor shadows on chest film.

F. Cardiac Catheterization

Catheterization is not diagnostic of heart failure itself but essential in detecting underlying heart disease.

VII. DIAGNOSIS

The diagnosis of heart failure depends on the history and physical examination because there is no specific diagnostic test for heart failure. In equivocal cases, electrocardiogram, echocardiography, cardiac catheterization, chest X-ray, or radionuclide angiography may be helpful.

VIII. DIFFERENTIAL DIAGNOSIS

There are many disorders which may mimic heart failure. Needless to say, the differential diagnosis is extremely important. Heart failure should be differentiated from the following disorders.

1. Pulmonary embolism
2. Bronchial asthma

  3. Chronic obstructive pulmonary disease

  4. Renal disorders

  5. Hepatic disorders

IX. TREATMENT

The proper management depends on the nature of underlying heart disease, the severity of heart failure, and the rapidity of its progression. Generally the treatment of heart failure includes the following.

  1. Control of the heart failure state: this is done by reduction of cardiac workload by rest and vasodilators, removal of fluid retention by diuretics, and enhancement of myocardial contractility by positive inotropic agents.

  2. Removal of precipitating factors.

  3. Identification and management of the underlying heart disease: this can be performed by specific diagnostic tests and therapeutic approaches. In some cases, a specific surgery may be necessary (e.g., coronary artery bypass surgery, correction of congenital cardiac defect, etc.).

A. Rest

Physical and mental rest are critical in the treatment of heart failure. The degree and duration of rest depend on the severity of heart failure. In many patients with mild heart failure, simple bed rest and mild sedation may result in recovery from cardiac failure. The hazards of phlebothrombosis and pulmonary embolism, that may occur with bed rest, should be reduced with anticoagulants, leg exercises, and elastic stockings. In any case, absolute bed rest is rarely required and heavy sedation is not necessary. A small dose of tranquilizers such as flurazepam (15 to 30 mg) or triazolam (0.125 to 0.25 mg) is helpful. In patients with marked anxiety, diazepam (2 to 5 mg twice a day) may be helpful.

B. Diet

A low salt diet is required. However, after the advent of potent diuretics, strict sodium restriction does not play an important role because it may make the diet unpalatable and because the diuretics can remove body sodium effectively. Weight reduction through restriction of caloric intake, especially in obese patients, will reduce the load placed on the myocardium.

C. Digitalis

For rapid digitalization, intravenous digoxin can be started with an initial dose of 0.5 mg given slowly over 10 to 20 minutes, and additional doses of 0.125 or 0.25 mg may be given every 3 hours. Thus, a total dose is usually 1.5 mg or less. In the oral route, the initial dose is 0.50 to 0.75 mg with additional doses of 0.25 every 4 hours. In most cases, maximum effect is accomplished by administering 0.5 mg daily for 3 days and then by a maintenance dose of 0.125 to 0.5 mg daily depending upon the patient's response. The therapeutic serum level is 1 to 2 ng/ml. Smaller doses are necessary in patients with renal failure, COPD, and elderly individuals.

Though digitalis is beneficial in most patients with symptomatic heart failure, it is of little benefit in patients with mitral stenosis with normal sinus rhythm, pericardial tamponade, constrictive pericarditis, cardiomyopathy, or myocarditis. At present, digitalis is less commonly used in the treatment of CHF because many other new drugs are available. Digitalis intoxication is discussed in Chapter 18.

D. Diuretics

Removal of fluid from the body is an essential component in the treatment of heart failure because most symptoms of heart failure are due to fluid retention. Removal of fluid is mainly achieved by diuresis. There are a variety of diuretics and their mechanisms of action are various.

1. Thiazide Diuretics

These are commonly used diuretics in the treatment of mild heart failure because of their safety and effectiveness by mouth. They inhibit sodium and chloride reabsorption from distal tubule and ascending limb of the loop of Henle. By inhibiting sodium reabsorption in the distal tubule, they prevent normal dilution of tubular fluid. The resultant increased sodium in the collecting duct augments the sodium-potassium exchange channel, resulting in increased secretion of potassium.

The prototypes of thiazide diuretics are chlorothiazide and hydrochlorothiazide. Their average daily dosages are 500 to 1500 mg in 2 to 4 divided doses and 50 to 150 mg in 1 to 2 divided doses, respectively. They are not effective when the glomerular filtration rate is below 30 ml/min.

Excessive or chronic use of thiazide diuretics may produce hypokalemic metabolic acidosis. Hypokalemia is a predisposing factor of digitalis intoxication (see Chapter 18). Therefore, it should be corrected by an oral supply of potassium chloride or by combined therapy with potassium-sparing diuretics. Other side effects are hyperuricemia and hyperglycemia. Rarely, patients may develop skin rashes, thrombocytopenia, and granulocytopenia.

2. Metozalone

This is a quinazoline sulfonamide derivative. It has site-of-action and potency similar to that of thiazide diuretics. The average daily dose is 2.5 to 10 mg as a single dose. Side effects are also similar to those of thiazide diuretics. In contrast to the thiazide diuretics, this medication is effective when the glomerular filtration rate is less than 20 ml/min.

3. Loop Diuretics

Furosemide and ethacrynic acid are the most potent diuretics currently available and are usually used in the treatment of moderate to severe heart failure, refractory heart failure, or acute pulmonary edema. Though these diuretics are quite different chemically, they inhibit reabsorption of sodium, potassium, and chloride in the thick ascending limb of the loop of Henle. They have rapid onset with short duration of action. They are effective in patients with hypoalbuminemia, hyponatremia, hypochloremia, hypokalemia, or reduced glomerular filtration rate and even in patients in whom other diuretics are not effective. Furosemide has some carbonic anhydrase inhibitor effect. The usual daily dosage is 40 to 120 mg orally or 20 to 100 mg intravenously. After rapid intravenous administration, significant vasodilation occurs before the onset of diuresis. The usual oral doses of ethacrynic acid and bumetanide are 50 to 100 mg and 0.5 to 2 mg, respectively. Bumetanide can be administered every 4 hours up to a daily dose of 10 mg. Nonsteroidal anti-inflammatory drugs, including aspirin, blunt the natriuresis of loop diuretics because of their inhibition of the prostaglandin-induced rise in renal blood flow that accompanies and sustains the natriuretic response to the loop diuretics.

Side effects include hypochloremic alkalosis, hypokalemia, glucose intolerance, hyponatremia, azotemia, and, rarely, hypocalcemia.

4. Potassium-Sparing Diuretics

These include aldosterone-antagonist (spironolactone) and direct inhibitors of collecting duct sodium conductance (e.g., amiloride, triamterene). The major site of action of spironolactone is the distal tubule. It is ineffective in the absence of aldosterone. It promotes natriuresis, water excretion, and potassium retention by depressing aldosterone-dependent sodium-potassium exchange in the distal tubule. The usual dosage is 25 to 100 mg 3 to 4 times daily by mouth.

Triamterene and amiloride are noncompetitive inhibitors of aldosterone that block sodium reabsorption and secondarily inhibit potassium secretion, even in the absence of aldosterone. The usual dose of triamterene is 100 to 200 mg daily and that of amiloride is 5 to 10 mg.

Since the diuretic effect of potassium-sparing diuretics is not so strong, they are usually used to prevent the hypokalemia which often occurs with the use of other potent diuretics. Major side effects are hyperkalemia, hyponatremia, and gastrointestinal disturbances. Spironolactone can also produce gynecomastia.

E. Vasodilators

Patients with heart failure may have increased systemic or pulmonary arteriovenous pressure that causes pulmonary congestion and decreased cardiac output.

Venodilators increase venous capacitance and decrease venous pressure, and, by reducing left ventricular preload, relieve the symptoms of pulmonary congestion. Venodilators do not increase cardiac output and should not be used when the pulmonary venous pressure is normal. Arterial vasodilators decrease arterial resistance and increase cardiac output. These agents should not be used, however, when the systemic arterial pressure is less than 100 mm Hg. Balanced vasodilators produce both venous and arterial vasodilation and tend to relieve pulmonary congestion and improve cardiac output. Hypotension is a major side effect of all vasodilator drugs.

A choice of vasodilators depends upon the pathophysiologic status of the heart failure. If the major symptoms are related to pulmonary congestion, venodilators such as nitroglycerine or isosorbide dinitrate should be the drugs of choice to be added to the standard therapy. If the major symptoms are due to decreased cardiac output, arterial vasodilators such as hydralazine, minoxidil, or nifedipine should be considered as vasodilators of choice. When the patient has combined symptoms due to pulmonary congestion and reduced cardiac output, balanced vasodilators such as captopril, prazosin, or sodium nitroprusside or combination of arterial vasodilator and venodilator should be added to the standard therapy.

1. Nitroglycerine—Venodilator

    This relaxes vascular smooth muscle directly. Usual sublingual dose is 0.3 to 1.2 mg. Vasodilating effect usually begins within 2 minutes, with maximum effect in 8 minutes, and persists 15 to 30 minutes. Intravenously, the initial dose is 10 μg/min and may be increased by adding 10 μg/min every 5 minutes to a maximal dose of 100 μg/min. Transdermal patches may be used for prolonged duration of action, and the usual dose is 5 to 20 mg. Because of tachyphylaxis, a 12-hour nitrate-free period should be allowed between uses of transdermal patches.

2. Isosorbide Dinitrate—Venodilator

    The usual sublingual dose is 2.5 to 10 mg every 2 to 3 hours, and the oral dose is 20 to 60 mg every 4 to 6 hours. Side effects of nitrates include headache and postural hypotension.

3. Hydralazine—Arterial Vasodilator

    This dilates arteriolar smooth muscle directly and increases cardiac output markedly in patients with heart failure. The usual dose is 25 to 100 mg 3 to 4 times daily. Side effects include gastrointestinal disturbances, headache, flushing, and lupus-like syndrome. Combination therapy with nitrate and hydralazine is proven to improve survival in patients with mild to moderate heart failure.

4. Prazosin—Balanced Vasodilator

    This is an alpha-1 receptor blocker and can produce the same hemodynamic effects as those of combined hydralazine and isosorbide dinitrate. But, there are no sustained long-term effects because of hemodynamic tachyphylaxis. The initial dose is 0.5 to 1 mg and then may be increased up to 10 mg 3 to 4 times daily. Side effects include postural hypotension with first dose, headache, nausea, rash, urinary incontinence, and dry mouth.

A newly developed alpha blocker, terazosin has the same effect as prazosin. Its usual dose is 1 to 3 mg daily.

5. Angiotensin-Converting Enzyme (ACE) Inhibitor—Balanced Vasodilator

Currently captopril, enalapril, and lisinopril are available in the United States. They produce vasodilation by blocking angiotensin-II-induced vasoconstriction. They also inhibit aldosterone production and breakdown of bradykinin, increase circulating prostaglandin, and decrease circulating catecholamine. In patients with heart failure, ACE inhibitors reduce left ventricular filling pressure, right atrial pressure, and increase cardiac output with little or no effect on heart rate and arterial pressure. They improve exercise tolerance and survival in patients with severe heart failure.

The action of captopril begins 30 minutes after ingestion, reaches peak at 1 to 1½ hours and persists for 6 to 8 hours. Enalapril and lisinopril have slower onset and longer duration of action than captopril. The initial dose should be low in order to avoid or minimize their hypotensive effect. The initial dose of captopril is usually 12.5 mg and then increased to maintenance dose of 25 mg 3 times daily. Enalapril is usually given 2.5 mg as an initial dose and the maintenance dose is 5 to 10 mg twice daily. The maintenance dose of lisinopril is 10 to 20 mg once daily.

Side effects of captopril include neutropenia, proteinuria, skin rashes, taste change, and hypotension. Enalapril and lisinopril may cause headache, dizziness, fatigue, and hypotension but they are relatively mild and rare. ACE inhibitors should not be administered with potassium-sparing diuretics or in patients with intrinsic renal failure or bilateral renal artery stenosis.

6. Nifedipine—Arterial Vasodilator

This is a calcium channel blocker. It reduces systemic vascular resistance and increases cardiac output in patients with heart failure. The usual dose is 10 to 30 mg orally every 6 to 8 hours. Side effects include headache, hypotension, flushing, dizziness, and edema.

7. Minoxidil—Arterial Vasodilator

The drug produces a substantial increase in cardiac output but does not increase exercise tolerance in patients with heart failure. Side effects include sodium retention and hirsutism. The usual dose is 10 to 20 mg twice daily.

8. Sodium Nitroprusside—Balanced Vasodilator

This is a vascular smooth muscle relaxant and is the most

widely used vasodilator in the treatment of acute CHF because of its short action time. This should be given intravenously. The initial infusion rate is usually 10 μg/min, and then may be increased by increments of 5 to 10 μg/min every 5 minutes until the desired effect is achieved or until the occurrence of hypotension or other side effects. The maximum dose is 300 μg/min. Adverse effects include hypotension and cyanide poisoning with high dose.

F. Nonglycoside Inotropic Agents
  1. Sympathomimetic amine
    a) Dopamine.
        This endogenous catecholamine stimulates myocardial contractility through its action on beta 1 adrenoceptors. Dopamine-induced vasodilation is not related to activation of beta 2 receptors, but is related to the action on specific dopaminergic receptors. Larger doses of dopamine cause vasoconstriction through the action on serotonin-sensitive receptors and on alpha 1 receptors. The effect of dopamine is dose-dependent. With the infusion rate below 2 μg/kg/min, dopamine induces renal, mesenteric, and coronary vasodilation. When the dose is increased to 2 to 5 μg/kg/min, it exerts a positive inotropic effect with little change in heart rate and a reduction or no change in total peripheral resistance. With the infusion rate of 5 to 10 μg/kg/min, arterial pressure and heart rate increase and renal blood flow may decrease.

        In patients with refractory heart failure whose blood pressure is normal, infusion usually begins at a low rate (0.5 to 1.0 μg/kg/min) and is increased gradually until the urine output, diastolic blood pressure, or heart rate is increased. Dopamine is widely used for the treatment of acute heart failure after cardiac surgery.
    b) Dobutamine.
        This is a synthetic cardioactive sympathomimetic amine that stimulates beta 1, beta 2, and alpha adrenoceptors. Myocardial contractility is augmented by the stimulation of alpha and beta 1 receptors. There is little change in systemic vascular resistance because of the stimulation of each of these receptors in systemic vascular bed. This does not activate dopaminergic receptors and does not release norepinephrine from adrenergic nerve endings. Dobutamine is not a renal vasodilator. The usual dose ranges from 2.5 to 10 μg/kg/min and maximum dose is 30 μg/kg/min.
  2. Phosphodiesterase Inhibitors.
      The membrane-bound phosphodiesterase is responsible for the breakdown of cyclic AMP to AMP, and the inhibition of this enzyme increases intracellular cyclic AMP, resulting in positive inotropic and vasodilator effects. They do not

inhibit Na^+-K^+-ATPase and do not act on adrenergic or histaminergic receptors.

a) Amrinone.

This is a bipyridine derivative. The vasodilating effect may offset the positive inotropic effects, resulting in little change in myocardial oxygen consumption. It is useful in patients with refractory heart failure with the combined treatment of digitalis, diuretics, and vasodilators. It is available only for intravenous use because of severe gastrointestinal intolerance after oral administration. The usual maintenance dose is 5 to 10 µg/kg/min after the initial bolus of 0.75 mg/kg. It is particularly useful in patients with myocardial depression after cardiac surgery or in patients with acute exacerbation of chronic heart failure. Adverse effects include gastrointestinal intolerance, fever, liver function abnormalities, and reversible thrombocytopenia.

b) Milrinone.

This drug is similar to amrinone except that it is more potent than amrinone and has a shorter duration of action and tolerance with oral administration. The usual oral dose is 5 to 7.5 mg every 6 hours daily.

The value and safety of phosphodiesterase inhibitors await further studies.

G. Heart Transplantation

Since the first heart transplantation in humans in 1967, increased expertise and progressive improvements in long-term result have occurred. This means that heart transplantation can be considered earlier in the course of disease in potential recipients. The potential recipients must have end-stage heart disease with severe heart failure and a life expectancy of less than 1 year. Candidates should be stable psychologically, under 55 years of age, still in good general condition, and should have a history of compliance with medical therapy, and strong family support. Contraindications include pulmonary hypertension, parenchymal pulmonary disease, recent pulmonary infarction, donor-specific cytotoxic antibodies, active infection, insulin-requiring diabetes mellitus, coexisting liver or renal disease, active duodenal ulcer, drug addiction, psychosis, continued excessive alcohol consumption, clinically significant cerebral or peripheral vascular disease, and other malignant disease. The 1-year survival is 80%, 3 years 70%, and 5 years 55%. The major practical problems are limited donor supply, rejection of graft, infection, and the high cost of heart transplantation.

X. MANAGEMENT OF ACUTE PULMONARY EDEMA

Acute pulmonary edema is a life-threatening condition and requires prompt management with many nonspecific measures.

1. Oxygen: 100% oxygen should be given, occasionally with the aid of mechanical ventilation.
2. The patient should be in sitting position.
3. Morphine sulfate diminishes the patient's distress, reduces the work of breathing and diminishes the central sympathetic outflow resulting in vasodilation: 3 to 5 mg of morphine sulfate should be given intravenously over a 3-minute period and then may usually be repeated 2 to 3 times at 15-minute intervals, if necessary. Naloxone should be readily available in case of respiratory depression.
4. Diuretics: furosemide or ethacrynic acid, 40 to 80 mg or bumetanide, 1 to 2 mg is given intravenously over a 2-minute period. With furosemide diuresis, the effect starts within 5 minutes with the maximum effect in a half-hour, and its effect persists for about 2 hours. Furosemide has direct vasodilating effect that reduces preload and afterload.
5. Vasodilators: nitroprusside given intravenously at the rate of 20 to 30 µg/min until the systemic blood pressure falls below 100 mm Hg reduces preload and afterload. Sublingual nitroglycerine 0.3 to 0.6 mg is given to reduce preload.
6. Digitalis should be administered if it has not been given previously. Digoxin 0.75 mg may be given intravenously. This is most useful when supraventricular tachyarrhythmias, particularly AF or flutter, are associated with acute pulmonary edema.
7. Aminophylline: when the response to other measures is not prompt or if bronchospasm and wheezing are prominent, aminophylline should be administered. The usual dose is 250 to 500 mg intravenously. In addition to relaxing bronchospasm, it may increase cardiac contractility and renal blood flow.
8. Reduction of preload by rotating tourniquets.

XI. PROGNOSIS

The prognosis of heart failure is related to the underlying heart disease, the precipitating factors, and the severity of heart failure itself. If the underlying or precipitating causes are detected and treated properly, the prognosis will be improved significantly. Severity of symptoms, degree of exercise tolerance, depression of left ventricular function, and circulating catecholamine level are related to mortality. Ventricular arrhythmias are also closely related to sudden death that occurs commonly in patients with heart failure.

Although the overall prognosis of heart failure has improved after the advent of vasodilators, such as ACE inhibitors, and through the correction of underlying heart disease, it remains poor with the annual mortality ranging from of 10 to 50% depending upon the severity of heart failure.

ACKNOWLEDGMENT

The authors would like to express their sincere appreciation to Ms. Gudrun Loercher for her valuable assistance in the preparation of this chapter.

SUGGESTED READING

Braunwald, E.: Introduction—A symposium on amrinone. Am. J. Cardiol. *56* (No. 3):1B–2B, 1985.

Chalmers, J.P., West, M.J., Cyran, K.E., et al.: Placebo controlled study of lisinopril in congestive heart failure: a multicenter study. J. Cardiovasc. Pharmacol. *9* (suppl. 3):589, 1987.

Cleland, J.G.J., Dargie, H.J., and Ford, I.: Mortality in heart failure: clinical variables of prognostic value. Br. Heart J. *58*:572, 1987.

Cohn, J.N.: Current therapy of the failing heart. Circulation *78*:1099, 1988.

Cohn, J.N., Archibald, D.G., Ziesche, S., et al.: Effect of vasodilator therapy on mortality in chronic congestive heart failure: results of a Veterans Administration cooperative study (V-HeFT). N. Engl. J. Med. *314*:1547, 1986.

Colucci, W.S., Wright, R.F. and Braunwald, E.: New positive inotropic agents in the treatment of congestive heart failure. Mechanisms of action and recent clinical developments. N. Engl. J. Med. *314*:349, 1986.

Conradson, T.B., Ryden, L., Ahlmark, G., et al.: Clinical efficacy of hydralazine in chronic heart failure: One-year double-blind placebo-controlled study. Am. Heart J. *108*:1001, 1984.

Copeland, J.G., Emery, R.W., Levinson, M.M., et al.: Selection of patients for cardiac transplantation. Circulation *75*:2, 1987.

Creager, M.A., Faxon, D.P., Cutler, S.S., et al.: Contribution of vasopressin in vasoconstriction in patients with congestive heart failure; comparison with the renin-angiotensin system and the sympathetic nervous system. J. Am. Coll. Cardiol. *7*:758, 1986.

Fioretti, P., Benussi, B., Scardi, S., et al.: Afterload reduction with nifedipine in aortic insufficiency. Am. J. Cardiol. *49*:1728, 1982.

Fouad, F.M.: Left ventricular diastolic function in hypertensive patients. Circulation *75* (Suppl. I):48, 1987.

Fowler, M.B., Alderman, E.L., Oesterle, S.N., et al.: Dobutamine and dopamine after cardiac surgery: Greater augmentation of myocardial blood flow with dobutamine. Circulation *70* (Suppl. I): I–103, 1984.

Francis, G.S, Goldsmith, S.R., Levine, T.B., et al.: The neurohumoral axis in congestive heart failure. Ann Intern. Med. *101*:370, 1984.

Hartman, A. and Saeed, M.: Phosphodiesterase inhibition in positive inotropic therapy of congestive heart failure. J. Appl. Cardiol. *1*:361, 1986.

Jordan, R.A., Seth, L., Casebolt, P., et al.: Rapidly developing tolerance to transdermal nitroglycerin in congestive heart failure. Ann. Intern. Med. *104*:295, 1986.

Kannel, W.B.: Epidemiological aspects of heart failure. Cardiology Clin. *7*:1, 1989.

Kromer, E.P., Riegger, G.A.J., Liebau, G., et al.: Effectiveness of converting enzyme inhibition (enalapril) for mild congestive heart failure. Am. J. Cardiol. *57*:459, 1986.

Massie, B.M., Kramer, B.L., and Topic, N.: Long-term captopril therapy for chronic congestive heart failure. Am. J. Cardiol. *53*:1316, 1984.

McFate-Smith, W.: Epidemiology of congestive heart failure. Am. J. Cardiol. *55*:3, 1985.

Packer M.: Therapeutic options in the management of chronic heart failure: Is there a drug of first choice? Circulation *79*:198, 1989.

Packer, M., Medina, N., Yushak, M.: Hemodynamic and clinical limitations of long-term inotropic therapy with amrinone in patients with severe chronic heart failure. Circulation 70:1038, 1984.

Parmley, W.W.: Pathophysiology and current therapy of congestive heart failure. J. Am. Coll. Cardiol. 13:771, 1989.

Raine, A.G.E., Erne, P., Burgisser, E., et al.: Atrial natriuretic peptide and atrial pressure in patients with congestive heart failure. N. Engl. J. Med. 313:533, 1986.

Sica, D.A., Gehr, T.: Diuretics in congestive heart failure. Cardiol. Clin. 7:87, 1989.

The CONSENSUS Trial Study Group: Effects of enalapril on mortality in severe congestive heart failure: Results of the Cooperative North Scandinavian Enalapril Survival Study (CONSENSUS). N. Engl. J. Med. 316:1429, 1987.

Timmis, A.D., Smyth, P., Monaghan, M., et al.: Milrinone in heart failure: Acute effects on left ventricular systolic function and myocardial metabolism. Br. Heart J. 54:36, 1985.

van Trigt, P., Spray, T.L., Pasque, M.K., et al.: The comparative effects of dopamine and dobutamine on ventricular mechanics after coronary artery bypass grafting: A pressure-dimension analysis. Circulation 70 (Suppl. I): I–112, 1984.

Wilson, T.W., McCauley, F.A., and Wells, H.D.: Effects of low-dose aspirin on responses to furosemide. J. Clin. Pharmacol. 26:100, 1986.

Wong, D.G., Lamki, L., Spencer, J.P., et al.: Effect on non-steroidal anti-inflammatory drugs on control of hypertension by beta-blockers and diuretics. Lancet 1:997, 1986.

c h a p t e r

CARDIOGENIC SHOCK

Charles E. Rackley

I. DEFINITION

Cardiogenic shock is the clinical syndrome accompanying acute myocardial infarction (MI) characterized by arterial hypotension and evidence of impaired circulation to the skin, kidneys, and central nervous system. The definition of cardiogenic shock employed by the Myocardial Infarction Research Unit Program is an arterial blood pressure less than 90 mm Hg or a systolic fall of greater than 80 mm Hg in a patient previously known to have hypertension. In addition to hypotension, evidence of cold, clammy, cyanotic skin, reduced urine production, and altered sensorium must also be evident. Other precipitating causes of shock, such as primary cardiac arrhythmias or hypotension due to administration of pharmacologic agents to a patient with acute MI, must be excluded.

II. GENERAL CONSIDERATIONS

Cardiogenic shock is the most serious complication of patients sustaining acute MI, develops in 5% of patients hospitalized with acute MI, and is attended by a mortality rate exceeding 80%. Despite impaired cardiac performance and reduced circulation, certain patients with this complication of acute infarction survive. Pathophysiology, differential diagnosis, monitoring facilities, therapeutic interventions, assisted circulation, and emergency surgery must be considered in the approach to this clinical problem. While clinically evaluating the patient, the physician must simultane-

36

ously consider pathophysiology, differential diagnosis, appropriate laboratory studies, and optimal treatment. Initial therapy must be instituted while laboratory procedures are being performed and data collected. Therefore, knowledge of alterations in cardiac and circulatory function, clinical pathophysiological features of shock, monitoring systems, medical treatment, and indications for surgery are valuable to the physician.

III. CAUSES

Cardiogenic shock results from significant destruction of left ventricular myocardium. This destruction produces impairment of the mechanical performance of the left ventricle to the extent that cardiac output and arterial blood pressure are severely reduced. In addition to major disturbances in left ventricular mechanical performance, imbalances between blood volume and diastolic filling of the left ventricle may develop. Peripheral vascular tone is sometimes inappropriately affected by hormonal and neurogenic mechanisms.

IV. PATHOPHYSIOLOGY

Pathologic studies in patients who have expired from cardiogenic shock have demonstrated destruction of 40 to 50% of the total mass of the myocardium of the left ventricle. This is usually composed of a recent or a recent and previous MI. In addition to massive destruction of the myocardium, these patients often exhibit severe three-vessel coronary artery disease (CAD). Generally, the infarction produces transmural necrosis that involves the full thickness of the ventricular wall.

Cardiogenic shock can result from extensive subendocardial infarction limited to the endocardial layers of the left ventricle. Reduction of cardiac output and arterial blood pressure in the shock state further decrease coronary blood flow, which contribute to left ventricular dysfunction and extension of the infarcted area.

V. CLASSIFICATION

Although cardiogenic shock results from extreme mechanical dysfunction of the left ventricle, several hemodynamic subgroups have been identified: mechanical dysfunction, relative hypovolemia, and impaired peripheral vasomotor control mechanisms.

A. Mechanical dysfunction. In cardiogenic shock due to mechanical dysfunction, extensive destruction of ventricular myocardium severely impairs cardiac output and systolic emptying of the left ventricle.

B. Relative hypovolemia. In patients with relative hypovolemia, the shock state can develop while the filling pressure of the left ventricle is normal or slightly elevated. The hemodynamic alterations resemble the shock condition produced by blood loss or inadequate venous return to the heart.

C. Impaired peripheral vasomotor control mechanisms. The third category of shock may result from hormonal and neurogenic mechanisms that disproportionally alter peripheral vasomotor tone. Mechanical impairment of the left ventricle is less severe and survival rate is higher.

VI. SYMPTOMS AND SIGNS

The clinical features of patients presenting in cardiogenic shock are a history of recent chest pain, manifestations of reduced organ perfusion, and the electrocardiographic changes of acute MI. Cardiogenic shock can develop in the absence of chronic heart failure, and the physical findings of chronic volume overload may be absent.

A. Vital signs
   1. Vital signs generally reveal a normal temperature, tachycardia with a thready peripheral pulse, normal or increased respiratory rate, and significantly reduced blood pressure.
   2. In some patients there may be difficulty in obtaining blood pressure by the cuff technique.
   3. Bradycardia may be present in patients with inferior (diaphragmatic) MI and excessive vagal tone or complete atrioventricular (AV) block.

B. Inspection and palpation
   1. The patient is restless with altered sensorium, and the skin is pale, cyanotic, cool, and moist.
   2. Neck veins are flat but can be distended if right heart failure has been chronic.
   3. Neck vein distention, hepatic enlargement, and peripheral edema may be present if the patient has a history of chronic heart failure.

C. Auscultation
   1. If the patient has left ventricular failure and pulmonary edema, pulmonary rales are audible, but the lungs may be clear to auscultation.
   2. Heart sounds are often distant.
   3. Atrial and ventricular gallops or a summation gallop may be audible.
   4. Detection of a harsh systolic murmur at the apex or along the left sternal border suggests rupture of a papillary muscle or the ventricular septum.
   5. If an aortic diastolic murmur is present, this finding should be considered in the differential diagnosis.

D. Cardiac size
   Heart size may be normal or enlarged, depending on presence or absence of chronic left ventricular overload.

E. Peripheral pulses
   1. Peripheral pulses are diminished, thready, or not palpable.
   2. Disparity between the right and the left radial, brachial, or femoral pulses should suggest a dissecting aneurysm.

VII. LABORATORY FINDINGS
   A. Routine laboratory studies
      Since cardiogenic shock is usually a sudden complication of

acute MI, routine laboratory studies of the peripheral blood and urinalysis may be normal.

B. Serum electrolyte determinations

If the patient has a previous cardiac condition with a history of diuretic use, serum electrolytes should be determined.

C. Renal function tests

Evaluation of renal function is useful not only for detection of pre-existing renal disease but also to establish a baseline for comparison during management of shock.

D. Arterial blood gas determinations

Arterial blood gas determinations often reveal hypoxemia, normal CO_2, and varying degrees of acidosis.

E. Serum enzyme studies

Cardiac enzymes may not be elevated initially if the patient develops shock shortly after the acute MI. Two to 16 hours can elapse from the onset of chest pain before the cardiac enzymes are abnormally elevated.

F. Chest roentgenogram

1. Chest roentgenogram may reveal a normal cardiac silhouette if there is no prior history of heart failure or hypertension.
2. Cardiomegaly would suggest hypertension or heart failure secondary to coronary disease.
3. Acute MI can produce pulmonary vascular congestion and edema in the absence of cardiac enlargement.

G. Electrocardiogram (ECG)

The ECG is essential in documentation of a recent MI.

1. Abnormal Q waves, ST segments, and T-wave changes of myocardial necrosis confirm MI.
2. Although it is generally contended that Q waves are necessary and that transmural infarction is required to destroy sufficient myocardium to produce cardiogenic shock, cardiogenic shock can result from subendocardial infarction, showing only ST and T-wave abnormalities on the ECG.
3. The presence of conduction disturbances, such as left bundle branch block or complete AV block, may obscure the characteristic electrocardiographic findings of acute MI. However, in the absence of left bundle branch block or complete AV block, characteristic changes of MI usually accompany cardiogenic shock.

VIII. DIAGNOSIS

The diagnosis of acute MI is established by history of ischemic chest pain, enzymatic, and electrocardiographic abnormalities. Additional findings of hypotension and impaired skin perfusion, renal blood flow, and central nervous system function confirm the clinical diagnosis of cardiogenic shock.

Primary cardiac arrhythmias must be excluded as the precipitating cause of the shock, and this can be difficult because rhythm disturbances frequently develop as a result of cardiogenic shock and impaired coronary blood flow.

Administration of analgesics for the relief of MI pain can significantly reduce blood pressure. Therefore, cardiac arrhythmias and analgesics can cause hypotension in a patient with acute MI, and such mechanisms must be excluded in order to confirm the diagnosis of cardiogenic shock.

IX. DIFFERENTIAL DIAGNOSIS

Unless the history and clinical and electrocardiographic findings are unequivocal for recent MI and cardiogenic shock, other possible mechanisms must be considered. Shock due to any cause reduces coronary blood flow, and in a patient with preexisting CAD, hypotension can produce myocardial damage.

A. Hypovolemic shock
1. Hypovolemic shock can develop secondary to blood loss, and a common site of such loss is in the gastrointestinal tract of patients with peptic ulcer disease.
2. Internal bleeding can develop from trauma; occult sites for internal blood loss include the mediastinum and retroperitoneal space.
3. Dissection of the aorta produces intense pain similar to that of MI. Blood loss from a dissecting aorta can accumulate in the mediastinum, pleural space, or retroperitoneal space, producing shock syndrome. Rarely, the dissection may extend retrograde into the pericardium with cardiac tamponade. In addition to intense pain, blood loss, and cardiac tamponade, aortic dissection can occlude a coronary artery and produce MI.

B. Pulmonary embolism.

Pulmonary embolism can produce shock accompanied by obstruction of pulmonary blood flow, impaired filling of the left ventricle, and reduction in coronary blood flow.

C. Bacteremia.

Gram-negative bacteremia is a mechanism for the shock syndrome, but this condition is usually attended by chills and fever. Often bacteremia is secondary to urinary tract manipulation or surgical procedure.

D. Neurogenic shock

Shock can develop on a neurogenic basis from intense pain or trauma. However, significant blood loss must be considered under traumatic circumstances.

E. Anaphylactic shock

Anaphylactic shock can develop from insect bites, medications, or intravascular injections for various diagnostic procedures.

Finally, cardiogenic shock can result from any mechanism that reduces arterial pressure causing reduction of coronary blood flow in a patient with CAD.

X. COMPLICATIONS

The mortality rate is extremely high in cardiogenic shock as a complication of acute MI. The highest mortality is encountered in patients who have excessive destruction of left ventricular myocardium. The mortality is slightly lower when relative hypovolemia is an additional pathophysiologic mechanism in cardiogenic shock. Inappropriate peripheral vasomotor disturbances with minimal mechanical impairment of left ventricular function in cardiogenic shock have the most favorable prognosis. The development of a prominent precordial systolic murmur and thrill with the acute infarction and cardiogenic shock suggests a ruptured papillary muscle or ventricular septum. These mechanical complications can be managed with circulatory support systems and cardiac surgery.

Renal failure secondary to acute tubular necrosis may occur in patients who remain in cardiogenic shock for prolonged periods. Cerebrovascular accidents may be caused by reduced cerebral blood flow in a patient with cerebral vascular disease. Gastrointestinal disorders such as ischemia of the bowel with necrosis and bleeding can result from prolonged shock. Cardiovascular disorders such as cardiac arrhythmias as well as pulmonary edema and heart failure often accompany cardiogenic shock, and all of these cardiac disturbances can be attributed to a reduction in coronary blood flow.

XI. MANAGEMENT (Table 3–1)
   A. General therapeutic approach
      1. The initial management of the patient with cardiogenic shock requires the rapid establishment of an IV route for the administration of vasopressor agents.
      2. Several vasoactive medications are available, but dopamine and dobutamine are presently most reliable in the elevation of arterial blood pressure and restoration of vital organ perfusion.

Table 3–1. Drugs Commonly Used in Cardiogenic Shock

Agent	Concentration (mg/250 ml 5% D/W*)	Infusion Rate (Standard) μ/kg/min	Adverse Reaction
Dopamine	200	4	Nausea, vomiting, arrhythmia, angina, azotemia
Dobutamine	200	7.5	Tachycardia, arrhythmia, angina, nausea, headache
Norepinephrine	4	0.1	Bradycardia, headache, hypertension, extravasation can cause tissue necrosis
Epinephrine	4	0.1	Arrhythmia, headache, angina, anxiety
Isoproterenol	1	0.05	Nausea, vomiting, arrhythmia, tachycardia, angina
Metaraminol	50	As necessary to maintain BP	Sinus or ventricular tachycardia, arrhythmia

3. The filling pressure of the left ventricle should be elevated and an effective blood volume established for maximum action of the vasopressor agents. The Swan-Ganz catheter can provide this information in the shock patient.
4. Arterial systolic pressure should be maintained above 90 mm Hg by means of infusion of a vasopressor.
5. In addition to the prompt administration of vasopressors, a Foley catheter should be inserted to quantitate urine flow.
6. Patients generally maintain respiratory control in cardiogenic shock even though the arterial blood gases are significantly altered. If the patient does not exhibit spontaneous respirations, intubation and ventilatory support must be supplied.
7. Acute pulmonary edema can occur in cardiogenic shock syndrome, and phlebotomy is the most expedient method for reduction of blood volume.
8. Cardiac irritability requires IV lidocaine to control rhythm disturbances.
9. Metabolic acidosis quickly develops in cardiogenic shock, and infusion of sodium bicarbonate is required to restore acid-base balance.

These initial interventions can stabilize and sometimes restore arterial blood pressure and coronary blood flow.

B. Specific therapeutic measures
1. If facilities are available, a Swan-Ganz catheter should be introduced and advanced to the pulmonary artery for measurements of pulmonary artery end-diastolic or capillary wedge pressure and cardiac output.
2. An intra-aortic balloon should be inserted in the femoral artery for diastolic augmentation of cardiac output and coronary blood flow.
3. If severe mitral regurgitation or a ruptured ventricular septum is confirmed by the Swan-Ganz catheter, emergency cardiac surgery should be considered.
4. If rupture of the mitral apparatus, ventricular septum, or aortic dissection can be excluded, a thrombolytic drug should be administered, followed by systemic heparinization.
5. Coronary arteriography should be performed to identify potential lesions for angioplasty or bypass surgery.
6. The insertion of a Swan-Ganz catheter, intra-aortic balloon counter pulsation, emergency coronary arteriography, coronary angioplasty, and cardiac surgery require highly-trained cardiologists, cardiac surgeons, nurses, and technicians.

XII. PROGNOSIS

The prognosis, in patients who develop cardiogenic shock with acute MI, is determined by the extent of muscle damage from the acute, as well as the previous, MIs.

Patients who exhibit hemodynamic evidence of severe elevation in left ventricular filling pressure and reduction in cardiac index are in a high mortality category despite the use of available pharmacologic agents. Furthermore, these patients have a low probability of survival if emergency surgery and bypass grafting are performed.

Patients who present in shock with a normal or modestly elevated left ventricular filling pressure are relatively hypovolemic, and approximately one-third of these patients respond to expansion of the blood volume with low molecular dextran or albumin. Patients who reveal minimal alterations in left ventricular filling pressure and cardiac index with cardiogenic shock often respond promptly to vasopressor agents.

Although thrombolytic therapy offers rapid reperfusion in acute MI and shock, reported rates of recanalization have been low without any improvement in mortality. When facilities are available, angioplasty can be performed quickly and current success rates exceed 70%. However, survival statistics indicate patients with single vessel disease derive benefit from angioplasty, whereas bypass surgery should be considered when multivessel disease is found at catheterization. Technical advances in angioplasty and bypass surgery have significantly reduced the mortality when shock complicates myocardial infarction.

SUGGESTED READINGS

Katz, N.M., and Wallace, R.B.: Emergency coronary bypass surgery: indications and results. *In* C.E. Rackley and A.N. Brest (eds): Critical Care Cardiology, 2nd ed. Philadelphia, F.A. Davis, 1986.

Kent, K.M.: Transluminal coronary angioplasty. *In* C.E. Rackley and A.N. Brest (eds): Critical Care Cardiology, 2nd ed. Philadelphia, F.A. Davis, 1986.

Lee, L., Bates, E.R., Pitt, B., et al.: Percutaneous transluminal angioplasty improves survival in acute myocardial infarction complicated by cardiogenic shock. Circulation 78:1345, 1988.

Rackley, C.E., et al.: Cardiogenic shock in patients with myocardial infarction. *In* C.E. Rackley and R.O. Russell, Jr. (eds): Hemodynamic Monitoring in a Coronary Intensive Care Unit. Futura, NY, 1981.

Rackley, C.E., Russell, R.O., Jr., Mantle, J.A., et al.: Management of acute myocardial infarction. *In* C.E. Rackley and R.O. Russell, Jr. (eds): Coronary Artery Disease: Recognition and Management. Futura, NY, 1979.

Ratshin, R.A., Rackley, C.E., and Russell, R.O., Jr.: Hemodynamic evaluation of left ventricular function in shock complicating myocardial infarction. Circulation 45:127, 1972.

Satler, L.E., Kent, K.M., Green, C.E., et al.: Thrombolysis in acute myocardial infarction. *In* C.E. Rackley and A.N. Brest (eds): Critical Care Cardiology, 2nd ed. Philadelphia, F.A. Davis, 1986.

Swan, H.J.C., et al.: Hemodynamic spectrum of myocardial infarction and cardiogenic shock: A conceptual model. Circulation 45:197, 1972.

Weber, K.T., et al.: Left ventricular dysfunction following acute myocardial infarction: A clinico-pathologic and hemodynamic profile of shock and failure. Am J Med 54:697, 1973.

Zalewski, A. and Goldberg, S.: Interventional therapy in acute myocardial infarction. *In* C.J. Pepine and A.N. Brest (eds): Acute Myocardial Infarction. Philadelphia, F.A. Davis, 1989.

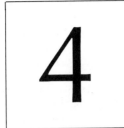

PULMONARY EMBOLISM

Se Woong Seo and Edward K. Chung

I. GENERAL CONSIDERATIONS

Any materials that are carried to and have impact on pulmonary circulation can cause pulmonary embolism. Although many materials such as fat emboli, amniotic fluid, bone marrow particles, tumor emboli, or air emboli may cause pulmonary embolism, blood clots from the venous system are by far the most common source. Therefore, the discussion in this chapter will primarily deal with pulmonary embolism due to venous thrombi.

Pulmonary embolism has been recognized since the pioneering work of Virchow in 19th century. However, the exact incidence of pulmonary embolism is not clearly known because the diagnosis of pulmonary embolism depends almost entirely upon clinical suspicion and because there is no generally reliable confirming test. It has been estimated that the total incidence of symptomatic pulmonary embolism in the United States is approximately 630,000 annually. In about two-thirds, pulmonary embolism is not diagnosed and the mortality rate in this group is about 30%. When pulmonary embolism is diagnosed and treated, the mortality rate falls to less than 10%. This information emphasizes the need for prevention, early recognition, and management of pulmonary embolism.

II. CAUSES

Pulmonary embolism is considered a complication of venous thrombosis, and therefore the etiology of pulmonary embolism is that of venous thrombosis. Virchow summarized factors that predispose to venous thrombosis as Virchow's triad: (1) damage to the blood vessel wall; (2) hypercoagulability; and (3) venous stasis. In practice, some or all of these factors may work together in producing venous thrombosis.

Trauma or surgery to legs, infection or inflammation of legs or systemic venous hypertension may cause stasis and damage to the vessel wall. Immobility, prolonged bed rest, obesity, or congestive heart failure are likely to produce venous stasis. Pregnancy, oral contraceptives, and malignancy may cause hormone-induced hypercoagulability and venous stasis.

Deficiency of antithrombotic proteins such as antithrombin III, protein C, protein S, or deficiency of plasminogen activator may predispose to pulmonary embolism through the production of hypercoagulability.

Most pulmonary emboli come from the thrombi in the deep veins of the thigh. Venous thrombi generally begin in the deep veins of the calf and propagate proximally to the popliteal, and occasionally, to the iliac veins. In 45 to 70% of patients with prolonged bed rest or after elective surgery, thrombi are detected in the soleal veins. In women, the pulmonary emboli may come from the thrombus in the pelvic venous system during or after pregnancy and delivery.

Uncommon factors that predispose to pulmonary embolism include systemic lupus erythematosus, nephrotic syndrome, polycythemia vera, paroxysmal nocturnal hemoglobinuria, and homocystinuria.

III. PATHOLOGY AND PATHOPHYSIOLOGY

In most patients, pulmonary embolism is produced by multiple emboli, and both lungs are affected. The right lung is more commonly affected than the left. The lower lobe vessels are more commonly involved than the upper lobe vessels.

The hemodynamic and respiratory response of pulmonary embolism depends upon the extent of pulmonary vascular obstruction, the time elapsed following embolization and the presence or absence of pre-existing cardiopulmonary disease.

In patients without pre-existing cardiopulmonary disease, pulmonary arterial pressure begins to rise when pulmonary vascular bed is obstructed by 25% or more, and the mean pulmonary arterial pressure is usually below 20 mm Hg unless more than 50% of the pulmonary vascular bed is obstructed. The pressure seldom rises above 40 mm Hg. As the pulmonary arterial pressure increases, the right ventricle begins to dilate and there may be tricuspid regurgitation. The right ventricle may become hypokinetic; right atrial pressure increases and jugular veins are distended. The cardiac output is decreased and cardiogenic shock may develop. A mean pulmonary arterial pressure above 40 mm Hg indicates chronic right ventricular hypertrophy secondary to recurrent pulmonary emboli or other diseases. When there is a pre-existing cardiopulmonary disease, relatively small emboli obstructing small pulmonary artery segments can exert severe hemodynamic change. After embolization, reflex pulmonary vasoconstriction and release of neurohumoral factors, such as serotonin or thromboxan A_2 from platelets, may also contribute to the increase of pulmonary arterial pressure.

Intrapulmonary dead space is produced by embolic obstruction. Through the reflex stimulation of the ventilation by pulmonary emboli, minute ventilation and alveolar ventilation are increased so that hypocapnia is produced. The release of vasoconstrictive substances from platelet aggregates within the clot, and hypocapnia secondary to the alveolar hyperventilation produces constriction of terminal bronchioles. Loss of alveolar surfactant and production of focal areas of edema in the vicinity of occluded pulmonary arteries contribute to the production of atelectasis, alveolar collapse, and fluid accumulation. Arterial hypoxemia is common. Several mechanisms may contribute to hypoxemia, and may include ventilation-perfusion inequality, low cardiac output with a decreased mixed venous O_2 saturation, and obligatory perfusion through hypoventilated lung zone because of elevated pulmonary arterial pressure. Rarely, increased pulmonary arterial pressure causes right to left shunt through a patent foramen ovale. This may be an another factor causing arterial hypoxemia and may produce paradoxical embolization.

IV. CLINICAL MANIFESTATIONS

Clinical features of pulmonary embolism are diverse, and range from no symptoms to sudden death. The clinical presentations of pulmonary embolism may be divided into 4 categories: (1) submassive pulmonary embolism; (2) massive pulmonary embolism; (3) pulmonary infarction; and, (4) chronic pulmonary hypertension.

A. Submassive Pulmonary Embolism

Submassive pulmonary embolism is the most common, and defined as involving less than 50% of the pulmonary arterial tree with no elevation of right ventricular and pulmonary arterial pressure. The primary symptoms are unexplained dyspnea, tachypnea, and tachycardia: occasionally, anxiety and pleuritic chest pain accompany them. Syncope is uncommon. Most of these patients may have one or more predisposing factors for deep venous thrombosis. The lungs are clear. The ECG and chest x-ray are normal. Arterial hypoxemia is common. Differential diagnosis includes left ventricular failure, pneumonia and hyperventilation syndrome.

B. Massive Pulmonary Embolism

This can be defined as sufficient obstruction of pulmonary arterial blood flow leading to an increase in right ventricular afterload and pulmonary arterial pressure. The most common features are hypotension, syncope, acute cor-pulmonale, or cardiogenic shock. Sudden cardiac death may occur. Patients frequently have tachycardia, tachypnea, and cyanosis with distended neck veins. A distended liver and peripheral edema may also occur if enough time has elapsed. Right-sided S_3 gallop and a parasternal heave are usually present. Predisposing factors of deep venous thrombosis may be present. The lungs are clear. The ECG often shows S_1, Q_3, T_3 pattern, acute right bundle branch block, signs of right ventricular strain, right axis deviation, P-pulmonale, sinus tachycardia, and various atrial tachyarrhythmias.

In most cases, massive pulmonary embolism occurs slowly. Dyspnea, tachypnea, pleuritic chest pain, and anxiety are common. The clinical features of shock are less common. Systemic hypotension is a consistent feature but is often mild. Differential diagnosis may include septic shock, cardiac tamponade, constrictive pericarditis, and right ventricular infarction.

C. Pulmonary Infarction

Because of dual blood supply from the pulmonary artery as well as bronchial artery and direct contact of the tissue with alveolar gas, pulmonary infarction is uncommon. However, bronchoconstriction and vasoconstriction that accompany pulmonary embolism may produce pulmonary infarction. Nearly all patients have severe pleuritic chest pain, cough, and mild fever. Hemoptysis may occur. Patients often have pleural or pleuropericardial friction rub. These symptoms and signs may persist for hours or several days. Chest x-ray will show pulmonary infiltrates and usually pleural effusion. Differential diagnosis should include viral or bacterial pneumonia.

D. Chronic Pulmonary Hypertension

Chronic recurrent pulmonary embolism may cause chronic pulmonary hypertension. This is a rare condition and has a poor prognosis. Patients usually have a long history of progressive dyspnea, exercise intolerance, and occasional syncope. They may have no predisposing factors for venous thrombosis. On physical examination, a loud pulmonary valve closure sound and pulmonary regurgitation or tricuspid regurgitation murmur may be heard. The lung fields are clear despite the presence of dyspnea, cyanosis, peripheral edema, and ascites. Occasionally these findings are subtle.

V. DIAGNOSIS

Various informations obtained from history and physical examination are not sufficient in the diagnosis of pulmonary embolism. Likewise, routine laboratory studies, chest x-ray, ECG, and arterial blood gas analysis show nonspecific findings.

A. Arterial Blood Gas

In most patients with acute pulmonary embolism, arterial blood gas analysis shows hypocapnia and respiratory alkalosis because of tachypnea. Hypoxemia will be observed in patients with massive pulmonary embolism and in patients having dyspnea due to pulmonary embolism. A PaO_2 less than 50 mm

Hg suggests massive pulmonary embolism in patients without underlying cardiopulmonary disease. But in patients with underlying cardiopulmonary disease, submassive pulmonary embolism may be associated with severe hypoxemia.

B. Electrocardiogram

In massive pulmonary embolism, electrocardiograms may show acute cor-pulmonale pattern such as S_1, Q_3, T_3, right bundle branch block, P-pulmonale, right axis deviation, or right ventricular strain pattern. These ECG changes are transient and resolve as right ventricular failure resolves. In patients with submassive pulmonary embolism, ECG may be normal or nonspecific. The main value of the ECG is to diagnose acute myocardial infarction that may mimic the clinical picture of pulmonary embolism.

C. Chest X-Ray

In submassive pulmonary embolism, the chest x-ray may show no abnormality. Abnormal findings that may be observed are small ill-defined wedge-shaped areas of consolidation, linear atelectasis, elevation of hemidiaphragm of affected side, and small pleural effusion due to pulmonary infarction. In massive pulmonary embolism, a relative local hyperlucency with markedly diminished pulmonary vascular markings is observed. An engorged hilar artery, sudden appearance of a plump vessel, or abrupt tapering or termination of a vessel may be seen on plain film. These findings are not diagnostic, however. The principal role of the chest x-ray is in the detection of other diseases that may mimic pulmonary embolism and in the proper interpretation of the lung scan.

D. Lung Scanning

Ventilation-perfusion lung scan is a sensitive test for pulmonary embolism. For perfusion scan, technetium[99m] labeled macroaggregated albumin or albumin microspheres are administered intravenously. In ventilation scan, xenon[133] is inhaled but other isotopes, such as krypton[81m] or technetium[99m] diethylene triamine penta-acetate in aerosols, can be used. The ventilation scan is done before the perfusion scan for technical reasons.

A normal perfusion scan shows a homogeneous distribution of radioisotope with an image that reveals the anatomic shape of the lungs and rules out the possibility of pulmonary embolism except trivial sized pulmonary embolisms. If there is a pulmonary embolus, the radioisotopic particles cannot reach the vessels distal to the embolus resulting in a perfusion defect on the image. Abnormal perfusion scan is nonspecific and can only be interpreted with careful review of the chest x-ray or with ventilation lung scans. If there is no corresponding abnormality on the chest x-ray, single segmental defect or multiple sub-segmental defects reveal low probability for pulmonary embolism. If the chest x-ray shows normal and the defects are segmental or larger, the probability of pulmonary embolism is very high. When there are corresponding abnormalities on chest x-ray, the probability may be indeterminate even though there are perfusion defects. Perfusion defects can be produced by other causes such as chronic obstructive lung diseases, lung cancer, or pulmonary hypertension. The specificity of perfusion lung scan is increased by the use of ventilation scan because pulmonary emboli do not usually disrupt regional ventilation. In the presence of multiple large segmental defects on perfusion scan with no defect in ventilation scan (ventilation-perfusion mismatch), the probability of pulmonary embolism is high (up to 90%). If there are corresponding defects on ventilation scan (ventilation-perfusion match), the probability is low (less than 10%). Intermediate probability shows multiple subsequential perfusion defects with ventilation mismatch or multiple segmental or larger perfusion defects with ventilation match.

In estimating the probability of pulmonary embolism, physicians should consider the clinical features and the presence or absence of predisposing factors for deep venous thrombosis.

E. Pulmonary Angiography

Pulmonary angiography is the most accurate procedure for the diagnosis of pulmonary embolism. It involves insertion of a catheter into the pulmonary artery usually by a percutaneous approach via the femoral vein. After the catheter is advanced to a proper location, contrast medium is injected and cine films or rapid sequence films are taken. After the injection of contrast material, pulmonary arterial pressure and systemic arterial pressure should be measured.

The most specific angiographic finding is the filling defect. Abrupt termination or cut offs of pulmonary arterial branches are highly suggestive of the diagnosis. Other abnormal findings, such as oligemic lung segment, asymmetrical filling, and delayed filling or clearing, are less reliable.

Pulmonary angiography is an invasive procedure and may produce some complications such as allergic reactions or febrile reaction to contrast materials, cardiac perforation, and arrhythmias. Thus, this procedure should be reserved for patients with intermediate probability or undetermined lung scan or when anticoagulation therapy, thrombolytic therapy, or vena caval interruption is being considered. The contraindications to this procedure include severe systemic reaction to contrast material, significant ventricular arrhythmias, and coexisting life-threatening disease.

F. Venography

Venography of the lower extremities is a useful test for identifying the source of emboli in patients with nonspecific findings of lung scan who have a positive impedance plethysmography.

VI. TREATMENT

Anticoagulation therapy prevents further clot deposition. Thrombolytic therapy accelerates restoration of pulmonary blood flow by the lysis of clot. When anticoagulation and thrombolytic therapy are ineffective or contraindicated, inferior vena caval interruption or pulmonary embolectomy should be considered. Supportive measures include supplemental oxygen therapy, analgesics for pleuritic chest pain, and hemodynamic and ventilatory support.

A. Anticoagulation Therapy

Intravenous heparin for 7 to 10 days is the initial therapy of choice for pulmonary embolism. Before the initiation of heparin therapy, a careful history of bleeding, recent surgery, drug therapy, underlying disease, and other risk factors should be obtained. The dosage regimen for achieving optimal heparinization is empirical. For submassive pulmonary embolism, the usual initial dose is a 5000-unit intravenous bolus followed by a continuous intravenous infusion at 1000 units per hour. In patients with massive pulmonary embolism, the initial dose is usually a 10,000 unit bolus followed by an infusion of 1500 units per hour. For maintenance therapy, partial thromboplastin time (PTT) should be maintained 1.5 to 2.5 times the control level and should be checked every 4 hours until the desired infusion rate is obtained.

A major complication of heparin is bleeding. If there is life-threatening or intracranial bleeding, protamine sulfate should be administered and the heparin discontinued. The incidence of major bleeding is higher in intermittent intravenous or subcutaneous heparin than in continuous heparin therapy. Other complications include thrombocytopenia that is rarely associated with thrombosis, accelerated osteoporosis during long-term heparin therapy, and aldosterone depression.

After 4 to 5 days of heparin therapy, oral anticoagulation is continued with warfarin. Warfarin inhibits the vitamin K-dependent coagulation factors (factors II, VII, IX and X). Initial dose is usually 10 mg daily for 3 days. For maintenance therapy, the prothrombin time (PT) should be in the range of 1.2 to 1.5 times the control. The optimal duration of warfarin therapy is unknown but generally advised to continue for 3 to 6 months or until the predisposing factors have resolved.

A major complication of warfarin is bleeding. Life-threatening bleeding requires immediate treatment with fresh frozen plasma (usually 2 units) to normalize the PT. In the case of bleeding, vitamin K, usually 10 mg, may be administered subcutaneously or intramuscularly, and warfarin should be discontinued. Another complication is skin necrosis. Warfarin should not be used during pregnancy because of its teratogenic effect.

Absolute contraindications of anticoagulation include recent hemorrhagic cerebrovascular accident and recent neurosurgery, spinal or ocular surgery. Relative contraindications include other recent surgery, major trauma, recent gastrointestinal bleeding, severe hypertension, severe renal or hepatic failure, and other bleeding diatheses.

B. Thrombolytic Therapy

Urokinase (UK) converts circulating endogenous plasminogen to plasmin directly, but streptokinase (SK) forms a complex with plasminogen and then converts plasminogen to plasmin. Plasmin lyses the fibrin clots in pulmonary emboli. SK is relatively inexpensive but can produce febrile and allergic reactions.

For SK, the usual dose is 250,000 IU over 30 minutes followed by 100,000 IU per hour for 24 hours. For UK, it is 4400 IU/kg over 10 minutes followed by 4400 IU/kg per hour for 12 to 24 hours. Laboratory monitoring may be performed by measuring the fibrin degradation products, thrombin time, whole blood euglobulin lysis time, PT or PTT, but the most sensitive and widely available test is the thrombin time. Though fibrinolytic therapy produces a more rapid resolution of pulmonary emboli and an earlier return toward normal hemodynamics, there is no evidence that this therapy improves the patient's mortality.

Absolute contraindications include active internal bleeding, active intracranial disease processes, cerebrovascular accident within 2 months, neurologic or ophthalmologic surgery, and head injury. Relative contraindications include major surgery, invasive procedures, delivery, cardiopulmonary resuscitation, and severe hypertension. A major complication is bleeding.

Tissue type plasminogen activator (t-PA) has been used in several trials and has shown dramatic thrombolytic effect in pulmonary embolism. T-PA is more fibrin-specific and less hemorrhagic than UK or SK. But its effectiveness in reducing mortality and recurrent pulmonary embolism is not known.

C. Vena Caval Interruption

Vena caval interruption is considered in patients who have absolute contraindications to anticoagulation therapy, when adequate anticoagulation does not prevent recurrent emboli, or when a severe internal bleeding develops during anticoagulation therapy. This does not promote resolution of emboli. Methods of vena caval interruption include ligation, external clipping of inferior vena cava, and percutaneous intravenous umbrella or filters. Except in the case of septic embolism, percutaneous devices are preferred.

D. Pulmonary Embolectomy

Emergency pulmonary embolectomy is considered in patients with severe massive pulmonary embolism and when there is contraindication to fibrinolysis in the presence of occluded central pulmonary arteries on pulmonary angiogram. This procedure is associated with high mortality rate. Elective pulmonary embolectomy for symptomatic, unresolved pulmonary emboli in large pulmonary artery branches has proved relatively safe and effective. In patients with chronic pulmonary embolism and pulmonary hypertension, surgical embolectomy may produce a considerable symptomatic and hemodynamic improvement. Aspiration embolectomy is also used to remove emboli.

VII. PREVENTION

The best management strategy for pulmonary embolism is the prevention and treatment of deep venous thrombosis. The predisposing factors should be identified and, if possible, corrected or removed. Low dose subcutaneous heparin (5000 units per 12 hours) appears to prevent venous thrombosis effectively in many patients with predisposing factors for deep venous thrombosis following general surgery, urologic or gynecologic surgery, and in patients with low output heart failure. Protective effect of low-dose heparin is not clear in patients undergoing orthopedic surgery. In these cases, adjusted dose of heparin or warfarin may be required. Other preventive measures include leg exercise, elastic stockings, dextran, and external leg compression.

VIII. PROGNOSIS

If diagnosis and treatment are done promptly, prognosis of pulmonary embolism is excellent. Most death from pulmonary embolism occurs because it is not recognized and treated. In a small number of patients, however, death occurs due to recurrent embolism or severe underlying diseases. In massive pulmonary embolism, clinical signs and symptoms of acute cor-pulmonale may subside rapidly because of fragmentation, dislocation and fibrinolysis of emboli, or pulmonary vasoconstrictive reflexes. On rare occasions, chronic recurrent pulmonary embolism may lead to chronic cor-Pulmonale. Its prognosis is very poor.

SUGGESTED READINGS

Alpert, J.S., Smith, R., Carlson, J., et al: Mortality in patients treated for pulmonary embolism. JAMA 236:1477, 1976.

American College of Chest Physicians and the National Heart, Lung, and Blood Institute National Conference on Antithrombotic Therapy. Arch. Intern. Med. 146:462, 1986.

Bell, W.R., Simon, T.L., and DeMets, D.L.: The clinical features of submassive and massive pulmonary emboli. Am. J. Med. 62:355, 1977.

Bell, W.R. and Simon, T.: Current status of pulmonary thromboembolic disease: pathophysiology, diagnosis, prevention and treatment. Am. Heart J. 103:239, 1982.

Braun, S.D., Newman, G.E., Ford, K., et al.: Ventilation-perfusion scanning and pulmonary angiography: Correlation in clinical high-probability pulmonary embolism. A.J.R. 143:977, 1984.

Collins, R., Scrimgeour, A., Yusuf, S., et al.: Reduction in fatal pulmonary embolism and venous thrombosis by perioperative administration of subcutaneous heparin: overview of results of randomized trials in general, orthopedic, and urologic surgery. N. Engl. J. Med. 318:1162, 1988.

Dalen, J.E. and Alpert, J.S.: Natural history of pulmonary embolism. Prog. Cardiovasc. Dis. 17(4):259, 1975.

Goldhaber, S.Z., Kessler, C.M., Heit, J., et al.: A randomized controlled trial of recombinant tissue plasminogen activator versus urokinase in the treatment of acute pulmonary embolism. Lancet 2:293, 1988.

Goldhaber, S.Z., Markis, J.E., Kessler, C.M., et al.: Perspectives on treatment of acute pulmonary embolism with tissue plasminogen activator. Semin. Thromb. Hemost. 13:221, 1987.

Goldhaber, S.Z., Savage, D.D., Garrison, R.J. et al.: Risk factors for pulmonary embolism: The Framingham Study. Am. J. Med. 74:1023, 1983.

Hull, R.D., Carter, C.J., Jay, R.M., et al.: The diagnosis of acute, recurrent, deep-vein thrombosis: A diagnostic challenge. Circulation 67:901, 1983.

Hull, R.D., Hirsh, J., Carter, C.J., et al.: Diagnostic value of ventilation-perfusion lung scanning in patients with suspected pulmonary embolism. Chest 88:819, 1985.

Hull, R.D., Raskob, G.E., Hirsh, J., et al.: Continuous intravenous heparin compared with intermittent subcutaneous heparin in the initial treatment of proximal-vein thrombosis. N. Engl. J. Med. 315:1109, 1986.

Hyers, T.M., Hull, R.D., and Weg, J.G.: Antithrombotic therapy for venous thromboembolic disease. Chest 89:26s, 1986.

Jeffrey, P.C., Immelman, E.J., Banatar, S.R.: Deep-vein thrombosis and pulmonary embolism: As assessment of the accuracy of clinical diagnosis. S. Afr. Med. J. 57:643, 1980.

Kelton, J.G., and Hirsh, J.: Bleeding associated with antithrombotic therapy. Semin. Hematol. 17:259, 1980.

Kessler, C.M., Druy, E. and Goldhaber, S.Z.: Acute pulmonary embolism treated with thrombolytic agents: current status of t-PA and future implications for emergency medicine. Ann. Emerg. Med. 17(11):1216, 1988.

Stein, P.D., Dalen, J.E., McIntyre, K.M., et al.: The electrocardiogram in acute pulmonary embolism. Prog. Cardiovasc. Dis. 17:247, 1975.

Stein, P.D., Willis, P.W., III, and DeMets, D.L.: History and physical examination in acute pulmonary embolism in patients without preexisting cardiac or pulmonary disease. Am. J. Cardiol. 47:218, 1981.

Sutton, G.C., Hall, R.J.C., and Kerr, I.H.: Clinical course and late prognosis of treated subacute massive, acute minor and chronic pulmonary thromboembolism. Br. Heart J. 39:1135, 1977.

The Urokinase Pulmonary Embolism Trial. Circulation (Suppl 2) 47:1, 1973.

Tissue plasminogen activator for the treatment of acute pulmonary embolism. A collaborative study by PIOPED Investigators. Chest 97:528, 1990.

Tsao, M.S., Schraufnagel, D., and Wang, N.S.: Pathogenesis of pulmonary infarction. Am. J. Med. 72:599, 1982.

Urokinase Pulmonary Embolism Trial Study Group. Urokinase-Streptokinase Embolism Trial. JAMA 229:1606, 1974.

Vaughan, D.E., Goldhaber, S.Z., Kim, J., et al.: Recombinant tissue plasminogen activator in patients with pulmonary embolism: Correlation of fibrinolytic specificity and efficacy. Circulation 75:1200, 1987.

Wessler, S.: Prevention of venous thromboembolism: rationale, practice, and problems. NIH Consensus Development Conference on Prevention of Venous Thrombosis and Pulmonary Embolism, National Institutes of Health, Bethesda, MD, 1986.

chapter

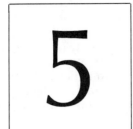

ACUTE CORONARY CARE

Edward K. Chung

I. GENERAL CONSIDERATIONS

Coronary care unit (CCU) was introduced into clinical medicine in the late 1950s, and the mortality rate in patients with coronary artery disease (CAD) was reduced significantly with the development of direct current (DC) shock and closed chest cardiopulmonary resuscitation (CPR) in the 1960s. In the 1960s, the development of hemodynamic monitoring in patients with acute myocardial infarction (MI) also contributed significantly to better understanding and treatment of hypovolemia as a correctable cause of cardiogenic shock. The survival rate of patients with CAD further improved following the development of counter-pulsation in the treatment of pump failure (see Chapters 2 and 3).

In the 1970s, a well-organized training program of medical, as well as nonmedical, personnel in CPR and the development of mobile CCUs provided significant contributions toward reducing the mortality rate. In addition, a new idea, using pharmacologic methods for myocardial preservation by improvement of nutrient supply to myocardium along with reduction of myocardial oxygen requirements with use of beta-adrenergic blockers and unloading agents, was introduced in the 1970s.

Reperfusion of the myocardium through early coronary artery bypass surgery (CABS) in patients with acute MI was the major step to improve the survival rate (see Chapter 20). In 1976, intracoronary fibrinolysis in acute MI was reported, and the catheter-directed reperfusion was performed by mechanically opening the artery and then using intracoronary thrombolytic agents.

In recent years, remarkable changes in the treatment of acute MI and unstable angina have been observed, especially in the fields of thrombolytic therapy and coronary angioplasty (see Chapters 6 and 7). New life-saving devices, including an automatic implantable cardioverter-defibrillator (AICD) and an antitachycardia artificial pacemaker, further contributed considerably to the improvement of the survival rate in high-risk patients with CAD (see Chapters 13 and 14).

For the best therapeutic results, the general public should be educated properly and continuously in the recognition of acute coronary events so that proper coronary care can be administered promptly without unnecessary delay. Patients with suspected or known CAD should be evaluated rapidly and transferred to a nearby hospital equipped to manage acute MI. All high-risk patients suffering from cardiac arrest, ventricular tachyarrhythmias, severe bradyarrhythmias, or cardiogenic shock should be taken to a medical institution equipped with cardiac catheterization and cardiac surgery facilities as soon as possible.

Every patient with suspected acute MI should be evaluated in the emergency room (ER) as soon as the patient enters the ER. Unnecessary delays in evaluation and treatment related to hospital administrative procedures, such as establishing medical insurance coverage, must be absolutely avoided.

When the diagnosis of acute MI is certain judging from clinical manifestations, characteristic ECG changes, and other supportive findings, the initial therapy, including appropriate use of thrombolytic therapy, should begin by the well-trained physician and staff in the ER. On the other hand, when the diagnosis of acute MI is equivocal, consultation with an immediately available cardiologist should be obtained as soon as possible.

In rural communities with limited medical facilities, plans should be developed with nearby medical centers for rapid telephone consultation and appropriate patient transfer to a tertiary medical institution. By and large, protocols for the initiation of thrombolytic therapy in the rural community hospital before transfer are appropriate and have been shown to be safe and effective (see Chapter 6).

A. Oxygen

Oxygen should be administered for all patients with suspected or proven acute coronary event at least in the first few hours. Oxygen therapy should be continued during transportation to the hospital, even if there is evidence of chronic pulmonary disease; however, lower flow rates may be appropriate in these patients. Oxygen therapy may *not* be fully effective to correct significant hypoxemia in patients with severe congestive heart failure (CHF), pulmonary edema, or other serious complications of acute MI. Under these circumstances, endotracheal intubation and mechanical ventilation are often necessary.

B. Nitroglycerin

Sublingual nitroglycerin (NG) should be administered for every patient suffering from coronary ischemic pain unless the initial systolic blood pressure (BP) is less than 90 mm Hg. A single sublingual NG tablet may be tried in the hospital even if the systolic BP is less than 90 mm Hg, provided that evidence of ongoing ischemic pain exists and an intravenous (IV) line has been established. NG should be avoided, however, when the patient shows marked bradycardia or tachycardia, especially if relative hypotension is present. It is essential to observe vital signs frequently for several minutes after the initial dose.

In the management of the early stage of acute MI, long-acting oral nitrates should be avoided. Intravenous NG infusion is preferable for more precise minute-to-minute control, although sublingual or transdermal NG can be administered. Intravenous NG can be effectively titrated by frequent measurement of BP and the heart rate. Hemodynamic monitoring is extremely valuable if high doses of vasodilating agents are used in order to detect the BP instability and the adequacy of the left ventricular filling pressure.

The most serious potential complication of NG therapy in patients with acute MI is systemic hypotension leading to the worsening of myocardial ischemia. NG should be carefully titrated in patients with diaphragmatic (inferior) MI and/or right ventricular MI. Severe hypotension can be produced during NG therapy under these circumstances because such patients are particularly dependent on adequate right ventricular preload to maintain cardiac output. Needless to say, NG therapy should be discontinued immediately when severe hypotension with bradycardia is produced. Leg elevation, rapid fluid administration, and atropine are appropriate therapies under this circumstance.

It has been shown that intravenous NG may reduce infarct size in some patients, and the best results can be achieved when NG is given early. In addition, NG may reduce susceptibility to ventricular fibrillation (VF) during both acute myocardial ischemia and reperfusion. In some reports, intravenous NG reduced mortality by 10 to 30%. The value of NG is also well known when acute MI is complicated by CHF or pulmonary edema.

1. NG Dosage:

When titrating intravenous NG, begin with a 15 μg bolus injection and a pump-controlled infusion of 5 to 10 μg/min and increase the dosage by 5 to 10 μg/min every 5 to 10 minutes while carefully monitoring hemodynamic and clinical responses. The titration end points are the control of clinical symptoms or a decrease in mean arterial pressure of

10% in normotensive patients, or 30% in hypertensive patients (never a systolic BP less than 90 mm Hg), an increase in heart rate more than 10 beats/min (not usually more than 110 beats/min), or a decrease in pulmonary artery end-diastolic pressure of 10 to 30%. High doses above 200 μg/min are often associated with an increased risk of hypotension, and alternative therapy should be considered in this circumstance.

Prolonged IV infusion may result in relative nitrate tolerance. As tolerance develops, the infusion rate can be increased, but if the high doses above 200 μg/min are required, another vasodilator, such as a calcium channel blocker, should be substituted. The combination of IV NG with a beta-adrenergic blocker is well tolerated in some patients, and the risk of undesired tachycardia may be reduced.

II. ANALGESIA

It has been well documented that the chest pain of acute MI is caused by continuing ischemia of the living jeopardized myocardium rather than to the effects of complete myocardial necrosis. Thus, all available anti-ischemic interventions should be carried out. They include the use of oxygen, nitrates, beta-adrenergic blocking agents and intra-aortic balloon counterpulsation (in some cases), in addition to reperfusion. Of course effective analgesia should be administered promptly as soon as the diagnosis of acute MI is made.

The agents available to suppress the pain of acute MI include morphine sulfate, hydromorphone, and meperidine. Meperidine is highly recommended for diaphragmatic MI because of its vagolytic properties. Morphine sulfate is considered to be the drug of choice to suppress the chest pain of acute MI except in patients with documented allergic reaction to the agent. Morphine sulfate is administered intravenously in small repeated doses of 2 to 5 mg every 5 to 30 minutes as needed. In some cases, relatively large cumulative doses of 2 to 3 mg/kg are required.

Side effects of morphine may include bradycardia and respiratory depression with aggravation of hypoxemia, especially in patients with chronic lung disease. Leg elevation, fluids, and atropine will correct the hemodynamic effects produced by morphine. Respiratory depression can be reversed with naloxone.

III. DIRECT CURRENT SHOCK

In patients with acute MI, approximately 65% of deaths occur during the first hour of the heart attack, and most deaths are caused by VF. When defibrillaton is successful within 8 minutes of cardiac arrest, 40% of patients will live to be discharged from the hospital. As many as 85% of episodes of VF will be terminated by a single shock of 200 J. Detailed descriptions regarding DC shock and AICD are found in Chapter 13. When VF is refractory to the conventional anti-arrhythmic drug therapy as a preventive measure, and when

VF recurs repeatedly following acute MI, the use of AICD should be strongly considered.

IV. ATROPINE

It is well documented that atropine sulfate reduces vagal tone, enhances the sinus node automaticity and facilitates the A-V conduction via its parasympatholytic (anticholinergic) activity. Atropine is useful to reduce nausea and vomiting as an adjunct to morphine administration. The drug is particularly beneficial during the first few hours of acute MI in the treatment of marked sinus bradycardia associated with reduced cardiac output and signs of peripheral hypoperfusion (e.g., arterial hypotension, confusion, fainting episodes, grayish pallor, etc.) or VPCs. Under this circumstance, leg elevation and the IV administration of atropine may be lifesaving in many cases.

A. Indications:
1. Atropine is the drug of choice for symptomatic Wenckebach (Mobitz type I) AV block particularly in acute diaphragmatic MI.
2. Marked sinus bradycardia with evidence of low cardiac output and peripheral hypoperfusion or frequent VPCs.
3. Bradycardia and hypotension following administration of NG.
4. For nausea and vomiting associated with morphine administration.
5. Ventricular asystole in some cases.
6. Complete AV (AV nodal) block in acute diaphragmatic MI (occasional cases).

B. Dosage
1. The recommended dosage of atropine for bradycardia is 0.5 mg IV, repeated if needed every 5 minutes, to a total dose of no more than 2 mg.
2. Atropine may be useful in ventricular asystole. The recommended dose is 1 mg IV, to be repeated in 5 minutes (while CPR continues) if asystole persists. The total cumulative dose should not exceed 2.5 mg over 2.5 hours.
3. The peak action of atropine given IV is observed within 3 minutes.

C. Side Effects:
1. Repeated administration of atropine may produce adverse CNS effects, including hallucination and fever.
2. Atropine may cause marked sinus tachycardia which often increases ischemia.
3. Following IV administration of atropine, VT or VF may occur on rare cases.
4. On rare occasions, a paradoxic effect (e.g., bradycardia and depression of AV conduction) may be observed when atropine in doses of less than 0.5 mg is given, or when administered other than IV. These effects are considered to be due

either to central reflex stimulation of the vagus or to peripheral parasympathomimetic effect on the heart.

Needless to say, artificial pacing should be the treatment of
choice when symptomatic sinus bradycardia or AV block are refractory to the drug therapy (see Chapter 14).

V. ECG AND HEMODYNAMIC MONITORING

As soon as the diagnosis of acute MI is suspected or established,
continuous ECG monitoring must be carried out. All medical technicians and nurses working in the ER or CCU, as well as in the
pre-hospital setting, should be capable of establishing ECG monitoring as well as diagnosing and initiating proper therapy for life-
threatening cardiac arrhythmias. In patients with suspected or
known unstable hemodynamic status, hemodynamic monitoring
is essential.

A. ECG Monitoring:

ECG monitoring should be continuous and uninterrupted
until the patient's condition becomes stable without significant
arrhythmias, and the responsible medical staff have discharged
the patient from the CCU. In most patients, a single anterior
chest lead provides adequate ECG monitoring.

1. Recommendation for ECG Monitoring:
   a) During the initial 48 to 72 hours in patients with acute
      MI.
   b) Hemodynamic instability, persistent ischemia, or signif-
      icant arrhythmias even after 72 hours following the onset
      of acute MI.
   c) Patients with suspected acute MI during the initial 12 to
      36 hours.
   d) Following insertion of a temporary transvenous artificial
      pacemaker.
   e) Patients with recurrent serious arrhythmias (continuous
      ECG monitoring).
   f) Following coronary angioplasty, thrombolysis or coro-
      nary artery bypass surgery (CABS).

B. Balloon Flotation Right Heart Catheter Monitoring

In the treatment of patients with acute MI who have an
unstable hemodynamic state, including low cardiac output,
hypotension, cardiogenic shock and pulmonary edema, the
balloon flotation catheter is extremely valuable. The balloon
flotation catheter is a relatively safe device associated with a
low risk of serious complications, including pulmonary hemorrhage or infarction.

1. Recommendations for Balloon Flotation Right Heart Catheterization:
   a) Severe or progressive CHF.
   b) Cardiogenic shock or progressive hypotension.
   c) Mechanical complications of acute MI (e.g., ventricular
      septal defect, papillary muscle rupture).
   d) As a diagnostic tool when there is suspicion of an intra-

cardiac shunt, acute mitral regurgitation or pericardial tamponade.
C. Arterial Pressure Monitoring

The necessary equipment and properly trained medical as well as paramedical staff to monitor intra-arterial pressure are essential for all CCUs. Arterial pressure monitoring is indispensable in the management of all hypotensive patients and patients with cardiogenic shock. By and large, intra-arterial catheters should *not* remain in the same arterial site for prolonged periods of time because of the risk of arterial thrombosis. The catheters should be changed within 48 hours (the maximum duration is less than 72 hours in certain situations).
1. Recommendations for Intra-arterial Pressure Monitoring:
    a) All patients with severe hypotension with systolic BP less than 80 mm Hg or cardiogenic shock.
    b) All patients receiving vasopressor agents.
    c) Patients receiving intravenous nitroprusside or other powerful arterial dilating agents.
    d) Patients receiving intravenous inotropic agents.
    e) Patients with life-threatening cardiac arrhythmias (usually VT or VF).
VI. LIDOCAINE

Lidocaine is the drug of choice for the management of ventricular tachyarrhythmias associated with acute MI. Prophylactic administration of lidocaine in patients with suspected or proven acute MI has been recommended, but is still controversial.
A. Recommendations for Lidocaine Administration:
    1. Frequent VPCs (30 or more beats/hr).
    2. VPCs with the R-on-T phenomenon.
    3. Multiformed or multifocal VPCs.
    4. Grouped VPCs.
    5. VT or VF in association with defibrillation and CPR as needed.
Detailed descriptions regarding lidocaine are found elsewhere in this book (see Chapter 12).
VII. ARTIFICIAL PACEMAKERS

In the treatment of clinically significant and drug resistant bradyarrhythmias associated with acute MI, artificial pacing is indicated. By and large, temporary pacing is required because most bradyarrhythmias are transient in nature. When the conduction system has irreversible damage (e.g., complete infra-nodal AV block) secondary to acute MI, needless to say, permanent artificial pacing is indicated. In addition, anti-tachycardia pacing is occasionally needed for patients with drug-resistant and/or DC shock-resistant VT. Furthermore, the prophylactic artificial pacing is highly recommended in certain cases with acute MI (e.g., acute bifascicular block consisting of RBBB with left anterior or posterior hemiblock).

Detailed descriptions regarding the use of artificial pacemakers in acute MI are found elsewhere in this book (see Chapter 14).

VIII. BETA-BLOCKING AGENTS

There are two major goals when beta-blocking agents are used in patients with acute MI. The two goals are as follow:

1. Limitation of myocardial damage or mortality, or both, when administered during the first few hours of acute MI.
2. Reduction of the risk of reinfarction or mortality, or both, when administered after completed MI.

A. Limitation of Myocardial Damage or Mortality, or Both:

Beta-blocking agents can potentially reduce myocardial oxygen demand during the first few hours of acute MI by reducing heart rate and arterial pressure or myocardial contractility or both, and have a favorable influence on myocardial blood flow distribution. The prolongation of diastole resulting from a reduction in heart rate may augment the amount of coronary blood flow reaching injured myocardium. Thus, the beta-blocking agents may increase the amount of myocardium salvaged by reperfusion if the agents are administered early enough in the course of acute MI.

1. Recommendation for Early Intravenous Beta-Blocking Agents:

   a) Patients, including those receiving thrombolytic therapy, with reflex tachycardia or systolic hypertension or both, without signs of CHF or contraindication.

   b) Patients with continuing or recurrent ischemic chest pain, tachyarrhythmias (e.g., AF with a rapid ventricular response) or an enzyme elevation thought to be due to recurrent injury in the absence of known contraindications.

   c) Postinfarction angina while awaiting study in patients without contraindications.

   d) Non-Q wave MI.

B. Reduction of the Risk of Reinfarction or Mortality, or Both After Completed MI

It has been well documented that chronic beta-blockade therapy begun in the early phase of MI improves survival and reduces the incidence of reinfarction for at least the first several months after the acute coronary event. The improved survival appears to include a reduction in the frequency of sudden cardiac death. The absolute reduction in the 2-year mortality rate effected by long-term beta-blocking agent therapy in patients appears to be 2 to 3 percent. Cardioselective as well as nonselective agents have favorable effects in this aspect. Daily dosages showing beneficial effects are relatively high (e.g., 180 to 240 mg of propranolol and 20 mg of timolol).

1. Recommendations for Long-Term Beta-Blockade for Secondary Prevention in Patients Without Myocardial Revascularization:

   a) All but low risk patients who do not have known contraindications to beta-blocking agents.

   b) The beta-blockade therapy should begin with the first

few days of MI and should be continued for at least 2 years.

c) Many physicians recommend the long-term beta-blockade therapy even for low risk patients provided that there are no contraindications.

Detailed descriptions regarding the beta-blocking agents are found elsewhere in this book (see Chapter 12).

IX. CALCIUM CHANNEL BLOCKERS

It has been well documented that calcium channel blocking drugs are effective anti-ischemic agents in the treatment of stable and unstable angina pectoris resulting from fixed coronary artery stenosis as well as from coronary artery spasm. There are three calcium channel blockers available for clinical use, including verapamil, nifedipine and diltiazem. All three agents reduce systemic vascular resistance and, therefore, are highly effective as antihypertensive agents. Diltiazem and verapamil have potent effects on the AV node, producing slowing of the ventricular response to AF or flutter and terminating paroxysmal supraventricular tachyarrhythmias.

A. Recommendations for Use of Calcium Channel Blockers:
   1. Symptomatic treatment of postinfarction angina while awaiting cardiac catheterization and therapy based on angiographic findings.
   2. Following angioplasty, a calcium channel blocker to prevent coronary vasospasm.
   3. Diltiazem in patients with non-Q wave MI. The drug should be given during the first 48 hours and continued through the hospital phase and the first postinfarction year.
   4. A calcium channel blocker may be used for all patients with Q-wave MI in the treatment of postinfarction angina.

Detailed descriptions regarding calcium channel blockers are found elsewhere in this book (see Chapters 1, 6, 12).

X. THROMBOLYTIC THERAPY

Significant S-T segment elevation is observed approximately in 66% of patients with acute MI, and the process is considered to be due to an occlusive coronary clot. Clot-dissolving therapy using intravenous streptokinase and other thrombolytic agents has become a standard treatment of acute MI, particularly during the first 5 to 6 hours following the onset of acute coronary event. Most trials of thrombolytic therapy have excluded elderly patients with acute MI (age above 70 years), primarily because of a fear of hemorrhagic complications.

A. Recommendations for Thrombolytic Therapy:
   1. Patients younger than 70 years of age who are presented with chest pain due to acute MI associated with 1 mm or more S-T segment elevation in at least 2 contiguous ECG leads in whom treatment can be initiated within 6 hours after the onset of acute event.

2. Patients with acute MI more than 6 hours old, but with a "stuttering" pattern of chest pain.
3. Patients who suffer clinically apparent reinfarction in the days after administration of thrombolytic therapy.
4. Some physicians recommend thrombolytic therapy for older patients (age between 70 and 75 years) with the same clinical and ECG findings described in #1.

Detailed descriptions regarding thrombolytic therapy are found in Chapter 6.

XI. ANTICOAGULANTS AND PLATELET INHIBITORY AGENTS

During early phase of acute MI, the major goals of antithrombotic therapy are as follows:

1. Prevention of deep venous thrombosis and pulmonary embolism.
2. Prevention of arterial embolization.
3. Reduction of early recurrence or extension of MI and death.
4. Reduction of reocclusion and death after successful reperfusion with thrombolytic therapy.
5. Secondary prevention of late recurrence of MI and death.

A. Prevention of Deep Venous Thrombosis and Pulmonary Embolism

It has been demonstrated that the incidence of deep venous thrombosis in the lower extremities of patients with acute MI ranges from 17% to 38%. Deep venous thrombi are formed early following acute MI (50% or more within 3 days), and the incidence of thrombi increases after massive or recurrent MI with CHF or cardiogenic shock and prolonged bed rest, especially in elderly patients.

In several reports, low dose heparin started within 12 to 18 hours following an onset of acute MI and continued for 10 days has successfully reduced the incidence of venous thrombosis.

1. Recommendations:
   a) Immediate subcutaneous heparin (5000 U every 12 hours) for the first 24 to 48 hours, unless full dose anticoagulant therapy has been initiated in association with thrombolytic therapy, or for the prevention of systemic emboli.
   b) Continued low dose subcutaneous heparin in high risk patients (e.g., elderly people above age 70, massive MI, CHF, or cardiogenic shock, a previous history of thromboembolic phenomena, etc.) until fully ambulatory.

B. Prevention of Arterial Embolism

It has been demonstrated that the overall incidence of mural thrombus is approximately 20% of acute MI, but the incidence of clinically apparent systemic embolism is reported to be only 2%.

1. Recommendations:
   a) Immediate high dose subcutaneous or IV heparin in a dosage sufficient to prolong the activated partial thromboplastin time to 1.5 to 2.0 times control in patients with

massive anterior transmural MI. Heparin should be continued until discharge.

    b) Oral anticoagulants administered at a dose sufficient to prolong the prothrombin time to 1.3 to 1.5 times the control level after heparin in patients with a ventricular mural thrombus or a large akinetic region of the left ventricular apex. Anticoagulant therapy should be continued for at least 3 months.

    c) Long-term (indefinite period) oral anticoagulant therapy in patients with a diffusely dilated and poorly contractile left ventricle.

C. Reduction of Early Recurrence or Extension of MI and Mortality in Patients Not Receiving Thrombolytic Therapy

It has been reported that recurrence or extension of MI ranges from 14 to 30% (recognized by the enzyme elevation) which is comparable to the incidence of 17% found at autopsy. More than half of the early recurrences occur within 10 days, and the remainder occur within 14 to 18 days following the initial MI. It is interesting to note that the ECG site of early recurrent MI has been the same as the initial site in more than 85% of cases.

1. Recommendations:

    a) Short-term aspirin therapy started immediately and continued for at least 1 month at a dose of 160 mg/day. After 1 month, aspirin should be continued at a dose of 160 to 325 mg/day.

    b) Heparin administration followed by oral anticoagulant therapy for at least 1 month following acute MI, and prothrombin time should be prolonged to 1.3 to 1.5 times control level.

D. Reduction in Early Reocclusion and Mortality After Successful Reperfusion with Thrombolytic Therapy

Significant residual thrombus contributes to the stenosis visualized at angiography following thrombolysis, and reocclusion incidence has been reported to be 5 to 15%.

1. Recommendations:

    a) Aspirin should be started in dosage of 160 mg/day as soon as the patient is admitted to the CCU, and given daily until discharge, at which time it can be continued at a dose of 160 to 325 mg/day.

    b) Heparin should be administered together with or immediately following thrombolysis in order to maintain the activated partial thromboplastin time 1.5 to 2.0 times the control level for 24 to 72 hours.

E. Secondary Prevention of Late Recurrence of MI and Death

Ten large trials using platelet inhibitor drugs in post-MI patients (mostly within the first 2 years) have been conducted. A significant reduction in mortality and reinfarction rates (15% and 31%, respectively) has been documented when aspirin (300

to 1500 mg/day) was used alone or combined with dipyridamole.

1. Recommendations:

   a) Aspirin in dosages of 160 to 325 mg/day, as long as there
   are no significant side effects.

   b) Oral anticoagulant therapy with warfarin (prothrombin
   time 1.3 to 1.5 times the control value) rather than aspirin
   for long-term prevention of recurrent MI.

XII. PERCUTANEOUS TRANSLUMINAL CORONARY ANGIO-
PLASTY (PTCA)

PTCA must be performed only in the hospitals where sophisticated medical facilities with properly trained medical as well as
technical staff are available for the procedure.

PTCA is recommended for patients presenting within 6 hours
of onset of chest pain due to acute MI and who meet the criteria
for thrombolysis but in whom thrombolytic therapy is clearly contraindicated. In addition, PTCA is recommended for intermittent
continual pain, indicating the possibility of "stuttering" infarction,
especially when there are ECG changes, but without clear indication for thrombolytic therapy. Furthermore, PTCA is recommended when patients develop cardiogenic shock or CHF within
18 hours of acute MI. PTCA is also recommended for patients who
have had previous CABS in whom recent occlusion of a vein graft
is suspected.

Detailed description regarding PTCA are found in Chapter 7.

XIII. TREATMENT OF PUMP FAILURE AND CARDIOGENIC SHOCK

Needless to say, pump failure and cardiogenic shock are the
most serious complications of acute MI, and the mortality is, unfortunately, still high. Detailed descriptions regarding CHF and cardiogenic shock are found elsewhere in this book (see Chapters 2
and 3). When cardiogenic shock or pump failure become refractory
to pharmacologic therapy, the use of intra-aortic balloon counterpulsation or other circulatory assist devices should be strongly
considered.

1. Recommendations for Intra-Aortic Balloon Counterpulsation or Other Circulatory Assist Devices

   a) Cardiogenic shock or pump failure *not* responding
   promptly to pharmacologic therapy.

   b) Right ventricular MI associated with pump failure or
   shock *not* responding to volume infusion and appropriate pharmacologic therapy.

   c) Refractory post-MI angina for stabilization before and
   during angiography.

   d) Intractable recurrent tachyarrhythmia (usually ventricular) in patients with hemodynamic instability during
   the arrhythmia.

   e) Other clinical situations including ventricular septal
   defect (VSD), acute mitral regurgitation, persistent ische-

mic chest pain, and progressive CHF despite pharmacologic therapy.

XIV. SURGICAL THERAPY

Detailed descriptions regarding various surgical approaches to
cardiac emergencies are found in Chapter 20, and only a brief
summary will be discussed as follows.

1. Recommendation for Emergency or Urgent CABS in the
   Early Management of Acute MI
   a) Failed PTCA with persistent chest pain or hemodynamic
      instability.
   b) Post-MI angina with left main or 3-vessel disease or
      where PTCA is not indicated, with 2-vessel disease
      involving the proximal left anterior descending coronary
      artery, or 2-vessel disease with poor left ventricular func-
      tion.
   c) At the time of surgical repair for VSD or acute mitral
      regurgitation.
   d) Cardiogenic shock *not* suitable for PTCA.
2. Recommendation for Emergency or Urgent Cardiac Repair
   a) Papillary muscle rupture (emergency).
   b) VSD or free wall rupture (urgent).
   c) Aneurysmal infarction with intractable ventricular tachy-
      arrhythmias or pump failure (urgent), or both.
   d) Acute mitral regurgitation with intractable CHF (urgent).
   e) Intractable ventricular tachycardia (urgent).

XV. PRE-DISCHARGE EVALUATION

Before any patient with acute MI is ready to be discharged, one
must be certain that a given patient is stable clinically without any
significant complications or cardiac arrhythmias. Serial ECGs
should be stable without any acute or new abnormality, and the
cardiac enzyme elevation should *not* be present.

Low-level exercise ECG test is commonly performed and the
ambulatory (Holter monitor) ECG is often obtained 1 to 2 days
before the discharge. Some patients may require 2-dimensional
echocardiography, and occasionally, electrophysiologic study
(EPS). Detailed descriptions regarding the predischarge evaluation
are purposely omitted in this chapter, because those aspects are
beyond the scope of this book.

SUGGESTED READINGS

Bhandari, A.K., Hong, R., Kulick, D., et al.: Day to day reproducibility of electrically
inducible ventricular arrhythmias in survivors of acute myocardial infarction. J. Am.
Coll. Cardiol. *15*:1075, 1990.

Bolooki, H.: Surgical treatment of complications of acute myocardial infarction. JAMA
263:1237, 1990.

Coller, B.S.: Platelets and thrombolytic therapy. N. Engl. J. Med. *322*:33, 1990.

Conti, C.R.: Clinical trials and decisions for thrombolytic therapy in patients with acute myocardial infarction. Clin. Cardiol. *13*:307, 1990.

Conti, C.R.: Coronary artery spasm. Cardiovas. Reviews & Reports *12*:34, 1990.

Fisch, C., Beller, G.A., DeSanctis, R.W., et al.: Guidelines for early management of patients with acute myocardial infarction: A report of the American College of Cardiology/ American Heart Association Task Force. J. Am. Coll. Cardiol. *16*:249, 1990.

Frye, R.L., Gibbons, R.J., Schaff, H.V., et al.: Treatment of coronary artery disease. J. Am. Coll. Cardiol. *13*:957, 1989.

Grines, C.R. and DeMaria, A.N.: Optimal utilization of thrombolytic therapy for acute myocardial infarction: Concepts and controversies. J. Am. Coll. Cardiol. *16*:223, 1990.

Hammill, S.C. and Khandheria, B.K.: Silent myocardial ischemia. Mayo Clin. Proc. *65*:374, 1990.

Lavie, C.J., Gersh, B.J. and Chesebro, J.H.: Reperfusion in acute myocardial infarction. Mayo Clin. Proc. *65*:549, 1990.

Lavie, C.J., and Gersh, B.J.: Acute myocardial infarction: Initial manifestations, management and prognosis. Mayo Clin. Proc. *65*:531, 1990.

Moss, A.J. and Benhorin, J.: Prognosis and management after a first myocardial infarction. N. Engl. J. Med. *322*:743, 1990.

Mueller, H.S.: Reperfusion therapy in acute myocardial infarction: Present status and controversy. Clin. Cardiol. *13*:239, 1990.

Munger, T.M. and Oh, J.K.: Unstable angina. Mayo Clin. Proc. *65*:384, 1990.

Popma, J.J. and Dehmer, G.J.: Care of the patient after coronary angioplasty. Ann. Int. Med. *110*:547, 1989.

Ross, A.M.: The uncertain role of thrombolytic angioplasty within the treatment strategy for myocardial infarction. Am. J. Cardiol. *62*:21K, 1988.

Rowe, W.W., Simpson, R.J., Jr., Tate, D.A., et al.: Nonemergent cardiac catheterization and risk-stratified revascularization following thrombolytic therapy for acute myocardial infarction. Arch. Intern. Med. *149*:1611, 1989.

Sane, D.C., Califf, R.M., Topol, E.J., et al.: Bleeding during thrombolytic therapy for acute myocardial infarction: Mechanisms and Management. Ann. Int. Med. *111*:1010, 1989.

Schlant, R.C.: Thrombolytic therapy of patients with acute myocardial infarction. JAMA *264*:738, 1990.

Stein, B., Fuster, V., Israel, D.H., et al.: Platelet inhibitor agents in cardiovascular disease: An update. J. Am. Coll. Cardiol. *14*:813, 1989.

Stevenson, W.G., Linssen, G.C.M., Havenith, M.G., et al.: The spectrum of death after myocardial infarction: A necropsy study. Am. Heart J. *118*:1182, 1989.

Tate, D.A. and Dehmer, G.J.: New challenges for thrombolytic therapy. Ann. Int. Med. *110*:953, 1989.

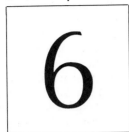

THROMBOLYTIC THERAPY IN ACUTE MYOCARDIAL INFARCTION

Andrew Zalewski and Yi Shi

The role of intracoronary thrombus in the pathogenesis of acute myocardial infarction was first proposed by Herrick in 1912. Recent angiographic studies have clearly demonstrated that occlusive thrombi are present in large epicardial coronary arteries in the majority of patients hospitalized within the first few hours after the onset of symptoms. DeWood and associates reported that 87% of patients with acute myocardial infarction had total coronary occlusion of the infarct-related artery if angiography was performed within 4 hours of symptoms, whereas the incidence decreased to 65% in patients undergoing cardiac catheterization more than 12 hours after symptom onset.

Experimental and clinical data suggest that the shift from reversible (i.e., ischemia) to irreversible myocardial damage (i.e., necrosis) occurs within the first few hours of myocardial infarction. Thus, the goal of early therapy in acute myocardial infarction is to achieve myocardial salvage via either the decrease in myocardial oxygen demand and/or coronary artery reperfusion. Large scale clinical trials with the early administration of beta-adrenergic blocking agents and of calcium antagonists have shown only limited effects on myocardial salvage.

In 1979, Rentrop and associates reported successful coronary reperfusion with intracoronary administration of streptokinase in evolving acute myocardial infarction. This observation dramatically increased the interest in thrombolytic therapy for acute myocardial infarction. Fur-

69

thermore, it became apparent that coronary reperfusion therapy is feasible not only in the experimental laboratory but also could be successfully used in patients with acute myocardial infarction.

I. MODALITIES OF CORONARY REPERFUSION

Several modalities are now available to accomplish coronary reperfusion in acute myocardial infarction. These include: surgical revascularization, coronary angioplasty and pharmacologic reperfusion. Only the last modality can be applied to a large population of patients. Pharmacologic reperfusion can be achieved via either intracoronary or intravenous administration of thrombolytic agents. Direct intracoronary administration of thrombolytic agents has now mostly historical importance since it involved significant delay in institution of therapy and required available cardiac catheterization facility. A more practical approach includes intravenous administration of a thrombolytic agent in the early hours of myocardial infarction which may enhance myocardial salvage.

A. Indications for Thrombolytic Therapy in Acute Myocardial Infarction

1. Duration of Symptoms. Persistent chest pain lasting more than 30 minutes accompanied by ST segment elevation is a major indication for intravenous thrombolytic therapy. Some controversy exists about how long after onset of chest pain reperfusion therapy is effective. Most experimental studies indicate that reperfusion beyond 6 hours of coronary occlusion does not result in myocardial salvage and is associated with extensive myocardial hemorrhage. In the clinical setting, however, episodes of spontaneous reperfusion in early hours of infarction ("stuttering" infarction) and uncertainty about the onset of chest pain sometimes prolong a window of time when thrombolytic therapy is advantageous. In addition, patients with a residual flow to infarcting zone (e.g., collateral circulation) may benefit from even delayed therapy. Thus, thrombolysis is recommended for patients with myocardial infarction within the first 6 hours of symptoms, and in those beyond that period of time if chest pain persists and surface electrocardiogram shows injury current (i.e., ST segment elevation) with preserved R-wave amplitude.

2. Electrocardiographic Changes. Sudden coronary artery occlusion results in ST segment elevation and a transient growth of R-wave amplitude in the surface electrocardiogram. These are typical electrocardiographic criteria for initiation of intravenous thrombolytic agent. In contrast, return of ST segment to the isoelectric line associated with loss of R-wave amplitude (QS pattern) is strongly suggestive of completed necrosis, where thrombolytic therapy is of questionable value.

The role of thrombolytic therapy in patients with chest pain and ST segment depression remains to be determined. It is most likely that this heterogeneous population of patients consists of those with 1) subtotal coronary occlusion, 2) ischemia at a distance (e.g., as a result of compromised collateral circulation in multivessel coronary artery disease), or 3) the left circumflex coronary occlusion manifested as isolated precordial ST segment depression. Only in the last group of patients is transmural myocardial ischemia present, and successful lysis of occlusive thrombus may improve the patient's prognosis. At present, no evidence exists that the benefit of thrombolysis outweighs the risk of bleeding complications in patients with unstable angina or nontransmural myocardial infarction. In addition, caution should be advised before thrombolytic therapy is used in patients with severe chest pain and no electrocardiographic changes. Severe chest pain in this subgroup of patients may be related to noncoronary events such as acute pericarditis or acute aortic dissection where thrombolytic therapy would cause devastating complications (e.g., cardiac tamponade, progression of dissection).

3. Hemodynamic Status. Most of the trials of thrombolytic therapy excluded patients with severe hemodynamic compromise reflected by cardiogenic shock and/or pulmonary edema. Since even marginal improvement in the left ventricular function may improve prognosis in this high risk patient group, thrombolytic therapy combined with emergency cardiac catheterization and possibly coronary angioplasty is recommended. Anecdotal observations suggest that coronary reperfusion in this subgroup sometimes exerts a strikingly beneficial effect.

4. Location of Myocardial Infarction. There is little controversy regarding the beneficial effect of thrombolytic therapy in patients with anterior wall myocardial infarction. Patients with inferior wall myocardial infarction demonstrate better left ventricular function and lower mortality than patients with anterior wall myocardial infarction. These differences can be explained by a smaller risk area and infarct size in the former group. Thus, not unexpectedly, benefit of thrombolytic therapy is more difficult to ascertain especially in elderly patients with inferior wall myocardial infarction. At present, it is our recommendation to administer intravenous thrombolytic agents in those patients with inferior wall myocardial infarction who 1) present early after onset of symptoms (i.e., 3 to 4 hours), 2) demonstrate electrocardiographic signs of large risk area (i.e., ST segment elevation in inferior leads with ST segment depression in precordial leads), or 3) have a history of an old anterior wall myocardial infarction which suggests that their systolic left ventricular function is markedly reduced. In contrast, in patients older than 70 years of age who present late after onset of symptoms (i.e., >3 hours) and/or are hypertensive, conventional medical therapy is probably more appropriate. These patients gen-

Table 6–1. Contraindications to Thrombolytic Therapy

1. Active internal bleeding
2. History of cerebrovascular accident
3. Recent (within 2 months) intracranial, intraspinal surgery, or trauma
4. Intracranial neoplasm, arteriovenous malformations, or aneurysm
5. Known bleeding diathesis
6. Severe uncontrolled hypertension
7. Central line (subclavian or internal jugular)
8. Recent trauma or CPR (within 10 days)
9. Hypertension: systolic BP > 180 mm Hg and or diastolic BP > 110 mm Hg
10. High likelihood of left heart thrombus, e.g., mitral stenosis with atrial fibrillation
11. Acute pericarditis
12. Subacute bacterial endocarditis
13. Hemostatic defects including those secondary to severe hepatic or renal disease
14. Significant liver dysfunction
15. Pregnancy
16. Diabetic hemorrhagic retinopathy, or other hemorrhagic opththalmic conditions
17. Septic thrombophlebitis or occluded AV cannula at seriously infected site
18. Advanced age, i.e., over 75 years old
19. Patients currently receiving oral anticoagulants, e.g., warfarin sodium
20. Any other condition in which bleeding constitutes a significant hazard or would be particularly difficult to manage because of its location

erally have an uneventful clinical course without thrombolytic therapy.

B. Contraindications to Thrombolytic Therapy

All thrombolytic agents cause a transient coagulation defect. This therapy is contraindicated in those patients who are at risk of developing external or internal bleeding or embolic complications as a result of clot lysis. Contraindications to thrombolytic therapy are listed in Table 6–1.

C. Markers of Coronary Artery Reperfusion

Coronary artery reperfusion following thrombolytic therapy sometimes can be diagnosed by clinical, electrocardiographic, or biochemical markers.

1. Clinical. Successful thrombolysis is usually manifested by an abrupt resolution of chest pain. In some patients, symptoms of Bezold-Jarisch reflex can be present (i.e., nausea, vomiting, hypotension, bradycardia). These symptoms are more common in patients with inferoposterior myocardial infarction.

2. Electrocardiographic. Sudden resolution of ST segment elevation accompanied by R wave loss are typical electrocardiographic manifestations of reperfusion. Q wave development is common despite successful and timely restoration of coronary blood flow. In some patients, partial regrowth

of R waves can be observed several weeks after myocardial infarction. In addition to changes in ST segment and QRS morphology, reperfusion is often associated with accelerated idioventricular rhythm. Accelerated idioventricular rhythm is a slow ventricular tachycardia that is usually well tolerated by patients and does not require specific therapy. Although the presence of accelerated idioventricular rhythm indicates reperfusion, its absence does not preclude it. Other electrocardiographic changes suggestive of reperfusion include sinus bradycardia, sinus pauses, or escape junctional rhythm, especially if accompanied by sudden relief of chest pain in patients with inferoposterior myocardial infarction.

3. Biochemical. Creatine kinase is released from infarcting myocardium. In patients with successful reperfusion, early peak of creatine kinase (approximately 13 hours after pain onset) is seen, as opposed to creatine kinase peak at 18 to 24 hours in those patients who fail reperfusion therapy. This marker, however, has only retrospective value, since creatine kinase determinations should be followed at 6 hour intervals for the first 48 hours to determine the shape of creatine kinase curve after myocardial infarction.

The above mentioned noninvasive markers of reperfusion have been found to have high specificity but low sensitivity in diagnosing the patency of the infarct-related vessel. Therefore, their absence does not allow us to distinguish between patients with successful reperfusion and those who failed thrombolysis.

D. Clinical Benefits of Thrombolytic Therapy in Acute Myocardial Infarction

The goal of reperfusion therapy is myocardial salvage leading to improved survival and preservation of the left ventricular function after myocardial infarction.

1. Survival. Several large studies unequivocally showed improvement in early survival in patients treated with intravenous thrombolytic agents such as streptokinase, an isolated plasminogen-streptokinase activator complex or tissue plasminogen activator. Early mortality after myocardial infarction ranged from 9.8 to 13% in placebo-treated patients compared with 6.3 to 10% in those treated with thrombolytic agents. This represents a reduction in mortality by 20 to 51% afforded by thrombolysis. Preliminary data suggest that this beneficial effect on survival is sustained for at least 1 year. The reduction in cardiac mortality after thrombolysis may depend on: 1) time of reperfusion after symptom onset, 2) the size of risk area, 3) choice of thrombolytic agents, and/ or 4) incidence of coronary reocclusion following thrombolysis.

Since infarct size is a time-dependent phenomenon, not surprisingly the biggest effect of thrombolysis on survival is seen with early (i.e., <3 hours) administration of thrombolytic agents. Delayed reperfusion salvages most of the subepicardial rim of the myocardium, thereby, improving less the survival rate.

The size of the risk area is determined by the amount of myocardium supplied by an occluded infarct-related coronary artery. In general, the left anterior descending coronary artery causing anterior wall myocardial infarction involves more myocardium than the right coronary or the left circumflex coronary occlusion responsible for inferior/posterior myocardial infarction. Thus, in the former group, which has a higher mortality, early thrombolysis may improve survival, while, in the latter group, the effects of this therapy are more difficult to prove since prognosis is relatively benign even without reperfusion.

Various thrombolytic agents have distinct pharmacologic properties, but their beneficial effects on survival have yet to be compared with each other. Preliminary results of large randomized trials have shown comparable effects of streptokinase and tissue plasminogen activator on survival following myocardial infarction (GISSI II study).

2. Left ventricular function. Preservation of left ventricular function after myocardial infarction not only improves long-term survival, but it may also improve quality of life by reducing the symptoms of pump failure. A modest increase in the left ventricular ejection fraction has been reported with intravenous administration of streptokinase or recombinant tissue plasminogen activator. There are several reasons that explain the small effect of thrombolytic agents on global left ventricular function. Delayed reperfusion therapy (i.e., >4 to 6 hours from symptom onset) or early reocclusion may prevent a more striking improvement in the ejection fraction. In addition, not uncommonly the global ejection fraction remains in low normal range as a result of hyperdynamic function of the portion of the left ventricle remote from the infarcted area. In patients with more severe left ventricular involvement, the phenomenon of "stunned" myocardium (i.e., prolonged systolic dysfunction following successful reperfusion) may obscure significant myocardial salvage if measurements of systolic left ventricular function are obtained early (i.e., days) after myocardial infarction.

3. Other potential benefits. Patients with widely patent infarct-related artery have better survival at 1 year than those who failed thrombolysis despite similar ejection fraction in both groups. Therefore, it has been postulated that even late reperfusion therapy may prevent left ventricular dilatation and remodeling without significant myocardial salvage. Reduction in the incidence of late ventricular fibrillation is another suggested benefit of late myocardial reperfusion.

E. Pharmacology of Thrombolytic Agents

Dissolution of the thrombus (i.e., thrombolysis) requires active protease plasmin which is formed by the action of plasminogen activators on its inactive precursor, plasminogen. Plasminogen circulates freely in the blood stream as well as binds to fibrin during thrombus formation. Plasmin degrades not only primary components of vascular thrombi fibrin, but also circulating fibrinogen and factors V and VIII.

1. Classification of thrombolytic agents. First-generation plasminogen activators include agents lacking fibrin selectivity, such as streptokinase or urokinase. Accordingly, they activate circulating and fibrin-bound plasminogen. This group of activators will significantly lower levels of fibrinogen and factors V and VIII.

Streptokinase is a protease produced by beta-hemolytic streptococci. Streptokinase activates plasminogen after forming a complex with plasminogen on a 1:1 basis. Thus, streptokinase-plasminogen complex is capable of activating other plasminogen molecules. Since the half-life of streptokinase is 23 minutes, longer fibrinolytic activity can be achieved by rapid infusion of a large dose. The recommended dose is 1.5 million units given intravenously over a one-hour period. Besides bleeding complications, streptokinase can cause allergic reactions such as fever, hypotension, nausea, and rash, and, rarely, anaphylactoid reaction.

Urokinase is a human enzyme initially obtained from urine. It directly activates plasminogen to plasmin. Because of a half-life of 16 minutes, urokinase is administered intravenously in a large dose, producing coagulation defects similar to those observed with streptokinase.

Second generation plasminogen activators include human proteins produced by endothelial cells, such as tissue plasminogen activator (tPA) and single-chain urokinase plasminogen activator (SCU-PA or prourokinase). These agents possess relative fibrin selectivity since they predominantly activate fibrin-bound plasminogen.

Tissue plasminogen activator can be obtained in large quantities using recombinant DNA technology. Currently used tissue plasminogen activator (Activase) is a single chain molecule which binds to fibrin at the site of a vascular thrombus. Because of a very short half-life (5 minutes), tPA is given in a continuous intravenous infusion. Recommended doses of currently available tissue plasminogen activator are 100 mg given as follows: 10 mg is infused over 2 minutes, 50 mg is infused for the next hour, and the remaining 40 mg is infused for an additional 2 hours. Thus, duration of therapy is a total of 3 hours. Others have recommended so called front-loaded regimen, which includes tissue plasminogen activator 15 mg intravenous bolus followed by 0.75 mg/kg over 30 minutes followed by 0.5 mg/kg given over 60 minutes. Because of relative fibrin-specificity, tissue plasminogen activator produces a smaller decrease in circulating fibrinogen in comparison with first generation plasminogen activators.

Single-chain urokinase plasminogen activator is a new investigational thrombolytic agent. Although it does not bind directly to fibrin, single-chain urokinase plasminogen activator activates fibrin-bound plasminogen. The half-life and other pharmacologic properties of single-chain urokinase plasminogen activator are similar to those of tissue plasminogen activator. Synergism between these 2 agents with potential for enhanced thrombolysis has been suggested.

Third generation plasminogen activators include newer proteins obtained either in the process of chemical modification (e.g., acylated plasminogen-streptokinase activator complex) or by recombinant DNA technology (e.g., mutant for tissue plasminogen activator).

Acylated plasminogen-streptokinase activator complex (APSAC, Eminase) has unique pharmacologic properties. Plasminogen component of acylated plasminogen-streptokinase activator complex binds to fibrin. Subsequent deacylation of the molecule allows for activation of plasminogen. Although acylated plasminogen-streptokinase activator complex is not as fibrin specific as tissue plasminogen activator, it activates circulating plasminogen less than the first generation of activators. In contrast to other thrombolytic agents, it has a longer half-life (90 minutes), which provides prolonged fibrinolysis even after 5 minutes of intravenous infusion. Recommended dose for acylated plasminogen-streptokinase activator complex is 30 units given intravenously over 2 to 5 minutes.

F. Choice of Thrombolytic Agent
   1. Reperfusion efficacy of intravenous tissue plasminogen activator seems to be superior to that of streptokinase in acute myocardial infarction. Combined data from 2 large trials indicate reperfusion rates of 79% and 53% after tissue plasminogen activator and streptokinase, respectively, with therapy started within 3 hours of symptoms. Similarly, if the infusion was started between 3 and 6 hours after the onset of pain, tissue plasminogen activator resulted in more frequent reperfusion (60%) than streptokinase (37%), as determined by coronary angiography at 90 minutes after onset of therapy. It remains to be determined whether early higher reperfusion efficacy afforded by tissue plasminogen activator can result in greater reduction of cardiac mortality or better preservation of the left ventricular function as compared with streptokinase therapy.
   2. Bleeding complications. Risk of bleeding is similar for all

thrombolytic agents. Hemorrhagic complications were initially observed in more than 30% of patients treated with either tissue plasminogen activator or streptokinase, with half of them defined as major bleeding events. If invasive procedures, such as cardiac catheterization, are deferred, risk of bleeding complications is reduced to about 5%. The incidence of cerebrovascular bleeding in patients treated with all thrombolytic agents is less than 1%. It is not surprising that even fibrin-specific agents, such as tissue plasminogen activator, are associated with bleeding complications. This is related to the inability of any thrombolytic agent to distinguish between coronary thrombus and a protective hemostatic plug in other vascular areas. Unexpected lysis of such hemostatic plug leads to untoward bleeding events. Incidence of bleeding complications can be reduced by careful patient selection, short duration of therapy, and avoidance of invasive procedures during the first 24 hours of therapy (e.g., cardiac catheterization, placement of central line, etc.). Serious bleeding requires immediate discontinuation of the thrombolytic agent.

3. Reocclusion following successful thrombolysis occurs in about 10 to 20% of patients. Theoretically, administration of agents with a longer half-life (e.g., acylated plasminogen-streptokinase activator complex, streptokinase) should be associated less frequently with rethrombosis than plasminogen activator with short half-life (e.g., tissue plasminogen activator). Reocclusion, however, is related to several additional factors, such as severity of a residual stenosis following thrombolysis and platelet activation by ruptured plaque in the infarct-related artery. To prevent reocclusion, patients receiving thrombolytic agents, especially tissue plasminogen activator, are placed on an intravenous infusion of heparin and oral aspirin. Invasive procedures, such as percutaneous transluminal coronary angioplasty, are usually deferred to allow for more complete lysis of an intracoronary thrombus.

II. CONCLUSIONS

Early coronary artery reperfusion improves prognosis in myocardial infarction. Successful lysis of intracoronary thrombus results in improved survival and better preservation of left ventricular function following myocardial infarction. Unresolved issues, however, include the role of adjunctive therapy (e.g., beta-blockers, free radical scavengers) and optimal identification of the patient who requires coronary angiography following thrombolysis. Recent advances in molecular biology will hopefully lead to the discovery of more effective (i.e., higher reperfusion efficacy) and safer (i.e., less bleeding complications) thrombolytic agents.

SUGGESTED READINGS

DeWood, M.A., Spores, J., Notske, R., et al.: Prevalence of total coronary occlusion during the early hours of transmural myocardial infarction. N. Engl. J. Med. 303:897, 1980.

Rentrop, K.P., Blanke, H., Harsch, K.R., et al.: Acute myocardial infarction: intracoronary application of nitroglycerin and streptokinase. Clin. Cardiol. 2:354, 1979.

Loscalzo, J. and Braunwald, E.: Drug therapy: tissue plasminogen activator. N. Engl. J. Med. *319*:925, 1988.

Verstraete, M., et al.: Randomized trial of intravenous recombinant tissue-type plasminogen activator versus intravenous streptokinase in acute myocardial infarction. Lancet *1*:842, 1985.

Chesebro, J.H., Knatlerud, G., Roberts, R., et al.: Thrombolysis in myocardial infarction (TIMI) trial. Phase I: a comparison between intravenous tissue plasminogen activator and intravenous streptokinase: clinical findings through hospital discharge. Circulation *76*:142–154, 1987.

Runge, M.S., et al: Plasminogen activators: the old and the new. Circulation *79*:217, 1989.

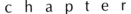

CORONARY ANGIOPLASTY

Michael P. Savage

Ischemic heart disease, caused by atherosclerosis of the epicardial coronary arteries, remains the leading cause of death in the industrialized world. Myocardial ischemia results from an imbalance in myocardial oxygen supply-and-demand and, therefore, all modes of therapy for coronary artery disease are designed to alleviate this imbalance. Pharmacologic treatments of angina act primarily by reducing myocardial oxygen demand. In contrast, coronary artery bypass surgery augments myocardial oxygen supply by direct revascularization. Through continued refinements, coronary bypass surgery has assumed an essential role in the treatment of ischemic heart disease. Nevertheless, operative morbidity and the chronic risk of graft occlusion have been persistent limitations of the surgical approach. The introduction of the technique of percutaneous transluminal coronary angioplasty (PTCA) by Andreas Gruentzig represented a revolutionary departure from previous forms of therapy. Coronary angioplasty improves blood flow to ischemic myocardium by nonoperative dilatation of coronary artery stenoses using a distensible balloon catheter. This chapter will review the current state of the art of this evolving technique.

I. HISTORICAL DEVELOPMENT

The development of balloon angioplasty can be traced to a series of important historic milestones.

A. Balloon catheters have been used therapeutically for nearly 2 centuries. In 1819, Arnott devised balloon catheters made from catgut to relieve urethral strictures.

B. Initial developments in percutaneous dilatation of diseased blood vessels involved bougie-type catheters. In 1964, Dotter and Judkins performed the first percutaneous angioplasty procedures by employing a series of progressively wider dilators to enlarge the lumens of obstructed peripheral arteries.

C. Technical limitations imposed by the use of rigid catheters fostered the development of the expandable balloon catheter by Gruentzig in 1974. Following initial success with peripheral vascular dilatations, further miniaturization of the system led to experimental trials involving coronary arteries in animal models, human cadavers and, intraoperatively, in patients. In September 1977, after careful development of technique through these preliminary studies, Gruentzig performed the first percutaneous transluminal coronary angioplasty in man.

D. In response to increasing dissemination of the technique, an international registry was established in 1979 under the auspices of the National Heart, Lung, and Blood Institute (NHLBI) in order to monitor its safety and efficacy. By the time of closure to new patient entry in September 1982, data from 3079 procedures was enrolled.

E. Since the time of the initial NHLBI registry, continued technical refinements, particularly the development of steerable guidewires, have further advanced the therapeutic efficacy of coronary angioplasty.

II. TECHNICAL ASPECTS

Optimal performance of coronary angioplasty requires the coordinated efforts of cardiologists, cardiothoracic surgeons, laboratory technicians, and specialized nursing personnel. The operator should be facile with all aspects of diagnostic cardiac catheterization and coronary angiography. Moreover, the previous experience of the individual operator in performing PTCA is a significant determinant of the procedure's success or failure. Because of this "learning curve" effect, it is recommended that all cardiologists conducting the procedure do so initially under close supervision by physicians already skilled in PTCA. Finally, PTCA should be undertaken with the backup of a cardiac surgery team and operating room in the event of an acute ischemic complication during the procedure.

A. Equipment
 1. The radiographic equipment necessary for PTCA should include certain essential features:
   a) X-ray tube image intensifier units capable of steep cranial and caudal angulations. Biplane image intensifier systems are particularly helpful in cases with complex or difficult anatomy.
   b) High-resolution image intensifier capable of providing clear visualization of fine guidewires as small as 0.010 inch in diameter.
   c) Video recorder which projects a freeze-frame image of

the baseline coronary angiogram. When displayed simultaneously with ongoing manipulations, this image provides a continual reference or anatomic road map which facilitates appropriate positioning of the guidewire and balloon catheter.

d) An oscilloscopic monitor capable of displaying surface electrocardiographic leads, central aortic (guide-catheter) pressure, and distal coronary (dilatation-catheter) pressure simultaneously.

2. The working tools for PTCA include:
   a) The guiding catheter: The role of the guide catheter is to provide for contrast injection and to provide the necessary coaxial support for passage of the dilatation (balloon) catheter into the atherosclerotic lesion.
      (1) Guiding catheters are a composite with three layers:
         (a) An inner layer of teflon which, because of its low coefficient of friction, permits unimpeded passage of the dilatation catheter through its lumen.
         (b) A middle layer of woven wire mesh which provides body and stability to the catheter and allows for torque control.
         (c) An outer layer of polyurethane polyethelene, or woven dacron which imparts catheter memory.
         (d) These catheters are available in a variety of preformed shapes and sizes.
   b) The dilatation catheter: Refinements in the dilatation apparatus have significantly improved the safety and efficacy of PTCA. The original catheter design (a nonsteerable balloon catheter at the end of which was a fixed 5 mm wire tip) has been all but abandoned. Current dilatation systems utilize an independent, steerable guidewire which is freely movable through a central lumen in the balloon catheter. The use of steerable guidewires and the development of low profile balloon catheters have made even severe distal lesions and tortuous arteries accessible to angioplasty.
      (1) Most dilatation catheters contain two lumens:
         (a) A central lumen allows passage of the guidewire and measurement of distal coronary artery pressure.
         (b) A second lumen that connects directly with the distensible balloon, is used for balloon inflation with a solution of saline and radiographic contrast.
      (2) The balloons are constructed of polyethylene or polyvinylchloride materials and are located at the distal end of the catheter.
         (a) The standard length of coronary angioplasty bal-

loons is 20 mm; shorter and longer balloons are also available.

(b) Inflated diameters range from 1.5 to 4.0 mm. The balloon size is selected to correspond with the diameter of normal arterial segments adjacent to the lesion.

(c) Further advances in catheter design have yielded catheters with extremely narrow deflated balloon profiles and more gradually tapered tips. These "low profile" catheters are useful for long, narrow lesions in which greater resistance to balloon passage may be encountered.

c) Guidewires

(1) Special guidewires are available in sizes varying from 0.014 to 0.018 inch in diameter. These steerable wires are advanced out of the dilatation catheter and across the stenosis into the distal segment of the diseased vessel. Once positioned beyond the stenosis, the guidewire serves as a track over which the dilatation catheter can be passed into the lesion.

(2) The introduction of movable, steerable guidewires was a major advance toward improving primary success rates and reducing the complications of PTCA. Anatomical obstacles often troublesome for the early fixed-guidewire catheters, such as distal and eccentric lesions or abruptly angulated branches, are now routinely overcome.

(3) Prior to the introduction of steerable catheter systems, failure to cross the stenosis occurred in 25% of all attempts and represented the most common cause of PTCA failure. With currently available guidewires and low-profile balloon catheters, PTCA failure due to inability to cross the stenosis is now rare except in the presence of a chronic total occlusion.

B. Procedure (See Fig. 7–1.)

1. Premedication is administered before the procedure to reduce coronary vasospasm and platelet deposition associated with coronary angioplasty:

a) Nifedipine 20 to 30 mg every 6 hours, or diltiazem 60 to 90 mg every 6 hours.

b) Dipyridamole (Persantine) 75 mg every 8 hours.

c) Aspirin 325 mg daily.

2. PTCA is performed on patients in the fasting sedated state under local lidocaine anesthesia.

a) PTCA may be undertaken by either the femoral or brachial approach.

(1) The percutaneous transfemoral approach is preferred by most operators. If an acute ischemic complication

requiring surgery occurs, it provides immediate vascular access for intraaortic balloon counterpulsation.

(2) The brachial approach can be useful for dilating stenoses in the right coronary artery and in bypass grafts.

b) A temporary pacemaker catheter is placed within the right atrium or ventricle.

c) The guiding catheter is then positioned in the coronary ostium and baseline angiograms are obtained.

(1) Heparin (10,000 units intravenously) is given to prevent thromboembolic complications. Surveillance of appropriate anticoagulation status is achieved by monitoring the activated coagulation time periodically throughout the procedure.

(2) Intracoronary nitroglycerin (200 mcg) is administered to prevent coronary artery spasm; infusion of intravenous nitroglycerin is also begun.

(3) Diagnostic angiography should be performed in the LAO and RAO projections which best display the lesion undergoing dilatation. Freeze frame road map images are selected and then projected by video monitor to aid correct positioning of the guidewire and balloon catheter. Important anatomic features should be given special attention when defining the diseased coronary:

(a) The severity, length, eccentricity and calcification of the stenosis.

(b) The presence of side branches arising from or near the lesion.

(c) Delineation of the distal vessel.

(4) Selection of the optimal guiding catheter is a critical factor affecting the outcome of the procedure:

(a) The guiding catheter must adequately seat in the coronary ostium to ensure the necessary support for passage of the guidewire-dilatation catheter system across the stenosis.

(b) Painstaking care must be paid to avoid wedging of the guide catheter which results in obstruction of coronary blood flow and may traumatize the coronary ostium.

d) After satisfactory seating of the guide catheter is achieved, the guidewire-balloon catheter system is then inserted through the guide.

(1) The steerable guidewire is then advanced across the stenotic lesion and into the distal artery. Thus, the guidewire serves to anchor the system and provides a guiderail over which the balloon catheter can gain access to the lesion.

(2) The balloon is then passed into the lesion and positioned so that it is symmetrically engaged across the

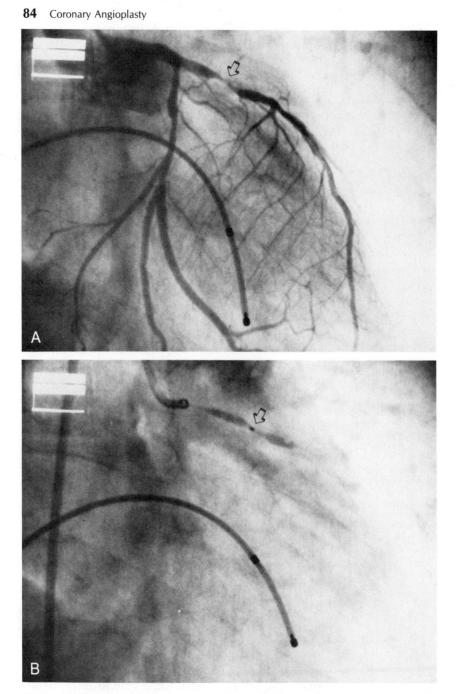

FIG. 7–1. Coronary angioplasty in a 54-year-old man with angina pectoris. *A*, Baseline coronary angiogram demonstrates a severe stenosis in the proximal left anterior descending coronary artery (arrow). *B*, During inflation, the dilatation catheter demonstrates a "dumbbell" appearance (arrow) due to indentation of the expanding balloon by the atherosclerotic lesion.

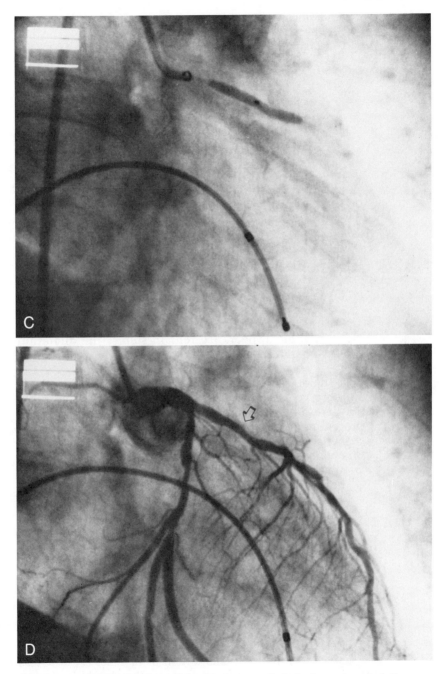

FIG. 7–1 (Continued). *C,* With further increase in inflation pressure, full expansion of the balloon is observed. Dilatation of the stenosis is indicated by loss of the previous "dumbbell" deformity. *D,* Post-PTCA angiogram demonstrates a widely patent left anterior descending coronary artery.

stenosis. The translesional pressure gradient may then be recorded prior to balloon inflation.

(a) Balloon inflation is performed with gradually increasing distending pressure while full expansion of the balloon is observed fluoroscopically. Balloon inflation pressures vary from 60 to 180 lb/in² depending upon the rigidity of the lesion.

(b) Initial inflation is generally for 30 to 60 seconds. Duration of inflation is determined by the ischemic response from transient coronary occlusion (i.e., chest pain and ST segment changes) and by the given therapeutic effect from the dilatation (i.e., the angiographic and hemodynamic results).

(c) Successful PTCA is defined as a residual stenosis of less than 50% and a residual translesional gradient below 20 mm Hg. Repeated inflations may be necessary (often at higher pressure or longer duration) to achieve a satisfactory result.

(3) Once a satisfactory result is achieved, the patient is observed for signs of abrupt reclosure over a 30 minute period. If the translesional gradient and angiographic appearance remain stable, the dilatation apparatus is removed and a final coronary angiogram is obtained.

3. Post-angioplasty Care. Following successful PTCA, patients are observed in a monitored unit for 24 hours. Generally, they are discharged from the hospital two days after the procedure.

a) Serial electrocardiograms and creatine kinase levels are obtained.

b) When an intimal dissection has occurred, intravenous heparin is continued overnight and the vascular sheaths are removed the following morning.

c) Since no intervention has been conclusively shown to reduce post-PTCA restenosis, all follow-up therapy is therefore empiric.

(1) Aspirin 325 mg daily is widely used despite its lack of efficacy in preventing restenosis in controlled clinical trials.

(2) Calcium-channel antagonists are continued in the subgroup of patients with documented variant angina.

d) Repeat exercise testing and/or angiography is recommended for all patients 6 months after PTCA to assess for restenosis. Coronary angiography should be undertaken sooner should anginal symptoms recur.

C. Mechanism of PTCA

The underlying principle of transluminal coronary angioplasty is the application of a radially directed force produced by balloon inflation within the diseased arterial segment. The complex histopathologic consequences of balloon angioplasty have been analyzed by several investigators. These morphologic studies have greatly enriched our understanding of the mechanisms of PTCA.

1. Initially, it was proposed that transluminal angioplasty worked by compression of atheromatous material within the intimal plaque. It is now appreciated that such lesions have minimal compactibility. Histologic studies in both animal and cadaver models have shown that balloon angioplasty does not significantly compress the volume of either the atheromatous plaque or the arterial wall.

2. Another potential mechanism for PTCA is the release of fragmented atheromatous material with embolization to the distal vessel. Although superficial endothelial desquamation may occur, release of plaque elements has not been found in experimental studies. Furthermore, distal embolization is rarely observed clinically. Plaque embolization, therefore, is not an important mechanism of transluminal angioplasty.

3. The probable mechanism of PTCA involves 2 fundamental processes: splitting of the intimal plaque, and stretching of the media and adventitia with distension of the arterial diameter.

   a) Balloon inflation within the stenotic lesion initially causes the splitting or cracking of the intimal plaque. The intimal split may extend down to the internal elastic membrane, producing a cleavage plane between intima and denuded media.

   b) Once intimal disruption has occurred, continued balloon expansion leads to stretching of the media and adventitia. Further deformation of the elastic components of the media results in loss of recoil and permanent widening of the vessel which remains after balloon deflation. Characteristic histologic correlates of this process have been described, and include straightening of elastic fibers and corkscrew deformity of smooth muscle cell nuclei.

   c) Thus, the net result of this "controlled injury" is the overall expansion of both the internal and external diameters of the involved artery. The enlarged lumen within the diseased segment allows greater coronary blood flow and amelioration of myocardial ischemia.

   d) The splitting of the intimal plaque accounts for the frequent hazy angiographic appearance of these lesions immediately following angioplasty. The split areas fill with angiographic contrast which produces the inhomogeneous and less radio-opaque appearance of the dye column at the site of coronary dilatation.

   e) The healing process of this lesion is less well understood.

An accelerated fibrocellular proliferation leads to a recurrent stenosis in up to one-third of patients following PTCA.

III. PATIENT SELECTION

The indications for PTCA continue to evolve and expand as a result of progressive refinements in equipment and technique.

A. Candidates for PTCA should fulfill the following selection criteria:
   1. Angina pectoris inadequately controlled by medical therapy.
   2. Objective evidence of myocardial ischemia demonstrated by resting electrocardiogram or stress testing.
   3. Discrete, high-grade stenosis in a single epicardial coronary artery.
   4. Eligibility for coronary artery bypass surgery in the event of unsuccessful angioplasty.

B. Decisions regarding applicability of PTCA must be individualized. Several clinical and angiographic factors should be considered which affect the likelihood for successful dilatation.
   1. Prior myocardial infarction with left ventricular dysfunction (patients undergoing PTCA who have had a prior myocardial infarction in the distribution of a contralateral coronary artery are at high risk of severe hemodynamic compromise should an acute ischemic complication occur).
   2. Lesion location (proximal lesions are ideal but even more distal lesions are routinely accessible using steerable low-profile equipment).
   3. Length of stenosis (lesions >10 mm in length are associated with a greater risk of both acute dissection and restenosis).
   4. Calcification (calcified lesions are more rigid which makes them resistant to dilatation and prone to dissection).
   5. Thrombus (the presence of intracoronary thrombus detected angiographically has been associated with an increased risk of abrupt closure during attempted PTCA).
   6. Vessel tortuosity (extreme tortuosity proximal to the stenosis will decrease the likelihood of crossing the stenosis with the balloon catheter; a stenosis located within a sharp bend in the vessel will increase the likelihood of an unstable dissection).
   7. Presence of side branches (diseased side branches originating at the site of the primary lesion carry a 14% risk of occlusion).

C. Originally confined to patients with proximal single-vessel disease, PTCA is increasingly applied in a number of more complex and high-risk settings.
   1. Total coronary artery occlusions.
   2. Multiple vessel coronary artery disease.
   3. Following coronary artery bypass grafting.
   4. Acute myocardial infarction.

D. Contraindications to PTCA include:
  1. Left main coronary artery disease.
     a) PTCA of the left main coronary artery is generally unwarranted because of unacceptable immediate and long-term risk of mortality. Coronary artery bypass surgery is the treatment of choice in such patients.
     b) Exceptions to this rule include patients with partial protection of left coronary branches via patent bypass grafts and patients with hemodynamic collapse due to acute left main occlusion in which PTCA may be attempted as a life-saving measure.
     c) Ostial stenoses involving the RCA and bypass grafts are amenable to PTCA, however, they are characteristically more resistant to dilatation and are associated with a high recurrence rate.
  2. Ineligibility for coronary artery bypass surgery either because of surgical contraindication or patient refusal.
  3. Diffusely diseased coronary arteries.
  4. Likelihood of incomplete revascularization with PTCA because of multiplicity or complexity of disease.
  5. Total coronary artery occlusion of long-standing duration (greater than 6 months).

IV. RESULTS

The salutary effects of coronary angioplasty have been established by an array of scientific studies demonstrating improvement in clinical, angiographic, and physiologic endpoints.

A. Angiographic and Clinical Results
  1. According to the NHLBI registry, primary PTCA success has been defined as a reduction in mean luminal diameter of the stenosis by at least 20%. From a more practical standpoint, a successful PTCA is defined by a residual stenosis of less than 50% of the normal luminal diameter, a residual translesional gradient of less than 20 mm Hg, and the absence of major complications (emergency surgery, myocardial infarction, and death).
  2. Of the initial 50 angioplasties performed in Zurich by Dr. Gruentzig, the procedure was successful in 32 patients (64%).
     a) Mean stenosis was significantly reduced from 84% to 34%.
     b) Mean translesional pressure gradient was reduced from 58 to 19 mm Hg.
     c) 29 patients (58%) remained clinically improved after a mean follow-up period of 9 months.
  3. The NHLBI Registry
     a) The initial NHLBI registry analyzed in detail the results of 3079 PTCA procedures performed before October, 1982.
     b) Demographic characteristics of the registry patients were as follows:

       (1) 77% male

       (2) Mean age 53.5 years

       (3) 63% were Canadian Heart Class III or IV

       (4) Extent of coronary artery disease

           (a) Single vessel in 72.5%

           (b) Multivessel in 25%

           (c) Left main in 2.5%

       (5) Lesions attempted

           (a) LAD in 62%

           (b) LCX in 7%

           (c) RCA in 26%

           (d) Left main in 1%

           (e) Bypass grafts in 4%

    c) PTCA was successful angiographically in 67% of patients.

    d) Patients with successful PTCA were followed for a one year period after the procedure.

       (1) 72% remained clinically improved without further procedure.

       (2) 14% required repeat PTCA

       (3) 12% underwent bypass surgery

       (4) 2% had a myocardial infarction or death

4. The initial NHLBI registry was an important step in establishing the indications and efficacy of PTCA during its infancy. The recent introduction of steerable guidewires, low-profile balloons, and greater technical expertise by more experienced operators have significantly improved the safety and efficacy of the technique. Currently, experienced centers now achieve overall success rates of approximately 90%.

B. Physiologic Correlates

To clinicians, the obvious effect of PTCA is the reduction in stenosis severity and relief of anginal symptoms. More sophisticated investigations have demonstrated the beneficial consequences of coronary angioplasty by objective measurements of coronary blood flow and ventricular function.

1. Serial exercise electrocardiographic studies (before and after PTCA) have shown significant enhancement of:

    a) Exercise capacity.

    b) Myocardial oxygen consumption.

    c) Normal ST segment response.

2. Several studies employing thallium 201 exercise scintigraphy have observed normalization of regional myocardial perfusion following PTCA. Moreover, exercise thallium 201 testing appears to be useful clinically in screening patients for recurrent stenosis.

3. Restoration of normal coronary vasodilatory reserve following PTCA has been demonstrated by analyses of coronary blood flow in response to rapid arterial pacing.

4. Similar benefit has been observed in left ventricular function. Serial exercise radionuclide studies have shown improve-

ment in both systolic and diastolic function following successful coronary angioplasty.

C. Long-term Efficacy

Because of the relatively recent introduction of PTCA, little data is available on long-term follow up after angioplasty. A recent report on Gruentzig's initial patients, followed 5 to 8 years after successful intervention, has contributed valuable information regarding this important issue. In 133 patients with initially successful PTCA, actual cardiac survival was 96% after 6 years. At the last followup evaluation, 67% were asymptomatic and exercise testing tests were negative in 90%. The efficacy of PTCA was confirmed by lasting improvements in exercise ECG testing and coronary arteriography.

D. Special Applications

PTCA continues to be extended to a number of more complex clinical settings.

1. Multivessel coronary artery disease.
   a) PTCA has been performed safely and effectively in selected patients with multivessel disease.
   b) "Staged" procedures involving PTCA of each individual lesion on separate days are frequently recommended in circumstances where large amounts of myocardium are at risk (e.g., two-vessel dilatation involving a proximal LAD and dominant RCA) or when the result of dilatation of the first lesion is suboptimal (e.g., because of an intimal dissection).
   c) The long-term benefits and comparative role to coronary bypass surgery remain unclear and are currently being evaluated by randomized, multicentered trials.
   d) Bypass surgery is currently preferable for most patients with triple-vessel disease in view of its proven benefits and the problematic rate of recurrence following transluminal angioplasty of multiple lesions.

2. Coronary artery bypass grafts.
   a) Whereas cardiac surgery provided the indispensable safety net which allowed the development of coronary angioplasty, PTCA has now evolved as an important therapeutic modality for patients with recurrent symptoms following bypass operations.
   b) A variety of angioplasty strategies have been successfully utilized.
      (1) Dilatation of the bypass graft itself.
      (2) Dilatation of the native artery following graft occlusion.
      (3) Dilatation of the native artery because of new disease distal to the graft anastomosis.
      (4) Dilatation of a nonbypassed artery because of interim progression of disease.
   c) PTCA can be performed in saphenous vein grafts with

primary success rates equivalent to PTCA in native coronary arteries. However, PTCA appears ill advised in older venous grafts with diffuse, irregular lesions because of the risk for thromboembolic complications.

d) Secondary recurrence (restenosis) is greater in saphenous vein bypass grafts than in native coronary arteries.

    (1) PTCA of stenoses of the proximal anastomosis or in the body of the graft are associated with a high recurrence rate (approximately 50%).

    (2) The optimal site for PTCA is the distal anastomosis since the restenosis rate is lower at this location.

3. Acute myocardial infarction.

a) In patients presenting within the first 6 hours of acute myocardial infarction, PTCA may be undertaken emergently as the primary method of myocardial revascularization.

    (1) Acute reperfusion rates of 80 to 90% can be achieved with PTCA alone.

    (2) Primary PTCA (without prior administration of thrombolytic drugs) has the potential advantage of a lower incidence of bleeding complications and thus is particularly useful when contraindications to thrombolytic therapy are present.

    (3) Use of primary PTCA in the treatment of acute myocardial infarction is limited by the need for immediate availability of a cardiac catheterization laboratory and an experienced interventional team.

b) PTCA can also be performed in the acute setting in conjunction with use of intravenous thrombolytic agents.

    (1) Urgent cardiac catheterization has the advantage of identifying those patients with persistent occlusion of the infarct-related artery who might benefit from rescue angioplasty.

    (2) PTCA immediately following intravenous thrombolytic therapy, however, carries an increased risk of bleeding complications and a higher rate of emergency coronary bypass surgery.

c) In patients with acute myocardial infarction treated with thrombolytic agents, PTCA is more commonly performed on an elective basis prior to hospital discharge.

    (1) Successful intracoronary thrombolysis with coronary reperfusion usually uncovers a significant atherosclerotic lesion which remains following clot dissolution. Since this residual stenosis frequently instigates subsequent coronary reocclusion, thrombolysis is best considered a temporary measure which often necessitates a more definitive revascularization procedure.

    (2) The presence of post-infarction angina, or ischemia

on a predischarge stress test are indications for coronary angioplasty.

4. Chronic total occlusions.

   a) PTCA can also be successfully performed in chronically occluded coronary arteries.

   b) Most series report primary success rates of 50 to 70% in patients with total coronary artery occlusion. This is significantly lower than the success rate for nonoccluded vessels.

   c) The most important factor affecting a favorable outcome in this group is a short duration of complete occlusion. The yield from PTCA is substantially better when performed within 12 to 20 weeks from the estimated time of closure. PTCA is rarely successful in older occlusions.

   d) Restenosis occurs more frequently following angioplasty of chronic total occlusion.

   e) PTCA can be attempted with a relatively lower risk of acute ischemic complications in this setting since the target artery is already completely obstructed.

V. COMPLICATIONS

   A. Frequency

      1. The frequency of major complications from the early NHLBI registry were as follows:

         a) Myocardial infarction (5.8%).

         b) Emergency bypass surgery (6.6%).

         c) Death (0.9%).

      2. Benefiting from the refinements in guidewires and balloon catheter technology, most experienced centers currently sustain significantly fewer complications than those reported by the initial registry. In patients undergoing single vessel angioplasty, the incidence of acute myocardial infarction and emergency surgery have been reduced to 2 to 4%.

   B. Risk Factors

      1. Clinical features associated with greater morbidity and mortality during PTCA include:

         a) Age greater than 60 years.

         b) Acute myocardial infarction.

         c) History of unstable angina.

         d) Prior coronary artery bypass surgery.

         e) Left ventricular dysfunction.

      2. Angiographic risk factors:

         a) Left main coronary artery disease.

         b) Severely stenotic lesions.

         c) Nondiscrete lesions.

         d) Intracoronary thrombus.

   C. Pathophysiologic Mechanisms

      1. Most acute ischemic complications during PTCA are the result of untoward subintimal dissection.

2. Acute compromise in coronary blood flow may also occur by several other mechanisms.
   a) Obstruction or injury of the coronary ostium induced by the guiding catheter.
   b) Coronary artery spasm.
   c) Coronary artery thrombosis.
   d) Side branch occlusion.
3. Embolism of atherosclerotic material and coronary artery rupture occur only rarely.
D. Management
   1. The potential for acute myocardial ischemia necessitates the immediate availability of skilled surgical backup as a prerequisite to the performance of PTCA. New Q-wave infarction develops in at least one-third of PTCA patients who require emergency coronary artery bypass surgery. Intra-aortic balloon counterpulsation and autoperfusion catheters with multiple sideholes have been important adjunctive modalities in patients requiring emergency surgery.
   2. Abrupt reclosure occurring after an initially successful dilatation can often be treated with nonoperative interventions.
      a) Nitroglycerin and calcium blockers are effective in both preventing and treating coronary spasm following PTCA.
      b) In some patients, the lesion can be recrossed with the balloon catheter and redilated.
      c) Intracoronary streptokinase has been utilized successfully in selected patients with thrombotic occlusion post-PTCA.
      d) Definitive surgical revascularization should not be unnecessarily delayed in the presence of severe coronary dissection or in the setting of refractory myocardial ischemia.
VI. RESTENOSIS
   After initial successful coronary angioplasty, patients may develop recurrent stenosis of the lesion particularly within the first few months following the procedure.
   A. Frequency
      1. Restenosis is generally defined as a recurrent stenosis of 50% or more as determined by follow-up angiography. Based on this definition, the restenosis rate reported by most series is 30–40%.
      2. In those patients with angiographic evidence of restenosis, 76 to 95% have recurrent symptoms.
      3. Restenosis typically develops within the first 6 months after PTCA with its peak incidence during the third month. It is unusual for restenosis to develop after this initial 6 month period.
   B. Risk Factors
      1. Prediction of restenosis is difficult in any individual patient. Several studies, however, have examined the relationship

of various clinical and anatomic factors to the development of restenosis in an attempt to identify potential risk factors.

2. Clinical variables associated with greater likelihood of restenosis following successful PTCA include:
   a) Diabetes mellitus.
   b) Recent onset of angina.
   c) Variant angina.
3. Anatomic features associated with restenosis include:
   a) Lesions in the left anterior descending artery.
   b) Stenoses located at the proximal anastomosis or body of saphenous vein bypass grafts.
   c) Chronic total occlusions.
   d) Suboptimal result from primary PTCA due to residual stenosis and/or translesional pressure gradients.

C. Mechanism
   1. The healing process following the controlled injury produced by balloon angioplasty is poorly understood.
   2. Several mechanisms have been postulated to account for recurrent stenosis including accelerated atherosclerosis, elastic recoil of the dilated arterial segment, hemorrhage into disrupted plaque, and superimposed thrombosis.
   3. Recent pathologic studies involving postmortem specimens indicate that restenosis is due to intimal proliferation of fibrocellular tissue with subsequent obstruction of the vessel's lumen. This fibrocellular material appears to result from the proliferation of smooth muscle cells in response to balloon induced vascular injury.
   4. In contrast to spontaneous atherogenesis, restenosis does not appear to be influenced by serum lipids.

D. Management
   1. Prevention of restenosis.
      a) Although antiplatelet drugs have been effective in experimental animal models of restenosis, in humans, no intervention has been conclusively shown to reduce the restenosis rate following coronary angioplasty.
      b) Calcium channel blockers may reduce the frequency of restenosis in the specific subgroup of patients with coronary vasospasm.
   2. Treatment of restenosis.
      a) Repeat PTCA can generally be performed in patients with restenosis and recurrent evidence of myocardial ischemia.
      b) Compared with initial angioplasties, repeat PTCA is associated with higher success rates and lower complication rates. The favorable results in these patients is attributed to the fact that they are a preselected group well suited for successful dilatation.
      c) However, the potential for restenosis is not diminished by repeated angioplasty procedures.

VII. FUTURE DIRECTIONS

Gruentzig's introduction of percutaneous balloon angioplasty in 1977 was the fuse igniting an explosion in the field of interventional cardiology. In the ensuing decade, rapid advances have been made in technique, equipment and clinical application. Accordingly, achieving an initially successful result is no longer the major challenge of coronary angioplasty. The future horizons for PTCA will be to improve long-term efficacy, to extend the role of angioplasty in patients with more complex disease, and to incorporate new technological methods of nonoperative revascularization for ischemic heart disease.

A. The Problem of Restenosis

1. With improvements in primary success rate, the high recurrence of stenosis following initial dilatation has become the most vexing problem of coronary angioplasty.

2. Likelihood of restenosis is partially dependent upon the initial functional result of PTCA. Lesions with a residual stenosis of greater than 30% or a translesional gradient of greater than 15 mm Hg post-PTCA are more likely to develop restenosis.

3. The effects of a variety of drug interventions on restenosis have been evaluated by prospective randomized trials.

   a) Agents demonstrated to have no influence on the restenosis rate include aspirin, persantine, coumadin, nifedipine, diltiazem, and corticosteroids.

   b) Randomized trials of n-3 fatty acids in patients undergoing PTCA have yielded mixed results.

B. Applicability in Multivessel Disease

1. The role of PTCA in patients with double and triple vessel disease remains uncertain.

2. Restenosis is particularly problematic when multiple lesions are dilated. Thus, future attempts to modify restenosis will have significant impact on this group of patients.

3. Randomized trials are in progress to compare the efficacy of coronary angioplasty and bypass surgery in patients with multivessel disease.

C. New Modalities

1. Laser angioplasty.

   a) An active area of research is the use of laser (light amplification stimulated emission of radiation) energy for recanalization of obstructed arteries.

   b) The biologic effect of laser is mediated by tissue absorption of photon energy which results in either thermal or photochemical vaporization of atherosclerotic plaque.

   c) A variety of delivery systems have been devised for laser angioplasty.

      (1) Bare optical fibers: the "laser beam" approach has been limited by a high incidence of vessel perforation

because of the difficulty of controlling the direction of the beam as its exits from the fiberoptic.

(2) Modified metal-capped fiberoptic tips: these "laser probe" devices use argon laser to heat a blunt metal cap at the end of the fiberoptic.

(3) Laser balloon: these balloon catheters are loaded with a Nd:YAG optical fiber with the goal of performing "thermal welding" of the intimal dissection flaps commonly created by balloon dilatation.

(4) As alternatives to the expensive laser systems, other sources of thermal energy, such as microwaves, are being developed.

d) Current clinical status of laser angioplasty.

(1) The laser probe device has been FDA approved for use in peripheral vascular lesions not amendable to conventional angioplasty.

(2) Use of laser angioplasty in the coronary circulation remains promising but still experimental. Complications including coronary spasm, thrombosis, and restenosis have been observed in initial clinical trials. Complication rates appear lower with use of the excimer or "cool" laser systems.

2. Coronary atherectomy.

a) Transluminal atherectomy refers to the physical removal of atheroma using a percutaneous catheter system.

b) Directional atherectomy catheters are constructed as a cylindrical tube with a longitudinal opening on one side through which a cap shaped rotary cutter excises and extracts the atheroma.

c) Transluminal atherectomy has been successfully performed in peripheral and coronary arteries. Further follow-up is necessary to better assess the clinical role of this interesting modality.

3. Intracoronary stenting.

a) Coronary stents are devices made of a stainless steel mesh which are delivered via a modified balloon catheter system.

b) Deployed after initial balloon dilatation of the lesion, stents function as an intracoronary scaffold permanently implanted within the vessel wall.

c) A variety of stents are currently undergoing clinical trials, including both self-expandable and balloon-expandable designs.

d) Investigational indications for coronary stenting include abrupt closure and chronic restenosis.

ACKNOWLEDGMENT

The author wishes to thank Ms. Laraine Bartlett for her excellent secretarial assistance.

SUGGESTED READINGS

ACC/AHA Task Force Report. Guidelines for percutaneous transluminal coronary angioplasty. A report of the American College of Cardiology/American Heart Association Task Force on assessment of diagnostic and therapeutic cardiovascular procedures. J. Am. Coll. Cardiol. 12:529, 1988.

Austin, G.E., Ratliff, N.B., Hollman, J., et al.: Intimal proliferation of smooth muscle cells as an explanation for recurrent coronary artery stenosis after percutaneous transluminal coronary angioplasty. J. Am. Coll. Cardiol. 6:369, 1985.

Blackshear, J.L., O'Callaghan, G.O., and Califf, R.M.: Medical approaches to prevention of restenosis after coronary angioplasty. J. Am. Coll. Cardiol. 9:834, 1987.

Block, P.C., Myler, R.K., Stertzer, S., et al.: Morphology after transluminal angioplasty in human beings. N. Engl. J. Med. 305:382, 1981.

Bredlau, C.E., Roubin, G.S., Leimgruber, P.P., et al.: In-hospital morbidity and mortality in patients undergoing elective coronary angioplasty. Circulation 72:1044, 1985.

Castaneda-Zuniga, W., Formanek, A., Tadavarthy, M., et al.: The mechanism of balloon angioplasty. Radiology 135:565, 1980.

Detre, K., Holubkov, R., Kelsey, S., et al.: Percutaneous transluminal coronary angioplasty in 1985–1986 and 1977–1981. N. Engl. J. Med. 318:265, 1988.

Douglas, J., Gruentzig, A., King, S.B., III, et al.: Percutaneous transluminal coronary angioplasty in patients with prior coronary bypass surgery. J. Am. Coll. Cardiol. 2:745, 1983.

Goldberg, S., ed.: Coronary Angioplasty. Philadelphia: F.A. Davis Company, 1988.

Gruentzig, A.P., Senning, A., and Siegenthaler, W.E.: Nonoperative dilatation of coronary artery stenosis. N. Engl. J. Med. 301:61, 1979.

Gruentzig, A.R., King, S.B. III, Schlumpf, M., et al.: Long-term follow-up after percutaneous transluminal coronary angioplasty. The early Zurich experience. N. Engl. J. Med. 316:1127, 1987.

Holmes, D.R., Holubkov, R., Vlietstra, R.E., et al.: Comparison of complications during percutaneous transluminal coronary angioplasty from 1977 to 1981 and from 1985 to 1986: The National Heart, Lung, and Blood Institute Percutaneous Transluminal Coronary Angioplasty Registry. J. Am. Coll. Cardiol. 12:1149, 1988.

Kereiakes, D.J., Selmon, M.R., McAuley, B.J., et al.: Angioplasty in total coronary artery occlusion: Experience in 76 consecutive patients. J. Am. Coll. Cardiol. 6:526, 1985.

Leimgruber, P.R., Roubin, G.S., and Hollman, J.: Restenosis after successful coronary angioplasty in patients with single-vessel disease. Circulation 73:710, 1986.

Meier, B., King, S.B., Gruentzig, A.R., et al.: Repeat coronary angioplasty. J. Am. Coll. Cardiol. 4:463, 1984.

O'Neill, W., Timmis, G.C., Bourdillon, P.D., et al.: A prospective randomized clinical trial of intracoronary streptokinase versus coronary angioplasty for acute myocardial infarction. N. Engl. J. Med. 314:812, 1986.

Proceedings of th National Heart, Lung and Blood Institute workshop on the outcome of percutaneous transluminal coronary angiplasty. Am. J. Cardiol. 53:IC, 1984.

Rosing, D.R., Cannon, R.D., Watson, R.M., et al.: Three year anatomic, functional, and clinical follow-up after successful percutaneous transluminal coronary angioplasty. J. Am. Coll. Cardiol. 9:1, 1987.

Rothbaum, D.A., Linnemeier, T.J., Landin, R.J., et al.: Emergency percutaneous transluminal coronary angioplasty in acute myocardial infarction: a 3 year experience. J. Am. Coll. Cardiol. 10:264, 1987.

Sanborn, T.A.: Laser angioplasty. What has been learned from experimental studies and clinical trials? Circulation 78:769, 1988.

Savage, M.P., Dervan, J.P., Zalewski, A., et al.: Percutaneous transluminal coronary angioplasty in patients with prior myocardial infarction: angioplasty at a distance from the prior infarct zone. Am. Heart J. 114:1102, 1987.

Schwartz, L., Bourassa, M.G., Lesperance, J., et al.: Aspirin and dipyridamole in the prevention of restenosis after percutaneous transluminal coronary angioplasty. N. Engl. J. Med. 318:1714, 1988.

Sigwart, U., Puel, J., Mirkovitch, V., et al.: Intravascular stents to prevent occlusion and restenosis after transluminal angioplasty. N. Engl. J. Med. *316*:701, 1987.

The TIMI Study Group. Comparison of invasive and conservative strategies after treatment with intravenous tissue plasminogen activator in acute myocardial infarction. Results of the thrombolysis in myocardial infarction (TIMI) phase II trial. N. Engl. J. Med. *320*:618, 1989.

Topol, E.J.: Coronary angioplasty for acute myocardial infarction. Ann. Int. Med. *109*:970, 1988.

Topol, E.J., Califf, R.M., George, B.S., et al.: A randomized trial of immediate versus delayed elective angioplasty after intravenous tissue plasminogen activator in acute myocardial infarction. N. Engl. J. Med. *317*:581, 1987.

Zalewski, A., Savage, M., and Goldberg, S.: Protection of the ischemic myocardium during percutaneous transluminal coronary angioplasty. Am. J. Cardiol. *61*:54G, 1988.

c h a p t e r

DIAGNOSTIC APPROACH TO CARDIAC ARRHYTHMIAS

Edward K. Chung

In the analysis of cardiac rhythm disturbances, it is essential to use well-designed ECG calipers. The calipers should be made so that the 2 legs can be set in any position, and the opposing surfaces of the 2 legs should be flat so that any rapid or slow rate may be measured. The end of each leg should be sharply pointed.

For a detailed analysis of cardiac arrhythmias, it is preferable to have a long rhythm strip of lead II, or sometimes leads III or aVF, because these leads show the P wave most clearly. Occasionally, lead V_1 shows the P wave more clearly than the above mentioned leads. Ideally, long rhythm strips of leads II and V_1 should be used for detailed analysis. A rhythm strip should be taken immediately following the original 12-lead ECG when any cardiac arrhythmia is suspected or found because certain arrhythmias are very transient in nature and may change within a few seconds or minutes. When the cardiac arrhythmia is a rapid one, long strips should be obtained during various procedures such as carotid sinus massage in order to clarify the fundamental mechanism involved. At times, it is necessary to take a long rhythm strip with a double speed and/or double standardization in order to magnify the P waves, if they are believed to be present.

In selected cases, electrophysiologic study (EPS) may be necessary to diagnose various cardiac arrhythmias more accurately, especially in dealing with tachyarrhythmias with broad QRS complexes. The diagnostic approach to cardiac arrhythmias is summarized as follows:

1. Evaluation of the atrial activity
2. Evaluation of the QRS configuration
3. Evaluation of the Ashman's phenomenon
4. Evaluation of the R-R cycles
5. Evaluation of the post-ectopic pause
6. Evaluation of the coupling interval
7. Evaluation of the heart rate
8. Evaluation of the response to CSS
9. Exercise ECG testing, Holter monitor ECG and EPS in selected cases.

When the suspected cardiac arrhythmias are not recorded by repeated 12-lead ECGs, the ambulatory ECG (Holter monitor ECG) should be taken for 24 to 72 hours. In addition, exercise ECG testing may be indicated in selected cases when any cardiac arrhythmia is considered to be related to the physical exercise. Furthermore, the exercise ECG testing often provides a clinical guideline to determine the nature of a given arrhythmia in conjunction with the proper therapeutic approach.

Although there are many kinds and types of cardiac arrhythmias, various cardiac arrhythmias may be classified as follows:

1. Disturbances of impulse formation
2. Conduction disturbances
3. Combination of #1 and #2
4. Artificial pacemaker-induced rhythm.

Various conduction disturbances may be expressed as *Heart Blocks*, but there are many types depending upon the site of the heart blocks. Not uncommonly, two or more sites may show conduction disturbances simultaneously. For instance, SA block and AV block often coexist in a patient with acute diaphragmatic MI. Various conduction disturbances are summarized as follows:

1. SA block
2. Intra-atrial block
3. AV block
4. Intra His block
5. Intraventricular block: LBBB, RBBB, hemiblock, bifascicular block, trifascicular block, nonspecific (diffuse)
6. Exit block
7. Combined conduction disturbances

When any physician wishes to interpret a cardiac arrhythmia accurately, clinical significance of a given arrhythmia should be considered. In particular, the presence or absence of significant underlying heart disease is extremely important for the proper diagnostic as well as therapeutic approach to various arrhythmias. In general, underlying causes of various cardiac arrhythmias are summarized as follows:

1. Cardiac diseases (e.g., CAD, RHD)
2. Noncardiac diseases (e.g., hyperthyroidism)
3. Electrolyte imbalances (e.g., hypokalemia, hyperkalemia)
4. Drug-induced (e.g., digitalis toxicity)
5. Cocaine, coffee, alcohol, smoking, anxiety, etc.

One of the most important points to remember is to identify various

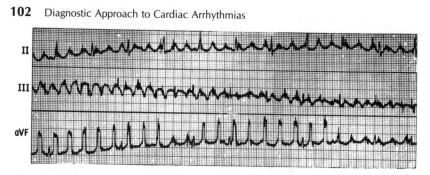

FIG. 8–1. ECG tracing showing artifacts caused by muscle tremors closely resembling atrial flutter or even ventricular tachycardia.

artifacts which may cause ECG findings very similar to true cardiac arrhythmias. The best example is muscle tremors from Parkinson's disease which commonly produces artifacts superficially mimicking various cardiac arrhythmias (Figs. 8–1 and 8–2).

Because of the ready availability of direct current (DC) shock for treatment of various ectopic tachyarrhythmias, a tendency to oversimplify the diagnosis of various tachyarrhythmias exists. However, it should be emphasized that DC shock is not only ineffective but also hazardous in the treatment of digitalis-induced tachyarrhythmias, particularly those of ventricular origin. Furthermore, the precise diagnosis of a given tachyarrhythmia enables one to employ the proper drug therapy. For instance, digitalis is often the drug of choice in the treatment of various supraventricular tachyarrhythmias, regardless of the configuration of the QRS complex, whereas the drug is either ineffective or even contraindicated in the treatment of ventricular tachyarrhythmias. A correct and precise diagnosis of the tachyarrhythmia is important when evaluating the total clinical picture of a given patient, because certain arrhythmias are almost

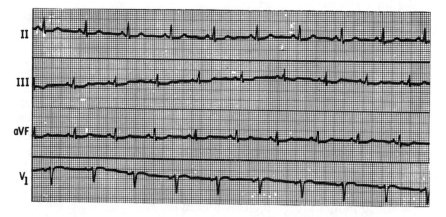

FIG. 8–2. ECG tracing taken on the same patient (Fig. 8–1) after elimination of the muscle tremors reveals normal sinus rhythm without any artifact.

pathognomonic features of certain clinical entities. For example, atrial tachycardia with varying AV block and nonparoxyxmal AV JT in the presence of AF during digitalization are almost pathognomonic features of DI.

Rapid heart action may originate from any portion of the heart. Thus, rapid heart action may be sinus in origin or it may be ectopic in origin. In addition, tachyarrhythmias may occur in paroxysmal and nonparoxysmal forms. The nonparoxysmal form may originate from a primary or any ectopic pacemaker, while paroxysmal tachyarrhythmias are always ectopic in origin. Since sinus tachycardia can be diagnosed without any difficulty in most instances, primarily ectopic tachyarrhythmias will be discussed. The main discussion will be focused on differential diagnosis between various supraventricular tachyarrhythmias with wide QRS complexes and ventricular tachyarrhythmias because of their practical importance.

It should be pointed out that any supraventricular tachyarrhythmias may coexist with any ventricular tachyarrhythmias, leading to double or even triple ectopic tachyarrhythmias. On the other hand, multifocal supraventricular tachyarrhythmias, such as a combination of AF or flutter with independent AV JT or double AV JT, may occur. Needless to say, these multifocal tachyarrhythmias are rare forms of AV dissociation.

Although it has been known for many years that the differential diagnosis between supraventricular and ventricular tachyarrhythmias is extremely important in view of their management and prognosis, it is often difficult or, at times, impossible to distinguish between them. The reason for this is that supraventricular tachyarrhythmias, regardless of the fundamental mechanism involved, may closely resemble ventricular tachyarrhythmias when the QRS complex is wide in the former. Because of the difficulty in distinguishing between them, various additional studies, such as esophageal and intracardiac ECGs including His bundle recording, have been utilized recently in order to identify the atrial activity in relation to the His bundle potential and ventricular activity.

Recently, new terms regarding VT have been used frequently. The term "nonsustained VT" is used when VT lasts 29 seconds or less. When VT persists more than 29 seconds, the term "sustained VT" is applied.

Although the differential diagnosis between supraventricular and ventricular tachyarrhythmias is not always possible in every instance, the following may be used to distinguish them:

1. Identification of the atrial activity
   a) Determination of the relationship between atrial and ventricular activities.
   b) Comparison between atrial and ventricular cycles.
2. Evaluation of the configuration of the QRS complexes during the tachyarrhythmia.
   a) Comparison of the QRS complexes during the tachyarrhythmia and isolated ectopic beats preceding or following the rapid heart action.
   b) Comparison of the QRS complex during the tachyarrhythmias and ventricular captured beats.

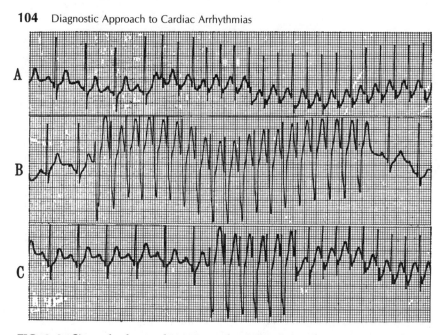

FIG. 8–3. Sinus rhythm and paroxysmal atrial tachycardia (rate: 210–220 beats/min) with aberrant ventricular conduction of varying degree. The Holter monitor ECG rhythm strips A, B, and C are *not* continuous.

        c) Determination of preexisting left or right bundle branch block (RBBB).

        d) Determination of preexisting Wolff-Parkinson-White (WPW) syndrome.

        e) Determination of aberrant ventricular conduction.

    3. Evaluation of the response to carotid sinus stimulation (CSS).

    4. Determination of the regularity of R-R cycles.

    5. Evaluation of the coupling intervals and the post-tachyarrhythmia pause.

    6. Determination of the heart rate.

    7. Identification of the His bundle potential in relationship to the ventricular activity.

I. IDENTIFICATION OF ATRIAL ACTIVITY

    Identification of the atrial activity is the first step in the determination of the origin of the tachyarrhythmias. When the P wave is definitely present, the relationship between the P wave and the QRS complex must be determined. When the ectopic P waves precede the QRS complexes, regardless of the configuration of the latter, the tachycardia is supraventricular in origin. In this circumstance, the tachycardia is atrial in origin if the axis of the ectopic P wave is similar to that of the sinus P wave (Fig. 8–3). On the other hand, AV junctional or reciprocating tachycardia can be diag-

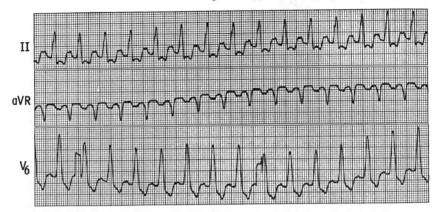

FIG. 8–4. Sinus tachycardia (rate: 125 beats/min) with first degree AV block and left bundle branch block. Slow VT is superficially simulated.

nosed when the retrograde P wave (inverted P wave in lead II and upright P wave in lead aVR) precedes the QRS complex, regardless of its configuration. When the QRS complex is wide and/or bizarre, either because of preexisting or rate-dependent bundle branch block or because of aberrant ventricular conduction, it closely mimics VT even if there are P waves preceding the QRS complexes (Fig. 8–3). VT may be closely simulated even in sinus tachycardia when there is bundle branch block (Fig. 8–4).

When the ectopic P waves, which are conducted in a retrograde fashion, follow the QRS complexes, the origin of the ectopic impulses may be either in the AV junction or in the ventricles. In this circumstance, AV JT is probably present when the QRS complex is narrow. However, VT may produce retrograde P waves which may resemble AV JT.

Comparison between atrial and ventricular cycles is important because atrial to ventricular conduction ratio may be 1:1, it may be any multiple of each other, or it may show Wenckebach phenomenon.

In the presence of regularly occurring P waves (either sinus or ectopic), the QRS complexes may independently originate from either the AV junction or the ventricles, leading to complete or incomplete AV dissociation. Thus, the presence of AV dissociation does not favor or exclude the diagnosis of AV JT or VT. In addition, AV JT or VT may develop in the presence of atrial tachyarrhythmias including AF, flutter, and tachycardia, leading to AV dissociation. In these circumstances, the comparison of the configuration of the QRS complex during the tachycardia and of a ventricular captured beat is often the only clue to distinguish between them. This aspect of the differential diagnosis will be discussed later in this chapter. The differential diagnosis between AV JT with a wide QRS complex and VT is one of the most difficult

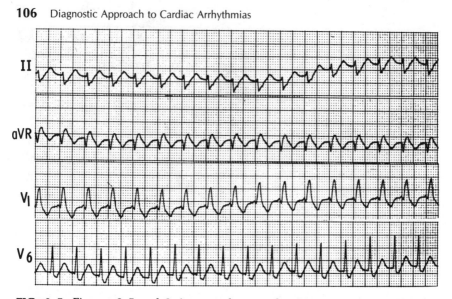

FIG. 8–5. Figures 8–5 and 8–6 were taken on the same patient on different occasions. Figure 8–5 shows a regular tachycardia (rate: 150 beat/min) with wide QRS complexes. This tachycardia can be diagnosed as either supraventricular (probable AV junctional) tachycardia with RBBB or VT. VT is definitely excluded because this patient had RBBB during sinus rhythm on another occasion (Figure 8–6).

problems in the interpretation of cardiac arrhythmias, because each may closely simulate the other. The most common cause of a wide QRS complex in an AV JT is preexisting bundle branch block (Figs. 8–5 and 8–6), which was described in detail previously.

II. EVALUATION OF CONFIGURATION OF QRS COMPLEX DURING TACHYARRHYTHMIAS

Evaluation of the configuration of QRS complexes during the tachycardia and comparison with that of isolated ectopic beats preceding or following the rapid heart action is often the only clue to identify the exact location of the ectopic impulse formation. This is true because the same ectopic focus is believed to be capable of producing isolated ectopic beats as well as tachyarrhythmias. For example, isolated APCs often lead to atrial group beats, AT, AF, or flutter, and these atrial tachyarrhythmias are often followed by isolated APCs upon termination of the rapid heart action (Fig. 8–3). This information is extremely valuable when the QRS complex is wide and/or bizarre during the tachyarrhythmia and isolated APCs resulting either from preexisting or rate-dependent bundle branch block or from aberrant ventricular conduction (Fig. 8–3).

The most practical point in the differential diagnosis is to compare the configuration of the QRS complex during the tachycardia

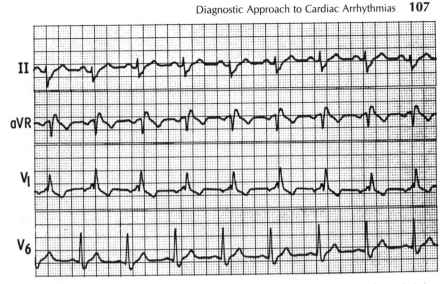

FIG. 8–6. Right bundle branch block during sinus rhythm (rate: 76 beats/min).

with isolated VPCs before and after the tachycardia. When the configuration of the QRS complexes of the isolated VPCs and tachycardia are identical, the diagnosis of VT is certain (Fig. 8–7).

Comparison of QRS configuration during the tachycardia and ventricular captured beats (or reciprocal beats) is another important aspect of the differential diagnosis in the presence of incomplete AV dissociation. When the QRS complexes of ventricular captured beats or reciprocal beats have the same configuration as that of the tachycardia, regardless of whether the QRS complex is narrow or wide, the tachycardia is AV junctional in origin.

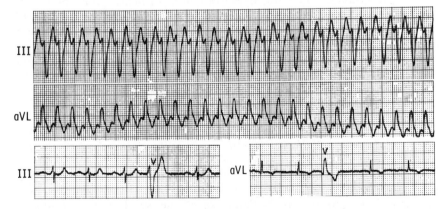

FIG. 8–7. Sinus rhythm with VPCs and paroxysmal VT (rate: 212 beats/min). Note that the configuration of an isolated VPC and VT is identical.

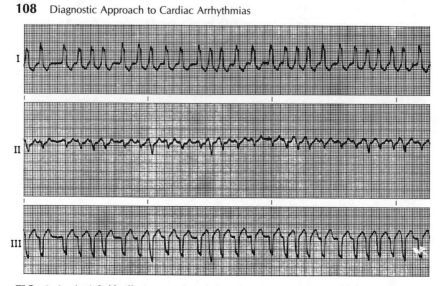

FIG. 8–8. Atrial fibrillation with left bundle branch block. This ECG finding superficially resembles VT.

Conversely, if the contours of the QRS complexes in the ventricular captured beats or reciprocal beats and the tachycardia are different, the diagnosis of VT can be made.

It should be emphasized that the presence of ventricular fusion beats supports the diagnosis of VT.

Determination of preexisting LBBB or RBBB is, at times, the only clue to distinguish between supraventricular and ventricular tachyarrhythmias, particularly when the atrial activity is not discernible or is independent of the QRS complex, and the QRS complex is wide and/or bizarre. Thus, when an electrocardiogram taken preceding or following an episode of rapid heart action shows left or right bundle branch block and the QRS contour is identical to that seen during the tachyarrhythmia, the diagnosis of ventricular tachycardia is definitely excluded (Figs. 8–5 and 8–6). Similarly, AF or flutter with preexisting or rate-dependent LBBB or RBBB also closely mimics ventricular tachycardia (Fig. 8–8). In these circumstances, grossly irregular R-R cycles with identification of fibrillation or flutter waves exclude VT.

Knowledge of a preexisting WPW syndrome is also helpful to differentiate various rapid heart actions. This syndrome is known to be associated with various supraventricular tachyarrhythmias with wide QRS complexes due to anomalous AV conduction, thus closely resembling ventricular tachyarrhythmias. A detailed description of the various supraventricular tachyarrhythmias associated with the Wolff-Parkinson-White syndrome is found in Chapter 9.

Recognition of aberrant ventricular conduction in supraventric-

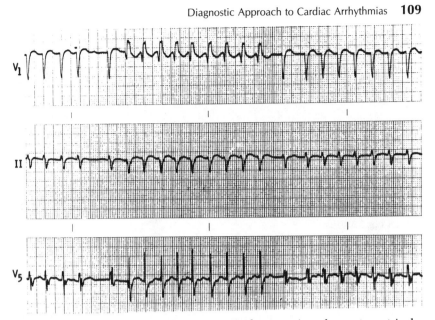

FIG. 8–9. Atrial fibrillation with consecutively occurring aberrant ventricular conduction initiated by Ashman's phenomenon. Ventricular tachycardia is closely simulated, but a lack of pause following many bizarre beats excludes its possibility.

ular tachyarrhythmias is extremely important in order to distinguish them from ventricular tachyarrhythmias. Aberrant ventricular conduction is favored by the following findings: RBBB pattern, absence of the post-tachyarrhythmia pause, varying coupling intervals, a long cycle preceding the coupling interval (Ashman's phenomenon), identical or similar initial vectors between the abnormal beat and the normally conducted beat, etc.

A. Ashman's Phenomenon

The most important factor for the production of aberrant ventricular conduction is Ashman's phenomenon (Figs. 8–9 and 8–10). Therefore, Ashman's phenomenon will be discussed in detail at this time. In 1945, Ashman had described the ECG finding that aberrant ventricular conduction tends to occur following a long ventricular cycle (R-R interval) preceding the coupling interval (the interval from a bizarre beat to the normal beat of the basic rhythm). It can be said that the longer the ventricular cycle (R-R interval), the longer the refractory period following it; the shorter the ventricular cycle, the shorter the refractory period.

1. Diagnostic criteria of Ashman's phenomenon

   a) Ashman's phenomenon may be recognized in any cardiac rhythm when aberrant ventricular conduction occurs following a long ventricular cycle (R-R interval).

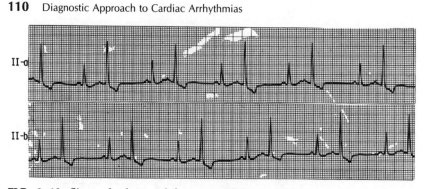

FIG. 8–10. Sinus rhythm and frequent APCs (atrial bigeminy) with aberrant ventricular conduction as a result of Ashman's phenomenon. Leads II-a and b are *not* continuous.

b) The aberrant ventricular conduction is more pronounced in a ventricular complex following the longest ventricular cycle as a result of marked Ashman's phenomenon.

c) Atrial or AV junctional bigeminy nearly always shows aberrant ventricular conduction in atrial or AV junctional premature beats because of Ashman's phenomenon. This is observed because atrial or AV junctional premature beats must follow a long ventricular cycle (postectopic pause) during atrial or AV junctional bigeminy (Fig. 8–10).

d) The P-R interval of atrial or AV junctional premature beat is often long during bigeminy, again as a result of Ashman's phenomenon. For the same reason, blocked APCs are common during atrial bigeminy (blocked atrial bigeminy).

e) Ashman's phenomenon is pronounced when the ventricular cycle becomes suddenly shortened following a long ventricular cycle, particularly in AF. As a result, aberrant ventricular conduction occurs (Fig. 8–9). It is not uncommon to observe consecutively occurring aberrant ventricular conduction once it is initiated by Ashman's phenomenon (Fig. 8–9). This ECG finding closely simulates VT.

f) Ashman's phenomenon may be encountered in MAT which leads to aberrant ventricular conduction.

g) Occasionally, a sinus beat (ventricular captured beat) during incomplete AV dissociation may show aberrant ventricular conduction as a result of Ashman's phenomenon.

h) The configuration of the QRS complex during aberrant ventricular conduction as a result of Ashman's phenomenon is commonly (about 80 to 85%) that of RBBB

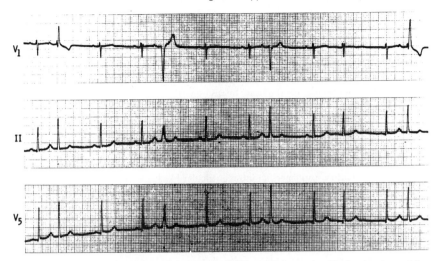

FIG. 8–11. Sinus rhythm and frequent APCs with occasional aberrant ventricular conduction as a result of Ashman's phenomenon. Note the 2 types of aberrant ventricular conduction—one with left bundle branch block pattern, and another with right bundle branch block pattern.

pattern (Figs. 8–9 and 8–10), and only 15 to 20% may show LBBB pattern. Not uncommonly, aberrantly conducted beats may reveal an ECG finding of bifascicular block pattern consisting of RBBB pattern and left anterior or posterior hemiblock pattern. At times, aberrantly conducted beats may show both LBBB pattern as well as RBBB pattern in the same ECG tracing (Fig. 8–11). The alternation of the QRS contour in aberrant ventricular conduction represents functional (not true) bundle branch block and/or hemiblock.

i) The secondary T wave change is observed in aberrantly conducted QRS complex. The T wave alteration in this circumstance is analogous to that of VPCs or L or RBBB.

Various ECG findings causing broad (bizarre) QRS complexes are summarized in Table 8–1, whereas various ECG findings which support (or favor) ventricular ectopy are summarized in Table 8–2. When the ectopic beat reveals incomplete RBBB pattern (not due to aberrant ventricular conduction), the impulse is considered to be originating from one of the fascicles of the left bundle branch system (Fig. 8–12).

III. EVALUATION OF RESPONSE TO CAROTID SINUS STIMULATION

The response to CSS is difficult depending upon the nature and origin of various tachyarrhythmias (Table 8–3). Sinus tachycardia

Table 8–1.   ECG Findings Causing Broad (Bizarre) QRS Complexes

Ventricular Ectopy
   Ventricular premature contractions
   Ventricular parasystole
   Ventricular tachycardia
   Ventricular escape beats or rhythm
   Ventricular fibrillation or flutter

Intraventricular Block
   Right bundle branch block
   Left bundle branch block
   Bifascicular or trifascicular block
   Diffuse (nonspecific) intraventricular block

Aberrant Ventricular Conduction
   Ashman's phenomenon
   Short coupling interval
   Very rapid supraventricular tachyarrhythmias of various
   origins or mechanisms

Wolff-Parkinson-White syndrome

Artificial pacemaker-induced ventricular beats or rhythm

is only transiently slowed by carotid sinus stimulation, and the original sinus rate returns soon after the procedure is over. At times, however, varying degree A-V block may be produced by CSS in sinus tachycardia.

When CSS is applied for AT, there may be three different responses. There may be no response at all, sinus rhythm may

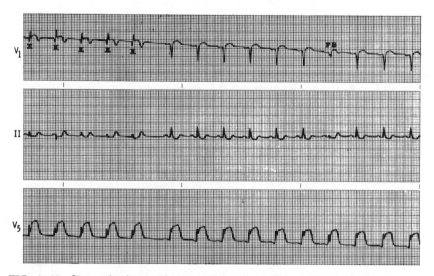

FIG. 8–12. Sinus rhythm with intermittent fascicular tachycardia (marked X) and a ventricular fusion beat (marked FB).

Table 8–2.   ECG Findings Support (or Favor) Ventricular Ectopy

Full compensatory pause during sinus rhythm (occasionally interpolated)—no disturbance on the sinus P-P cycle

Significant pause after a bizarre QRS complex in atrial fibrillation or flutter

No premature P wave preceding a bizarre QRS complex

Extremely broad and bizarre QRS complex

No evidence of Ashman's phenomenon

Left bundle branch block pattern or multiformed

Bizarre QRS complex in elderly or cardiac patients and/or in digitalis toxicity

be restored (Fig. 8–13), or there may be a slowing of the ventricular rate resulting from increase AV block, especially when the underlying cause is digitalis intoxication (DI). The response of AV JT to carotid sinus stimulation is similar to that of AT. That is, AV JT (usually paroxysmal) may convert to sinus rhythm, or it may not be influenced by the procedure. In reciprocating tachycardia, slow-

Table 8–3.   Cardiac Arrhythmias: Various Responses to Carotid Sinus Stimulation*

Arrhythmias	*Responses*
Sinus tachycardia	1. Transient slowing of sinus (atria) rate 2. Varying degree AV block (less common)
Atrial tachycardia	1. Termination 2. No response 3. Slowing of ventricular rate due to increased AV block (less common) 4. Increased atrial rate (less common)
Atrial fibrillation or flutter	Slowing of ventricular rate due to increased AV block
AV junctional tachycardia Paroxysmal	1. Termination 2. No response
Nonparoxysmal	No response
Ventricular tachyarrhythmias	No response (rare exceptions)
WPW syndrome	Vary
Parasystole	Vary

*Carotid sinus stimulation is not recommended in digitalis intoxication or in hypersensitive individuals.

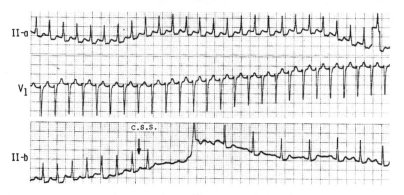

FIG. 8–13. Termination of supraventricular tachycardia by carotid sinus stimulation (indicated by arrow). Leads II-a and b are *not* continuous.

ing of the ventricular rate may be produced as a result of increased AV block by CSS.

When CSS is applied to AF or flutter, a slowing of the ventricular rate is invariably produced because of the increased AV block. Occasionally, a long ventricular standstill may result when CSS is applied to elderly patients with AF or flutter. In contrast to supraventricular tachyarrhythmias, VT, as a rule, does not respond to CSS. Thus, no response to the procedure does not diagnose or exclude supraventricular or VT. In other words, VT is excluded if there is any response to CSS.

IV. DETERMINATION OF REGULARITY OF R-R CYCLES

Although it has been said that VT often shows a slight irregularity of the R-R cycles, it is rather uncommon to recognize any appreciable irregularity except when VT transforms to VF. Conversely, supraventricular (atrial or AV junctional) tachycardia may produce a slight irregularity of the cardiac cycle, particularly in the initial portion of the paroxysm. Thus, slight irregularity of the R-R cycles is not a useful criterion for the differential diagnosis between supraventricular and VT.

Grossly irregular R-R cycles, regardless of the configuration of the QRS complex, are nearly always due to AF and, less commonly, may be due to atrial flutter or tachycardia with varying AV response or VF. When the QRS complex is wide and/or bizarre, owing either to preexisting or rate-dependent bundle branch block (Fig. 8–8) or to aberrant ventricular conduction (Fig. 8–9) or to anomalous AV conduction in Wolff-Parkinson-White syndrome, VT is closely simulated. On the other hand, when the R-R cycles show a regular irregularity, the tachycardia often arises from the AV junction, and the irregularity is often due to Wenckebach exit block or the periodic occurrence of reciprocal beats.

V. EVALUATION OF COUPLING INTERVALS AND POST-TACHYARRHYTHMIA PAUSE

In general, the coupling intervals are constant in VT or VPCs. Conversely, wide and/or bizarre QRS complexes due to aberrant ventricular conduction in AF always have varying coupling intervals (Fig. 8–9). In addition, VT is always followed by a post-tachycardia pause whereas aberrantly conducted beats in AF are *not* followed by a long pause (Fig. 8–9).

VI. DETERMINATION OF HEART RATE

Although various tachyarrhythmias produce different rate ranges, the heart rate is not a reliable index to use for the differential diagnosis of supraventricular and ventricular tachyarrhythmias because of the overlap of the heart rates. Nevertheless, a ventricular rate beyond 200 beats per minute usually favors supraventricular tachyarrhythmias, and a ventricular rate faster than 250 beats per minute nearly always indicates AF or flutter, regardless of the width of the complex.

VII. IDENTIFICATION OF HIS BUNDLE POTENTIAL IN RELATION TO VENTRICULAR ACTIVITY

Recently, study of the His bundle potential has been utilized in order to locate the precise origin of the ectopic focus or conduction defect. When the ventricular activity is preceded by a His bundle potential, the rapid heart action is due to a supraventricular tachycardia. Conversely, in ventricular tachycardia, the QRS complex is *not* preceded by the His bundle potential.

VIII. CONCLUSION

The differential diagnosis between supraventricular and ventricular tachyarrhythmias is often difficult and at times impossible because many features mimic each other. Yet, it is extremely important to distinguish between the two because their management and prognosis are different.

When the QRS complexes of supraventricular tachyarrhythmias are wide and/or bizarre, the following may be used to distinguish them from VT:

1. Determination of the relationship between atrial and ventricular activities.
2. Comparison of the QRS complexes during tachyarrhythmias with those of ventricular captured beats.
3. Comparison of the QRS complexes during tachyarrhythmias with those of isolated ectopic beats before or after the episode of rapid heart action.
4. Recognition of a preexisting or rate-dependent left or right bundle branch block.
5. Recognition of a preexisting WPW syndrome.
6. Recognition of an aberrant ventricular conduction and Ashman's phenomenon.
7. Evaluation of the response to CSS.
8. Determination of the regularity of the R-R cycles.

9. Identification of the His bundle potential in relationship to ventricular activity.

SUGGESTED READINGS

Akhtar, M.: Electrophysiologic bases for wide QRS complex tachycardia. PACE 6:81, 1983.

Akiyama, T., Richeson, J.F., Faillace R.T., et al.: Ashman phenomenon of the T wave. Am. J. Cardiol. 63:886, 1989.

Barold, S.S.: 12-Lead electrocardiography. Cardiol. Clin. 5:349, 1987.

Benditt, D.G., Epstein, M.L. and Benson, D.W., Jr.: Dual accessory nodoventricular pathways: role in paroxysmal wide QRS recipocating tachycardia. PACE 6:577, 1983.

Buxton, A.E., Waxman, H.L., Marchlinski, F.E. et al.: Right ventricular tachycardia: clinical and electrophysiologic characteristics. Circulation 68:917, 1983.

Caceres, J., Jazayeri, M., McKinnie, J., et al.: Sustained bundle branch reentry as a mechanism of clinical tachycardia. Circulation 79:256, 1989.

Chung, E.K.: Principles of Cardiac Arrhythmias, 4th ed. Baltimore, Williams & Wilkins, 1989.

Dailey, S.M., Kay, G.N., Epstein, A.E., et al.: Comparison of endocardial and epicardial programmed stimulation for the induction of ventricular tachycardia. J. Am. Coll. Cardiol. 13:1608, 1989.

Denes, P. and Ezri, M.D.: Clinical electrophysiology: a decade of progress. J. Am. Coll. Cardiol. 1:292, 1983.

Eldar, M., Belhassen, B., Hod, H., et al.: Exercise-induced double (atrial and ventricular) tachycardia: A report of three cases. J. Am. Coll. Cardiol. 14:1376, 1989.

Engel, T.R.: High-frequency electrocardiography: Diagnosis of arrhythmia risk. Am. Heart J. 118:1302, 1989.

Fisch, C., DeSanctis, R.W., Dodge, H.T., et al.: Guidelines for clinical intracardiac electrophysiologic studies. J. Am. Coll. Cardiol. 14:1827, 1989.

Fisch, C.: Evolution of the clinical electrocardiogram. J. Am. Coll. Cardiol. 14:1127, 1989.

Gibson, T.C. and Heitzman, M.R.: Diagnostic efficacy of 24-hour electrocardiographic monitoring for syncope. Am. J. Cardiol. 53:1013, 1984.

Gressard, A.: Left bundle branch block with left-axis deviation: an electrophysiologic approach. Am. J. Cardiol. 52:1013, 1983.

Griffin, J. and Most, A.S.: Torsade de pointes complicating acute myocardial infarction. Am. Heart J. 107:169, 1984.

Hess, D.S., Morady, F. and Scheinman, M.M.: Electrophysiologic testing in the evaluation of patients with syncope of undetermined origin. Am. J. Cardiol. 50:1309, 1982.

Horowitz, L.N.: Electrophysiologic Evaluation of Arrhythmias. Cardiol. Clin. 4:353, 1986.

Huycke, E.C., Lai, W.T. Nguyen, N.X., et al.: Role of intravenous isoproterenol in the electrophysiologic induction of atrioventricular node reentrant tachycardia in patients with dual atrioventricular node pathways. Am. J. Cardiol. 64:1131, 1989.

Josephson, M.E. and Wellens, H.J.J.: Tachycardias: Mechanisms, Diagnosis, Treatment. Philadelphia, Lea & Febiger, 1984.

Kapoor, W.N., Hammill, S.C. and Gersh, B.J.: Diagnosis and natural history of syncope and the role of invasive electrophysiologic testing. Am. J. Cardiol. 63:730, 1989.

Kessler, K.M., McAuliffe, D., Chakko, C.S., et al.: Multiform ventricular complexes: A transitional arrhythmia form? Am. Heart J. 118:441, 1989.

Klein, R.C. and Machell, C.: Use of electrophysiologic testing in patients with nonsustained ventricular tachycardia: Prognostic and therapeutic implications. J. Am. Coll. Cardiol. 14:155, 1989.

Kremers, M.S., Wells, P., Black, W. and Solo, M.: Differentiation of the origin of wide

QRS complexes by the net amplitude of the QRS in lead V₆. Am. J. Cardiol. *64*:1053, 1989.

Lemery, R., Brugada, P., Bella, P.D., et al.: Nonischemic ventricular tachycardia: Clinical course and long-term follow-up in patients without clinical overt heart disease. Circulation *79*:990, 1989.

Lemergy, R., Brugada, P., Bella, P.D., et al.: Ventricular fibrillation in six adults without overt heart disease. J. Am. Coll. Cardiol. *13*:911, 1989.

Lemery, R., Brugada, P., Jansseen, J., et al.: Nonischemic sustained ventricular tachycardia: Clinical outcome in 12 patients with arrhythmogenic right ventricular dysplasia. J. Am. Coll. Cardiol. *14*:96, 1989.

Levy, M.N.: Role of calcium in arrhythmogenesis. Circulation *80*:IV-23, 1989.

Lin, H.T., Mann, D.E., Luck, J.C., et al.: Prospective comparison of right and left ventricular stimulation for induction of sustained ventricular tachycardia. Am. J. Cardiol. *59*:559, 1987.

Meijler, F.L. and Fisch, C.: Does the atrioventricular node conduct? Br. Heart J. *61*:309, 1989.

Olshansky, B., and Waldo, A.L.: Atrial fibrillation: Update on mechanism, diagnosis and management. Mod. Conc. Cardiovas. Dis. *56*:23, 1987.

Pratt, C.M. Eaton, T., Francis, M. and Pacifico, A.: Ambulatory electrocardiographic recordings: The Holter monitor. Curr. Prob. Cardiol. *13*:519, 1988.

Proclemer, A., Ciani, R. and Feruglio, G.A.: Right ventricular tachycardia with left bundle branch block and inferior axis morphology: Clinical and arrhythmological characteristics in 15 patients. PACE *12*:977, 1989.

Prystowsky, E.N.: Indications for intracardiac electrophysiologic studies in patients with supra-ventricular tachycardia. Circulation *75*:III-119, 1987.

Prystowsky, E.N.: Electrophysiologic testing in patients with ventricular tachycardia: past performance and future expectations. J. Am. Coll. Cardiol. *1*:558, 1983.

Rahilly, G.T., Prystowsky, E.N., Zipes, D.P., et al.: Clinical and electrophysiologic findings in patients with repetitive monomorphic ventricular tachycardia and otherwise normal electrocardiogram. Am. J. Cardiol. *50*:459, 1982.

Rahimtoola, S.H., Zipes, D.P., Akhtar, M., et al.: Consensus statement of the conference on the state of the art of electrophysiologic testing in the diagnosis and treatment of patients with cardiac arrhythmias (Part I). Mod. Conc. Cardiovas. Dis. *56*:55, 1987.

Rahimtoola, S.H., Zipes, D.P., Akhtar, M., et al.: Consensus statement of the conference on the state of the art of electrophysiologic testing in the diagnosis and treatment of patients with cardiac arrhythmias (Part II). Mod. Conc. Cardiovas. Dis. *56*:61, 1987.

Schamroth L.: Premature ventricular contraction or ventricular extrasystole? Am. J. Cardiol *51*:1783, 1983.

Scheinman, M.M.: Interventional electrophysiology. Mayo Clin. Proc. *58*:832, 1983.

Scheinman, M.M. and Morady, F.: Invasive cardiac electrophysiologic testing: the current state of the art. Circulation *67*:1169, 1983.

Scher, D.L. and Arsura, E.L.: Multifocal atrial tachycardia: Mechanisms, clinical correlates, and treatment. Am. Heart J. *118*:574, 1989.

Schuger, C.D., Steinman, R.T. and Lehmann, M.H.: The excitable gap in atrioventricular nodal reentrant tachycardia: Characterization with ventricular extrastimuli and pharmacologic intervention. Circulation *80*:324, 1989.

Sung, R.J., Shen, E.N., Morady, F., et al.: Electrophysiologic mechanism of exercise-induced sustained ventricular tachycardia. Am. J. Cardiol. *51*:525, 1983.

Ward, D.E. and Camm, A.J.: Clinical Electrophysiology of the Heart. Baltimore, Edward Arnold, 1987.

Zipes, D.P. and Jalife, J.: Cardiac Electrophysiology and Arrhythmias. New York, Grune & Stratton, 1985.

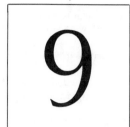

WOLFF-PARKINSON-WHITE SYNDROME

Edward K. Chung

The primary reason why every physician should be fully familiar with the Wolff-Parkinson-White (WPW) syndrome is the frequent occurrence of various ectopic tachyarrhythmias. In addition, the ECG findings in the WPW syndrome may closely resemble many other ECG abnormalities which are frequently misinterpreted in daily practice. The WPW syndrome was first recognized as a clinical entity by three physicians, Wolff, Parkinson, and White in 1930. The ECG findings that were found to be characteristic of this syndrome were described by Wilson in 1915, and by Wedd in 1921.

Since the WPW syndrome is a congenital cardiac anomaly, other congenital anomalies (cardiac or noncardiac) often coexist.

The WPW syndrome has been known as a benign syndrome, and there are no subjective manifestations or hemodynamic alterations as long as there is no ectopic tachyarrhythmia. The tachyarrhythmias may occur at any time and may begin at birth, during infancy, childhood, or adult life: 60 to 70% of the cases of WPW syndrome have been encountered in healthy individuals without organic heart disease.

For some reason, many physicians including cardiologists often fail to recognize the WPW syndrome. Besides frequent occurrence of various tachyarrhythmias, the WPW syndrome mimics other ECG abnormalities including true myocardial infarction (MI), RBBB, LBBB, hemiblocks, RVH, and LVH. VT is closely simulated when the WPW syndrome is associated with a very rapid supraventricular tachyarrhythmias (e.g., AF) with anomalous conduction. False positive exercise ECG test result is a common occurrence in individuals with WPW syndrome. Probably the most important clinical significance of the WPW syndrome is a danger of provoking VT or VF following administration of digitalis or verapamil when treating various supraventricular tachyarrhythmias, particularly AF. The reason for this is that digitalis or verapamil may enhance the conduction via an accessory pathway leading to faster ventricular rate. Under this circumstance, the faster ventricular rate may further provoke VT or VF and even sudden death. Thus, digitalis or verapamil is contraindicated in the treatment of various supraventricular tachyarrhythmias with anomalous conduction.

The true incidence of the WPW syndrome is difficult to assess, but it has been estimated to be between 0.15% and 0.2% in the general population. The syndrome occurs more frequently in men than in women, with an incidence of between 54% and 70% in males.

I. DIAGNOSTIC CRITERIA

Wolff-Parkinson-White syndrome can be diagnosed by 12-lead ECG, His bundle electrogram, or vectorcardiogram (VCG).

A. ECG Findings:

1. Typical ECG findings include a short P-R interval and prolonged QRS interval due to a delta wave (initial slurring of the QRS complex, Fig. 9–1).
2. Recognition of the delta wave is a key way to diagnose the syndrome. In some cases, however, the delta wave may not be obvious.
3. In addition, the P-R interval may be longer than 0.12 second, whereas the QRS interval may be narrower than 0.10 second in the proven WPW syndrome.
4. The actual values of the P-R and the QRS intervals in the WPW syndrome are greatly influenced by the preexisting values of these intervals.
5. The term *Lown-Ganong-Levine (LGL) syndrome* has been used when the ECG shows a short P-R interval and narrow QRS complex without a clear-cut delta wave associated with recurrent tachyarrhythmias. In reality, the LGL syndrome is considered to be a variant of the WPW syndrome.
6. The term *concealed bypass tract* is often mentioned in recent literature. It refers to the presence of bypass tract that is incapable of anterograde AV conduction, but the impulses can conduct retrogradely from ventricles to the atria. In this case, 12-lead ECG fails to reveal any evidence of WPW syndrome. During reciprocating tachycardia, ventriculo-atrial (VA) conduction often shows delayed VA activation under this circumstance.
7. It should be emphasized that many normal individuals may have a short P-R interval, particularly during stressful

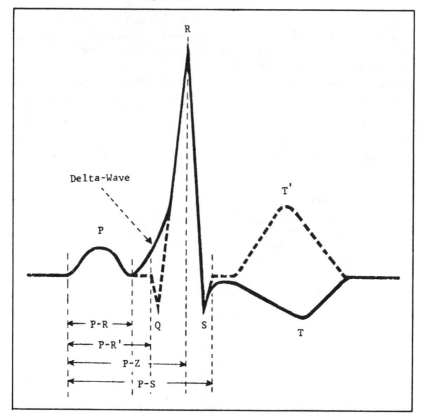

FIG. 9–1. Uninterrupted line indicates anomalous conduction in the Wolff-Parkinson-White syndrome; dotted line indicates normal conduction. P-R and P-R' intervals are AV conduction times in the Wolff-Parkinson-White syndrome and normal conduction, respectively. P-R interval is shorter than P-R' interval because of a delta wave. Note that P-Z and P-S intervals are constant during anomalous and normal conduction. T wave in Wolff-Parkinson-White syndrome is inverted because of secondary T wave change.

situations. Obviously, this isolated ECG finding is usually meaningless.

  B. VCG Findings

    A unique finding in the WPW syndrome is the initial conduction delay of the QRS sÊ loop, which can be readily recognized by any physician who is familiar with VCG.

  C. His Bundle ECG Findings

    In equivocal cases of WPW syndrome, His bundle ECG may be necessary to confirm the diagnosis. In the His bundle ECG of the WPW syndrome, the H-V interval is shorter than normal; the His bundle potential may occur simultaneously with the ventricular deflection or the His bundle potential may occur even later than the onset of the ventricular deflection. These findings are considered to occur because of a premature activation of a portion of the ventricles via anomalous conduction.

II. CLASSIFICATION

The WPW syndrome has been traditionally classified into 2 types, A and B, depending upon the direction of the delta wave. However, this classification is an oversimplification because many cases with WPW syndrome do not belong to either type A or B. The direction of the delta wave is primarily influenced by the location of the accessory pathway.

A. Type of WPW Syndrome

　1. In type A, the delta wave is directed anteriorly (commonly to the right and less commonly to the left).

　2. In general, lead V_1 shows R, RS, Rs, RSr' and Rsr' patterns, whereas leads V_5 and V_6 show Rs or R deflection (Fig. 9–2).

　3. Superficially, type A WPW syndrome resembles RBBB, right ventricular hypertrophy, and posterior MI.

　4. When the QRS complexes in all precordial leads are upright, a type A WPW syndrome should be considered as the first diagnostic possibility.

　5. In type A, a premature activation occurs in the left ventricle.

B. Type B WPW Syndrome

　1. In type B, the delta wave is directed posteriorly (commonly to the left and less commonly to the right).

　2. The left precordial leads (leads I, aVL and V_{4-6}) show tall R waves with delta waves, whereas leads V_{1-2} show negative QRS complexes (Q-S waves) with delta waves (Fig. 9–3).

　3. The ECG findings in type B WPW syndrome may closely resemble LBBB and LVH.

　4. At times, a pseudo-anteroseptal MI is produced in WPW syndrome, type B.

　5. In type B, a premature activation takes place in the right ventricle.

In both type A and B WPW syndrome, the delta wave is often directed inferiorly. This ECG finding commonly produces Q-S or Q waves in leads II, III and aVF which closely simulate diaphragmatic (inferior) MI (Fig. 9–2).

III. TACHYARRHYTHMIAS

The most significant clinical aspect of the WPW syndrome is, needless to say, the frequent occurrence of supraventricular tachyarrhythmias. The incidence of tachyarrhythmias in WPW syndrome has been reported to be 40 to 80%.

Recently, procainamide tests have been performed at various medical centers in order to determine the degree of risk when dealing with patients with frequent tachyarrhythmias in WPW

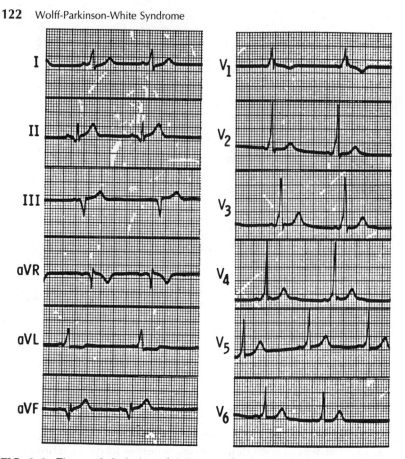

FIG. 9–2. Figures 9–2, 9–6, and 9–7 were obtained from the same patient (24-year-old man) on different occasions. Figure 9–2 shows sinus rhythm with the Wolff-Parkinson-White syndrome, type A. Diaphragmatic and posterior MI are superficially simulated.

syndrome. This is particularly true when the patient suffers from AF with very rapid ventricular response (Fig. 9–6).

It has been suggested that the rapid infusion of procainamide in a dose of 10 mg/kg intravenously over 5 minutes will produce complete block over an accessory pathway in patients whose bypass tracts have relatively long refractory periods (more than 270 msec), and would only be able to conduct at relatively slow or moderately rapid rates during AF. Under this circumstance, the refractory period refers to the ability of the accessory pathway to successfully conduct an atrial premature beat. Thus, it can be said that the shorter the refractory period, the greater is the likelihood of rapid conduction via an accessory pathway in AF or flutter. In this test, when the QRS complex reveals normalization without delta wave abruptly during a procainamide infusion of

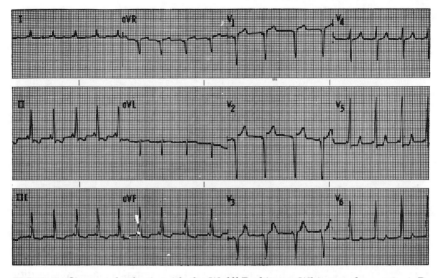

FIG. 9–3. Sinus arrhythmia with the Wolff-Parkinson-White syndrome, type B. Anteroseptal MI is closely simulated. This ECG tracing was obtained from an 11-year-old girl.

10 mg/kg or less, there is a minimum risk of developing rapid anomalous AV conduction even if AF or flutter occurs. Therefore, a possibility of sudden death will be very low under this circumstance.

It should be noted that the procainamide test is virtually useless when the delta wave is *not* obvious during anomalous AV conduction because a normalization of the QRS complex will be difficult or almost impossible to document during the test. The procainamide test may produce complications including marked hypotension and AV block of varying degrees.

A. Reciprocating Tachycardia

    1. Reciprocating tachycardia (the usual rate: 140 to 250 beats per minute), is found in the majority of cases (75 to 80% of all tachyarrhythmias).

    2. This type of tachycardia had been called paroxysmal atrial tachycardia until recently.

    3. At present, the term *reciprocating* or *reentrant* tachycardia is more commonly used because the tachycardia is considered to be caused by a re-entry phenomenon (Figs. 9–4 and 9–5). The term *circus movement* tachycardia has been frequently used in European literature to designate the same finding.

    4. In reciprocating tachycardia, the QRS complex is usually normal (narrow), and the broad QRS complex due to anomalous conduction is much less common.

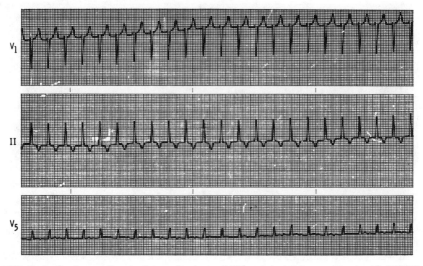

FIG. 9–4. Reciprocating tachycardia (rate: 143 beats/min) in a patient with WPW syndrome.

B. Atrial Flutter or Fibrillation
 1. Atrial flutter and fibrillation are rather uncommon in the WPW syndrome, and their incidence constitutes only 20 to 25% of all tachyarrhythmias.
 2. Among these two rhythm disorders, atrial flutter is extremely rare.
 3. The QRS complexes during AF or flutter in the WPW syndrome are extremely bizarre and broad in most cases (Fig. 9–6).
 4. The broad and bizarre QRS complexes are observed under this circumstance because of anomalous AV conduction caused by the nature of the WPW syndrome itself, plus aberrant ventricular conduction from very rapid ventricular rate (ventricular rate: 250 to 300 beats).
 5. VT or even VF is closely simulated when atrial flutter or fibrillation with anomalous AV conduction occurs (Fig. 9–6).
 6. In WPW syndrome, atrial flutter often exhibits 1:1 AV conduction, which results in extremely rapid ventricular rate.
 7. It should be remembered that atrial flutter or fibrillation in the WPW syndrome may lead to VT or VF (Fig. 9–7) and even sudden death, especially following the administration of digitalis or verapamil.
C. Ventricular Tachyarrhythmias
 1. Although the occurrence of VT has been reported in the WPW syndrome previously, in most if not all, cases AF

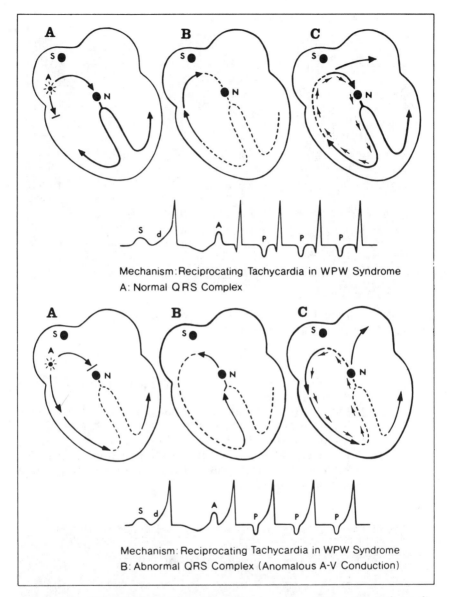

Mechanism: Reciprocating Tachycardia in WPW Syndrome
A: Normal QRS Complex

Mechanism: Reciprocating Tachycardia in WPW Syndrome
B: Abnormal QRS Complex (Anomalous A-V Conduction)

FIG. 9–5. *A,* Diagram illustrating the mechanism of a reciprocating tachycardia with a normal QRS complex in the Wolff-Parkinson-White syndrome. In diagram A, atrial premature impulse (marked A) is conducted to the AV node (marked N), but the atrial premature impulse is blocked in the anomalous pathway. The atrial premature impulse is then conducted to both ventricles by way of a bundle branch system (diagram A). In diagram B, the atrial premature impulse is conducted to the atria in retrograde fashion to produce an inverted P wave. In diagram C, the impulse is conducted in a clockwise fashion producing reciprocating (re-entry) cycle, and the same cycle may repeat indefinitely. Note that the QRS complex during the tachycardia is normal. (S = sinus node; d = delta wave; P = inverted P wave.) *B,* Diagram illustrating a reciprocating tachycardia with anomalous conduction in the Wolff-Parkinson-White syndrome. The reentry cycle is counterclockwise, which is exactly the reverse of that shown in diagram A.

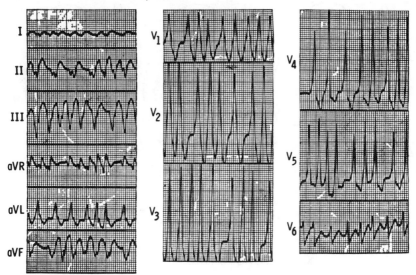

FIG. 9–6. Atrial fibrillation with anomalous AV conduction in a patient with the Wolff-Parkinson-White syndrome, type A.

or flutter with anomalous AV conduction had simply been misinterpreted.
2. On the other hand, a true incidence of VF has been reported in the WPW syndrome recently (Fig. 9–7).
3. Sudden death in the WPW syndrome is most likely caused by VF following atrial flutter or fibrillation with extremely rapid ventricular response, especially after administration of digitalis or verapamil.

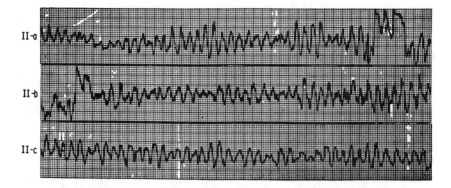

FIG. 9–7. Ventricular fibrillation is provoked following administration of digitalis in the treatment of atrial fibrillation with anomalous conduction in WPW syndrome (Figure 9–6). Leads II-a to c are continuous.

D. Other Arrhythmias

Besides the above-mentioned tachyarrhythmias, various other arrhythmias, such as VPCs, AV dissociation, ventricular or atrial parasystole, may simply coexist with WPW syndrome.

IV. OTHER CLINICAL SIGNIFICANCE

In addition to the frequent association of various supraventricular tachyarrhythmias, recognition of the WPW syndrome is extremely important because the QRS complex in WPW syndrome often resembles various other ECG findings.

A. The diagnosis of diaphragmatic (inferior) MI is frequently made erroneously in the WPW syndrome (either type A or B), because of Q or Q-S waves in leads II, III and aVF (Fig. 9–2). This ECG finding is observed when the delta wave is directed inferiorly.

B. Type B WPW syndrome may closely resemble anterior or anteroseptal MI (Fig. 9–3).

C. Because of the broad QRS complexes due to the delta waves in the WPW syndrome, LBBB or RBBB is closely simulated.

D. Type A WPW syndrome may also be misdiagnosed as true posterior MI or right ventricular hypertrophy because of the tall R waves in leads V_{1-3}.

E. At times, a pseudo-lateral MI is produced in WPW syndrome.

F. It is also common to observe tall R waves in leads I, aVL, and V_{4-6} with the secondary S-T, T wave changes in the WPW syndrome, type B. This ECG finding demonstrates a pseudo-LVH.

G. When the WPW syndrome is observed intermittently (Fig. 9–8), the ECG finding resembles VPCs or even short runs of VT.

H. Recently, it has been demonstrated that a false positive exercise ECG test is common in the WPW syndrome especially in type B. Therefore, there is no significant diagnostic value to obtain the exercise ECG test when the patient is known to have WPW syndrome.

V. DISORDERS ASSOCIATED WITH WPW SYNDROME

A. It has been demonstrated that patients with WPW syndrome often suffer from some form of psychoneurotic disorders and hyperthyroidism. The direct relationship between these disorders and the WPW syndrome is unknown, however.

B. Some patients with AF in WPW syndrome commonly suffer from RHD.

C. Congenital cardiac anomalies frequently associated with the WPW syndrome include Ebstein's anomaly, atrial septal defect (ASD), IHSS, and mitral valve prolapse syndrome (MVPS).

D. Occasionally, WPW syndrome may coexist with other abnormalities including true MI, LBBB, or RBBB (Figs. 9–9 and 9–10).

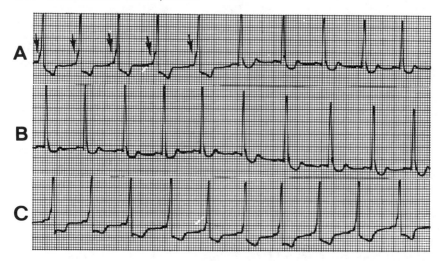

FIG. 9–8. These Holter monitor rhythm strips (A, B, and C are *not* continuous) show sinus rhythm with intermittent Wolff-Parkinson-White syndrome (arrows).

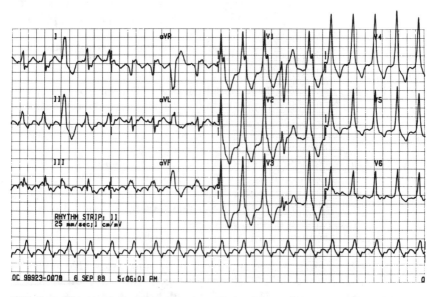

FIG. 9–9. Figures 9–9 and 9–10 were obtained from the same patient (70-year-old physician) with WPW syndrome on different occasions. Figure 9–9 shows atrial flutter with 2:1 AV conduction and occasional ventricular premature contractions associated with WPW syndrome, type A, coexisting with right bundle branch block.

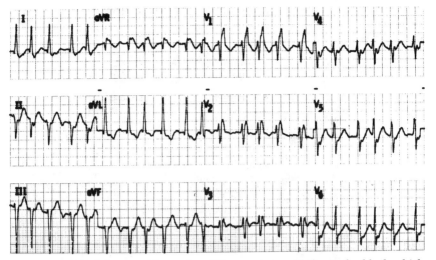

FIG. 9–10. Atrial flutter with varying AV response and bifascicular block which consists of right bundle branch block and left anterior hemiblock. The evidence of WPW syndrome is no longer present in this ECG tracing.

VI. MECHANISMS—ELECTROPHYSIOLOGIC STUDIES

Recently, electrophysiologic study (EPS) is performed frequently in patients with WPW syndrome for the diagnostic as well as the therapeutic purposes, especially in dealing with high risk patients. The indications as well as roles of EPS in WPW syndrome are summarized in Tables 9–1 and 9–2.

A. Reciprocating Tachycardia

1. Electrophysiologic and pathologic studies suggest that the WPW syndrome occurs because of a premature activation of a portion of the ventricles as a result of an anomalous AV conduction via an accessory pathway directly from the atria to the ventricles.

2. The remaining portion of the ventricular activation results from a varying degree of fusion of transmission via both

---

Table 9–1.   Indications of Electrophysiologic Study in WPW Syndrome

1. When the diagnosis of WPW syndrome is equivocal in suspected individuals with tachyarrhythmias.

2. Patients with known WPW syndrome and a family history of premature sudden death.

3. Asymptomatic WPW syndrome with high risk occupations or activities.

4. Before cardiac surgery (for other reasons) in patients with WPW syndrome.

5. Proper selection of antiarrhythmic drug(s) in patients with WPW syndrome associated with significant tachyarrhythmias.

6. Patients considered for nondrug therapy (e.g., antitachycardia pacing or surgery) because of life-threatening or drug-resistant tachyarrhythmias.

Table 9–2. Roles of Electrophysiologic Study in WPW Syndrome

1. Confirm the diagnosis of WPW syndrome.

2. Localize accessory pathway(s) by mapping

3. Determine the mechanism of tachyarrhythmias
   Reciprocating tachycardia (Orthodromic or antidromic)
   AF or atrial flutter.

4. Determine:
   The shortest R-R interval in AF
   The refractory period of accessory pathways (bypass tracts)
   The ease of AF induction and duration of AF.

5. Determine the effect of isoproterenol infusion on:
   The initiation of tachyarrhythmia(s)
   Refractory period of accessory pathway(s)
   Shortest R-R interval during anomalous conduction.

6. Evaluate the efficacy of treatment:
   Anti-arrhythmic agents
   Anti-tachycardia devices
   Catheter ablation
   Anti-arrhythmic surgery

    the normal AV conduction system as well as accessory pathway. In the majority of cases with WPW syndrome, the anomalous AV conduction is considered to occur through the Kent bundle.

3. On the other hand, a normal P-R interval with delta wave may result from slow conduction via the Kent bundle or conduction via the Mahaim tract.

4. Conduction through the James bundle, which is an AV nodal bypass tract, has been considered to be responsible for the LGL syndrome.

5. One of the important roles of the His bundle ECG is to diagnose WPW syndrome with accuracy, and to understand the exact mechanisms of tachyarrhythmias associated with the syndrome.

6. In equivocal cases, the His bundle ECG can confirm the diagnosis of WPW syndrome by recognizing shorter than-normal H-V interval, simultaneous occurrence of His bundle deflection, and ventricular deflection, or even the occurrence of ventricular deflection preceding the His bundle potential.

7. Electrophysiologic properties of both normal as well as anomalous AV pathways in the patients with WPW syndrome can be examined by the His bundle recordings and atrial stimulation.

8. The P-delta interval represents the duration of the anomalous pathway conduction time, whereas the AH interval

(simultaneously recorded) indicates normal AV conduction time.

9. The configuration of the QRS complex in WPW syndrome depends upon the degree of fusion in ventricular activation between the impulse conducted via the anomalous conduction and the normal AV conduction. The QRS complex is relatively narrow when the P-delta and A-H intervals are similar in duration, whereas the QRS contour is markedly bizarre when the A-H interval is long and the P-delta interval is short.

10. Refractory periods of both normal and anomalous pathways can be determined with the extrastimulus technique. It has been demonstrated recently that supraventricular tachycardia in WPW syndrome represents reciprocating tachycardia from a re-entry phenomenon.

11. The reason for the re-entry is that the marked discrepancy between the refractory periods in the normal and anomalous pathways predisposes to the initiation of the reciprocating tachycardia. Diagrammatic illustrations regarding the mechanisms of reciprocating tachycardia in this syndrome are found in Figure 9–5.

12. Once the re-entry is established, the impulse may be conducted antegradely to the ventricles via the normal pathway and retrogradely to the atria via the anomalous pathway (Fig. 9–5). In this case, the QRS configuration during the tachycardia is normal.

13. On the other hand, the re-entry impulse may be conducted antegradely to the ventricles via the anomalous pathway and retrogradely to the atria via the normal pathway. Under this circumstance, the QRS complex during the tachycardia is bizarre (Fig. 9–5).

14. Clinically, the majority of cases with reciprocating tachycardia in WPW syndrome shows normal QRS complexes because the re-entry cycle is carried out via antegrade normal AV conduction with retrograde anomalous conduction (Figs. 9–4 and 9–5).

15. The direction of the re-entry cycles depends upon the availability of either the normal or the anomalous pathway, whichever is in a nonrefractory period. A premature impulse (commonly atrial and less commonly AV junctional or ventricular) will be blocked in a pathway which is refractory, whereas it will be conducted antegradely in another pathway which is nonrefractory. The re-entry impulse, then will be conducted to the atria in retrograde fashion via the pathway which was previously refractory (Fig. 9–5).

16. The re-entry cycles may repeat once, twice, or even indefinitely. Reciprocating tachycardia is often terminated by

a properly timed atrial premature beat (either spontaneous or induced).
17. Multiple accessory pathways in WPW syndrome have been reported by this author previously, and the His bundle ECG analysis on double accessory pathways has been described recently.
B. Atrial Fibrillation and Flutter
1. The exact mechanism responsible for the initiation of AF in the WPW syndrome is not clearly understood.
2. It is considered that AF is triggered by the re-entry impulse which stimulates the atria during the atrial vulnerable period.
3. In AF or flutter in the WPW syndrome, the rapid atrial impulses may be conducted to the ventricles via normal or accessory pathways whichever is nonrefractory.
4. The QRS complexes during AF or flutter in this syndrome are frequently bizarre and wide because of anomalous conduction plus the common occurrence of aberrant ventricular conduction due to an extremely rapid ventricular rate (Fig. 9–6).
5. According to the electrophysiologic test results, when the shortest R-R intervals (ventricular cycles) during AF with anomalous AV conduction range from 210 to 250 msec., these individuals belong to a high-risk group. In other words, many patients with short R-R intervals develop serious symptoms (e.g., syncope or near syncope), and may lead to life-threatening ventricular tachyarrhythmias and even sudden death. The short refractory period (less than 270 msec) of the bypass tract is shown to have a similar clinical significance.

VII. PREVENTION AND TREATMENT OF TACHYARRHYTHMIAS

Needless to say, no treatment is indicated when the WPW syndrome is not associated with tachyarrhythmias. Similarly, a transient arrhythmia with a short duration also requires no therapy. Note, however, that EPS is strongly recommended even in asymptomatic WPW syndrome if there is a family history of premature cardiac death or if the individual is going to participate in any type of high risk occupations or physical activities (see Table 9–1). According to the EPS results, the prophylactic drug therapy may be indicated in some cases under these circumstances. Paroxysmal reciprocating tachycardia in WPW syndrome is often terminated by vagal maneuvers such as carotid sinus stimulation or Valsalva maneuver (Fig. 9–4). On the other hand, many patients with tachyarrhythmias in WPW syndrome require various anti-arrhythmic agents (Table 9–1) either acutely or as a long-term maintenance therapy. In urgent situations, especially in AF or flutter with extremely rapid ventricular response, DC shock may be needed. When tachyarrhythmias become refractory, an artificial pacemaker and even surgical therapy should be considered.

Table 9–3.   Effects of Drugs on Refractory Period in Normal and Anomalous Pathways

Drugs	A-V node	Accessory pathway
Propranolol	↑	0
Digitalis	↑	↓
Lidocaine	0	↑
Quinidine	↓	↑
Procainamide	0	↑
Phenytoin	↓	Variable
Amiodarone	↑	↑
Ajmaline	0	↑
Verapamil	↑	Variable

Upward arrow: increase in refractory period; *downward arrow:* decrease in refractory period; *zero:* no change in refractory period.

As far as the principles of therapy in WPW syndrome are concerned, therapy should be directed to change the conduction times in the normal AV and accessory pathways so that the re-entry cycle becomes impossible. This principle can be accomplished in the following ways: *(a)*, Equalizing the conduction times via the two pathways, either by accelerating the normal AV conduction, or by slowing the conduction in the anomalous pathway; or *(b)*, Inducing a functional or organic block in one or both pathways.

The equalization of the conduction times can be achieved by atropine or isoproterenol (Isurprel) intravenously by accelerating the normal AV conduction, but these methods provide only transient effects. Slowing the conduction in the accessory pathway seems to be a more physiologic approach. Various drugs can produce this slowing of the accessory pathway conduction (Table 9–3).

A. Drug Therapy

The His bundle ECG has provided significant contributions to the drug therapy for various tachyarrhythmias in the WPW syndrome. The drug of choice can be determined specifically according to the electrophysiologic properties of various antiarrhythmic agents for a given tachyarrhythmia in the WPW syndrome (Table 9–3). Procainamide and quinidine are found to be effective in the treatment of various supraventricular tachyarrhythmias (particularly AF) with anomalous conduction in WPW syndrome (Fig. 9–6), because these drugs effectively depress the conduction via the anomalous pathway (Table 9–3). These agents primarily produce a lengthening of the effective refractory period in the accessory pathway (Table 9–3). In addition, quinidine is considered to be effective because the drug is capable of suppressing atrial (less commonly AV junctional or ventricular) premature beats, which commonly initiate the paroxysmal reciprocating tachycardia in WPW syndrome (Figs. 9–4 and 9–5).

On the other hand, propranolol (Inderal) is considered to be the drug of choice in the treatment of reciprocating tachycardia with normal QRS complexes in WPW syndrome (Fig. 9–4), because the drug depresses the normal AV pathway. In addition, it has been demonstrated that digitalis depresses normal AV conduction, but it may accelerate the anomalous conduction via the accessory pathway in WPW syndrome. Therefore, digitalis is effective in the treatment of reciprocating tachycardia with normal QRS complexes, but the drug is contraindicated in the treatment of tachyarrhythmias, particularly AF or flutter, with anomalous AV conduction (Fig. 9–6). Propranolol (Inderal) is considered superior to digitalis.

Other beta-blocking agents have similar effects as propranolol in the treatment of various supraventricular tachyarrhythmias in WPW syndrome. Danger of provoking VT or VF following administration of digitalis or verapamil in the treatment of various tachyarrhythmias with anomalous conduction in WPW syndrome has been repeatedly emphasized because these agents often enhance the conduction via an accessory pathway so that the clinical situation deteriorates further (Figs. 9–6 and 9–7).

There are several new drugs, such as amiodarone and ajmaline, that are effective in the treatment of various supraventricular tachyarrhythmias in the WPW syndrome (Table 9–3). But some of these agents are not available in the United States for clinical use at the present time.

In addition, various other agents, including phenytoin (Dilantin), acetylcholine, neostigmine, atropine, amyl nitrite, and potassium salts, have been used in the past, but these drugs are not always effective in the treatment of rapid heart actions in the WPW syndrome.

B. Direct Current Shock
1. Direct current (DC) shock is the most effective treatment for any type of tachyarrhythmia associated with WPW syndrome.
2. In urgent situations, such as supraventricular tachyarrhythmias with extremely rapid ventricular response, especially in AF or flutter with anomalous conduction, DC shock is the treatment of choice.
3. Any drug resistant refractory tachyarrhythmias should be treated with DC shock under the usual precautions.
4. When the patient is taking digitalis, DC shock should be applied with extreme care because serious post-cardioversion arrhythmias, such as VT, may be provoked. In order to prevent post-cardioversion arrhythmias under this circumstance, phenytoin (125 to 250 mg) may be given intravenously a few minutes before the application of DC shock. In general, DC shock should be avoided if possible when the patient is taking digitalis.

5. For atrial flutter, a small amount of energy (5 to 50 ws) may be sufficient for its termination.
6. AF or other tachyarrhythmias usually require more energy (above 100 ws).
7. Immediate application of a defibrillator is the only life-saving measure available if the patient suffers from VF.
8. DC shock is effective whether the configurations of the QRS complexes during tachyarrhythmias are normal or wide (either due to anomalous conduction or due to aberrant ventricular conduction).
9. However, DC shock is *not* indicated when the paroxysmal tachyarrhythmia is of short duration or is easily converted to sinus rhythm spontaneously or by a simple procedure such as carotid sinus stimulation (Fig. 9–4).
10. It should be noted that most patients with the WPW syndrome require various drugs (e.g., propranolol or quinidine) as outlined as above following termination of the tachyarrhythmia in order to prevent its recurrence.

C. Artificial Pacemakers
1. In the treatment of drug-resistant and/or DC shock resistant tachyarrhythmias associated with WPW syndrome, the use of an artificial pacemaker should be considered. This is particularly true when the surgical approach is either contraindicated or declined by the patient.
2. The fundamental mechanism responsible for the termination of various tachyarrhythmias by artificial pacing is that the re-entry cycle of the tachycardia can be considered to be interrupted by the pacing stimuli.
3. Namely, an appropriately timed pacing-induced atrial or ventricular impulse may block the re-entry cycle either in the AV node or the anomalous pathway, so that the atria or ventricles become refractory to the re-entry (reciprocating) impulse.
4. Artificial pacing is found to be most effective when the pacing electrodes are close to the anomalous pathway.
5. The pacing can be carried out by the transvenous approach to the right ventricle or coronary sinus (near the left atrium and left ventricle), or transthoracic approach to the epicardium of any of the cardiac chambers.
6. In a specially designed pacemaker, as soon as the patient feels the tachycardia, the artificial pacing can be initiated as the fixed-rate unit by means of a magnet placed over the implanted battery-powered demand pacemaker.
7. The artificial pacing by a radiofrequency device is also found to be equally effective in terminating the reciprocating tachycardia in WPW syndrome. However, with this device, the development of AF is reported to be a potential risk when the rate of discharge is sufficiently high. It has been recommended that radiofrequency pacemakers

should only be used when the refractory properties of the anomalous pathway are known. No reported risk of the development of VF associated with the use of artificial pacemakers in the treatment of various tachyarrhythmias in the WPW syndrome exists.

D. Surgical Approach

1. The surgical approach is considered only in selected patients who suffer from recurrent supraventricular tachyarrhythmias which cause significant disturbances for their lives in any way (socially, physically or mentally), or life-threatening arrhythmias refractory to the usual drug therapy as outlined as above.

2. The rationale for surgical therapy is, obviously, to interrupt the re-entry cycle which is considered responsible for the tachyarrhythmias in WPW syndrome.

3. Electrophysiologically, the surgical approach will be the definitive means of therapy for the tachyarrhythmias in WPW syndrome. However, a successful surgical result is not always possible in every case.

4. Surgical treatment has been carried out in a relatively small number of patients, and the largest amount of data has been accumulated at the Duke University Medical Center.

5. It has been shown that the surgical results have been more favorable in patients with an anomalous pathway in the left or right ventricular free wall AV connections than in those with septal connections. In addition, there is a potential risk of damaging the normal AV conduction system in patients with septal connections.

6. In general, AF or flutter in WPW syndrome is difficult to control by various drugs and the surgical result is also not favorable.

7. It should be emphasized that the surgical approach should be attempted only at medical institutions where multichannel, high-fidelity equipment for recording along with facilities for cardiopulmonary bypass are available in the operating room. It requires a skillful electrophysiologist and surgical team who are fully familiar with the procedure.

8. The activation sequence of the human heart is measured by epicardial mapping for accurate demonstration of the area of pre-excitation. The epicardial mapping is performed by measuring local activation times at approximately 55 epicardial sites, and the point of the earliest epicardial pre-excitation is identified. The incision is made through the atrial wall at its attachment to the mitral or tricuspid valve annulus.

9. The alternative surgical treatment for the refractory tachyarrhythmias in WPW syndrome is the His bundle sec-

tion. In this case, implantation of the permanent pacemaker is necessary. This method can prevent reciprocating tachycardia, but AF via the anomalous pathway cannot be prevented.

SUGGESTED READINGS

Besson, D.W., Jr., Sterba, R., Gallagher, J.J., et al.: Localization of the site of ventricular preexcitation with body surface maps in patients with Wolff-Parkinson-White syndrome. Circulation 65:1259, 1982.

Boahene, K.A., Klein, G.J., Sharma, A.D., et al.: Value of a revised procainamide test in the Wolff-Parkinson-White syndrome. Am. J. Cardiol. 65:195, 1990.

Brodman, R., and Fisher, J.D.: Evaluation of a catheter technique for ablation of accessory pathways near the coronary sinus using a canine model. Circulation 67:923, 1983.

Brugada, P., Dassen, W.R., Braat, S., et al.: Value of the ajmaline-procainamide test to predict the effect of long-term oral amiodarone on the anterograde effective refractory period of the accessory pathway in the Wolff-Parkinson-White syndrome. Am. J. Cardiol. 52:70, 1983.

Burchell, H.B.: The surgical treatment of reentrant atrioventricular tachycardia (Wolff-Parkinson-White syndrome). Mayo Clin. Proc. 57:387, 1982.

Castellanos, A., Jr., Zaman, L., Molerio F., et al.: The Lown-Ganong-Levine syndrome. PACE 5:715, 1982.

Castellanos, A., Jr., Agha, A.S., Befeler, B., et al.: Double accessory pathways in Wolff-Parkinson-White syndrome. Circulation 51:1020, 1975.

Chia, B.L., Yew, F.C., Chay, S.O., and Tan, A.T.H.: Familial Wolff-Parkinson-White syndrome. J. Electrocardiol. 15:195, 1982.

Chung, E.K.: Wolff-Parkinson-White syndrome: Current views. Am. J. Med. 62:252, 1977.

Chung, E.K: Electrocardiography, Practical Applications with Vectorial Principles, 3rd ed. E. Norwalk, Conn., Appleton-Century-Crofts, 1985.

Chung, E.K.: Principles of Cardiac Arrhythmias, 4th Ed. Baltimore, Williams & Wilkins, 1989.

Chung, E.K., Walsh, T.J. and Massie, E.: Wolff-Parkinson-White syndrome. Am. Heart J. 69:116, 1965.

Cosio, F.G., Benson, D.W., Jr., Anderson, R.W., et al.: Onset of atrial fibrillation during antidromic tachycardia: association with sudden cardiac arrest and ventricular fibrillation in a patient with Wolff-Parkinson-White syndrome. Am. J. Cardiol. 50:353, 1982.

Dreifus, L.S., Haiat, R., Watanabe, Y., et al.: Ventricular fibrillation. A possible mechanism of sudden death in patients with Wolff-Parkinson-White syndrome. Circulation 43:520, 1971.

Dubuc, M., Kus, T., Campa, M.A., et al.: Electrophysiologic effects of intravenous propafenone in Wolff-Parkinson-White syndrome. Am. Heart J. 117:370, 1989.

Dye, C.L.: Atrial tachycardia in Wolff-Parkinson-White syndrome. Conversion to normal sinus rhythm with lidocaine. Am. J. Cardiol. 24:265, 1969.

Feld, G.K., Nademanee, K., Weiss, J., et al.: Electrophysiologic basis for the suppression by amiodarone of orthodromic supraventricular tachycardias complicating pre-excitation syndromes. J. Am. Coll. Cardiol. 3:1298, 1984.

Ferrer, M.I.: Pre-Excitation: Including the Wolff-Parkinson-White Syndrome and Other Related Syndromes. New York, Futura Co., 1976.

Gallagher, J.J., Gilbert, M., Svenson, R.H., et al.: Wolff-Parkinson-White syndrome: the problem, evaluation and surgical treatment. Circulation 51:767, 1975.

Goldstein, M., Dunnigan, A., Milstein, S. and Benson, D.W., Jr.: Bundle branch block during orthodromic reciprocating tachycardia onset in infants. Am. J. Cardiol. 63:301, 1989.

Goy, J.J., Kappenberger, L. and Turina, M.: Wolff-Parkinson-White syndrome after transplantation of the heart. Br. Heart J. 61:368, 1989.

Gulamhusein, S., Ko, P., Carruthers, G. and Klein, G.J.: Acceleration of the ventricular response during atrial fibrillation in the Wolff-Parkinson-White syndrome after verapamil. Circulation 65:348, 1982.

Gulamhusein, S., Ko, P., and Klein, G.J.: Ventricular fibrillation following verapamil in the Wolff-Parkinson-White syndrome. Am. Heart J. 106:145, 1983.

Harper, R.W., Whitford, E., Middlebrook, K., et al.: Effects of verapamil on the electrophysiologic properties of the accessory pathway in patients with the Wolff-Parkinson-White syndrome. Am. J. Cardiol. 50:1323, 1982.

Holmes, D.R., Jr., Osborn, M.J., Gersh, B., et al.: The Wolff-Parkinson-White syndrome: a surgical approach. Mayo Clin. Proc. 57:345, 1982.

Inoue, H., Matsuo, H., Takayanagi, K., et al.: Antidromic reciprocating tachycardia via a slow Kent bundle in Ebstein's anomaly. Am. Heart J., 106:147, 1983.

Jedeikin, R., Gillette, P.C., Garson, A., Jr., et al.: Effect of ouabain on the anterograde effective refractory period of accessory atrioventricular connections in children. J. Am. Coll. Cardiol. 1:869, 1983.

Josephson, M.E., Kastor, J.A. and Kitchen, J.G., III: Lidocaine in Wolff-Parkinson-White syndrome with atrial fibrillation. Ann. Int. Med. 84:44, 1976.

Kaplan, M.A., and Cohen, K.L.: Ventricular fibrillation in the Wolff-Parkinson-White syndrome. Am. J. Cardiol. 24:259, 1969.

Kerr, C.R., Prystowsky, E.N., Smith, W.M., et al.: Electrophysiologic effects of disopyramide phosphate in patients with Wolff-Parkinson-White syndrome. Circulation 65:869, 1982.

Klein, G.J., Guiraudon, G.M., Perkins, D.G., et al.: Surgical correction of the Wolff-Parkinson-White syndrome in the closed heart using cryosurgery: A simplified approach. J. Am. Coll. Cardiol. 3:405, 1984.

Klein, G.J. and Gulamhusein, S.S.: Intermittent preexcitation in the Wolff-Parkinson-White syndrome. J. Am. Coll. Cardiol. 52:292, 1983.

Lai, W.T., Huycke, E.C., Keung, E.C., et al.: Electrophysiologic manifestations of the excitable gap of orthodromic atrioventricular reciprocating tachycardia demonstrated by single extra-stimulation. Am. J. Cardiol. 63:545, 1989.

Langberg, J., Griffin, J.C., Herre, J.M., et al.: Catheter ablation of accessory pathways using radiofrequency in energy in the canine coronary sinus. J. Am. Coll. Cardiol. 13:491, 1989.

Lemery, R., Brugada, P. and Wellens, H.J.J.: Manifest and concealed accessory pathways: Behavior after catheter ablation of the atrioventricular conducting system. Am. Heart J. 118:188, 1989.

Lloyd, E.A., Hauer, R.N., Zipes, D.P., et al.: Syncope and ventricular tachycardia in patients with ventricular preexcitation. Am. J. Cardiol. 52:79, 1983.

Lown, B., Ganong, W.F. and Levine, S.A.: The syndrome of short P-R interval, normal QRS complex and paroxysmal rapid heart action. Circulation 5:693, 1952.

Massumi, R.A., Vera, Z. and Mason, D.T.: The Wolff-Parkinson-White syndrome. Mod. Conc. Cardiovasc. Dis. 42:41, 1973.

Masterson, M., Tarazi, R., Sterba, R., et al.: Preexcitation syndromes: surgical ablation therapy. Cleve. Clin. J. Med. 56:607, 1989.

Michelson, E.L.: Clinical perspectives in management of Wolff-Parkinson-White syndrome, Part 1: Recognition, diagnosis, and arrhythmias. Mod. Conc. Cardiovas. Dis. 58:43, 1989.

Michelson, E.L.: Clinical perspectives in management of Wolff-Parkinson-White syndrome, Part 2: Diagnostic evaluation and treatment strategies. Mod. Conc. Cardiovas. Dis. *58*:49, 1989.

Mitchell, L.B., Mason, J.W., Scheinman, M.M., et al.: Recordings of basal ventricular pre-excitation from electrode catheters in patients with accessory atrioventricular connections. Circulation *69*:233, 1984.

Morady, F., Sledge, C., Shen, E., et al.: Electrophysiologic testing in the management of patients with Wolff-Parkinson-White syndrome and atrial fibrillation. Am. J. Cardiol. *51*:1623, 1983.

Newman, B.J., Donoso, E., and Friedberg, C.K.: Arrhythmias in the Wolff-Parkinson-White syndrome. Prog. Cardiovasc. Dis. *9*:147, 1966.

Newman, D., Evans, G.T., Jr. and Scheinman, M.M.: Catheter ablation of cardiac arrhythmias. Curr. Probl. Cardiol. *14*:119–164, 1989.

Paul, T., Guccione, P. and Gerson, A., Jr.: Relation of syncope in young patients with Wolff-Parkinson-White syndrome to rapid ventricular response during atrial fibrillation. Am. J. Cardiol. *65*:318, 1990.

Portillo, B., Portillo-Leon, N., Zaman, L. and Castellanos, A., Jr.: Quintuple pathways participating in three distinct types of atrioventricular reciprocating tachycardia in a patient with Wolff-Parkinson-White syndrome. Am. J. Cardiol. *50*:347, 1982.

Proudfit, W.L. and Sterba, R.: Long-term status and survival in Wolff-Parkinson-White syndrome. Cleve. Clin. J. Med. *56*:601, 1989.

Prystowsky, E.N.: Diagnosis and management of the preexcitation syndromes. Curr. Probl. Cardiol. *13*:277–310, 1988.

Prystowsky, E.N., Browne, K.F. and Zipes, D.P.: Intracardiac recording by catheter electrode of accessory pathway depolarization. J. Am. Coll. Cardiol. *1*:468, 1983.

Prystowsky, E.N., Pritchett, E.L.C. and Gallagher, J.J.: Concealed conduction preventing anterograde preexcitation in Wolff-Parkinson-White syndrome. Am. J. Cardiol. *53*:960, 1984.

Saksena, S., Hussain, S.M., Gielchinsky, I. and Pantopoulos, D.: Intraoperative mapping-guided argon laser ablation of supraventricular tachycardia in the Wolff-Parkinson-White syndrome. Am. J. Cardiol. *60*:196, 1987.

Scheinman, M.: Catheter and surgical treatment of cardiac arrhythmias. JAMA *263*:79, 1990.

Schnittger, I., Lee, J.T., Hargis, J., et al: Long-term results of anti-tachycardia pacing in patients with supraventricular tachycardia. PACE *12*:936, 1989.

Sealy, W.C. and Wallace, A.G.: Surgical treatment of Wolff-Parkinson-White syndrome. J. Thorac. Cardiovasc. Surg. *68*:757, 1974.

Silberbach, M., Dunnigan, A. and Benson, D.W., Jr.: Effect of intravenous propranolol or verapamil on infant orthodromic reciprocating tachycardia. Am. J. Cardiol. *63*:438, 1989.

Suzuki, F., Kawara, T., Tanaka, K., et al.: Electrophysiological demonstration of antero-grade concealed conduction in accessory atrioventricular pathways capable only of retrograde conduction. PACE *12*:591, 1989.

Suzuki, F., Kawara, T., Sato, T., et al.: Fast-slow form of "Atrioventricular Nodal" reentrant tachycardia suggesting atrial participation in the reentrant circuit. Am. J. Cardiol. *63*:1413, 1989.

Wedd, A.M.: Paroxysmal tachycardia, with reference to normotropic tachycardia and the role of the extrinsic cardiac nerves. Arch. Intern. Med. *27*:57, 1921.

Wellens, H.J.J.: Wolff-Parkinson-White syndrome. Part I. Diagnosis, arrhythmias, and identification of the high risk patient. Mod. Conc. Cardiovasc. Dis. *52*:53, 1983.

Wellens, H.J.J.: Wolff-Parkinson-White syndrome. Part II. Treatment. Mod. Conc. Cardiovasc. Dis. *52*:57, 1983.

Wellens, H.J.J., Braat, S., Brugada, P., et al.: Use of procainamide in patients with the

Wolff-Parkinson-White syndrome to disclose a short refractory period of the accessory pathway. Am. J. Cardiol. *50*:1087, 1982.

Wellens, H.J.J., Brugada, P., Roy, D., et al.: Effect of isoproterenol on the anterograde refractory period of the accessory pathway in patients with Wolff-Parkinson-White syndrome. Am. J. Cardiol. *50*:180, 1982.

Wellens, H.J.J. and Durrer, D.: Effect of digitalis on atrioventricular conduction and circus movement tachycardias in patients with the Wolff-Parkinson-White syndrome. Circulation *47*:1229, 1973.

Wellens, H.J.J. and Durrer, D.: Effects of procaine amide, quinidine, and ajmaline in the Wolff-Parkinson-White syndrome. Circulation *50*:114, 1974.

Wellens, H.J.J., Janse, M.I., Van Dam, R.T., et al.: Epicardial mapping and surgical treatment in Wolff-Parkinson-White syndrome, type A. Am. Heart J. *88*:69, 1974.

Wolff, L., Parkinson, J. and White, P.D.: Bundle branch block with short P-R interval in healthy young people prone to paroxysmal tachycardia. Am. Heart J. *5*:685, 1930.

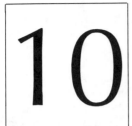

THERAPEUTIC APPROACH
TO CARDIAC ARRHYTHMIAS

Edward K. Chung

Because DC cardioverters and artificial pacemakers have become readily available (Chapters 13 and 14), the therapeutic results of the management of various arrhythmias have improved markedly in the past decade. The best therapeutic results can be obtained when a precise diagnosis of the arrhythmia is entertained because some drugs are more effective or even almost specific for certain arrhythmias. Digitalis, for instance, is usually the drug of choice for atrial fibrillation with a rapid ventricular response. Conversely, digitalis is ineffective or even contraindicated in the treatment of ventricular tachyarrhythmias (Chapter 18).

It is essential to eliminate the cause if it is still present. For instance, the most important and the first step in treating digitalis-induced arrhythmias is the immediate discontinuation of digitalis (Chapter 18). Another good example is that the first therapeutic approach to quinidine-induced polymorphous ventricular tachycardia (called "torsade de pointes") is to discontinue quinidine immediately. In addition, underlying etiological factors also significantly influence the therapeutic result. For example, ventricular tachycardia associated with acute MI is best treated with lidocaine (Xylocaine), whereas a digitalis-induced ventricular tachycardia responds best to phenytoin (Dilantin) or potassium (Chapter 18).

For alcohol-induced cardiac arrhythmias, immediate discontinuation of alcohol consumption is the most important therapeutic aspect. The term "holiday heart syndrome" describes the sudden occurrence of various tachyarrhythmias following consumption of large amounts of alcohol, because these episodes commonly follow holidays or weekends. At the present time, cocaine seems to be one of the most common contributing factors in the production of a variety of cardiac arrhythmias in young individuals.

Prevention of the recurrence of tachyarrhythmias is another important aspect of management. For this reason, maintenance therapy with digitalis and many anti-arrhythmic drugs (Chapter 12) is often necessary for long periods of time or even indefinitely. Quinidine is known to be the best agent for the prevention of recurrence of AF or flutter, whereas procainimide (Pronestyl) is known to be the best agent for the prevention of ventricular tachyarrhythmias in long-term therapy. Propranolol (Inderal) is the most effective agent in the treatment of catecholamine-induced arrhythmias and arrhythmias related to the WPW syndrome. Many new anti-arrhythmic agents are introduced in clinical medicine and some of them are still under investigation. These new anti-arrhythmic agents are discussed in Chapter 12. Various anti-arrhythmic agents have been classified into four major categories according to their electrophysiologic properties and their pharmacologic actions (Chapter 12).

Antibradyarrhythmic agents (Chapter 12) are less frequently used because of the ready availability of artificial pacemakers (Chapter 14). Commonly used antibradyarrhythmic agents include atropine and isoproterenol (Isuprel), especially during acute MI (Chapter 12).

Various anti-arrhythmic drugs are commonly used in conjunction with DC cardioverters and artificial pacemakers to deal with refractory cardiac arrhythmias (Chapters 13 and 14).

Because electrophysiologic studies have been carried out extensively, a specific anti-arrhythmic agent can now be used for a specific cardiac arrhythmia. For example, a reciprocating tachycardia with normal QRS complexes in the WPW syndrome is best treated with either propranolol (Inderal) or digitalis because these drugs block the normal AV conduction (Chapters 9 and 12). On the other hand, quinidine or other quinidine-like drugs are extremely effective in terminating atrial fibrillation with anomalous AV conduction in the WPW syndrome (Chapters 9 and 12).

Electrophysiologic investigative studies using an extrastimulation technique have shown that the best anti-arrhythmic agent for a specific tachyarrhythmia can be chosen according to its efficacy. For example, when ventricular tachycardia under a given clinical circumstance cannot be induced by the extrastimulation (arrhythmic-induction) technique following administration of a certain anti-arrhythmic agent (e.g., quinidine) in an electrophysiologic laboratory, that particular drug (quinidine) is the agent of choice for that clinical circumstance. This extrastimulation technique is useful when dealing with refractory ventricular tachycardia, and the technique is also beneficial for a long-term prophylactic anti-arrhythmic therapy.

I. GUIDE TO THE ANTI-ARRHYTHMIC THERAPY
   1. The purpose of the drug therapy for cardiac arrhythmias is

for the prevention of various untoward sequelae of the arrhythmias.

2. The common untoward sequelae of the arrhythmias include congestive heart failure (CHF), angina pectoris, fainting, dizziness, weakness, palpitations, skipped heartbeats, convulsion, feeling of impending death, cerebral ischemia, and even actual death.

3. The correct diagnosis of a given arrhythmia is essential. Three major categories of arrhythmias exist:
   a. Tachyarrhythmias, including premature contractions (extrasystoles) of various origins.
   b. Bradyarrhythmias.
   c. Bradytachyarrhythmias.

4. Careful consideration of indications and contraindications for various agents from electrophysiologic approaches (Chapter 12) is essential.

5. Familiarity with the recommended dosages of various anti-arrhythmic agents (Chapter 12) is necessary.

6. Prevention of side effects and toxicity of various agents is essential.

7. Elimination of the direct or indirect cause of a given arrhythmia, if possible, before any anti-arrhythmic agent is used.

8. When dealing with any unexplainable tachyarrhythmia, especially in young individuals, common underlying problems should be considered before initiating any anti-arrhythmic agent. Common underlying factors or disorders that frequently cause various cardiac arrhythmias include: (a) excessive usage of cocaine, coffee, tea, cola drinks, cigarette smoking, and emotional stress; (b) hyperthyroidism (thyrotoxicosis); (c) mitral valve prolapse syndrome; (d) Wolff-Parkinson-White (WPW) syndrome (Chapter 9).

9. Various anti-arrhythmic agents may show synergistic or antagonistic actions. The serum digoxin level, for example, often rises excessively when digoxin and quinidine are administered together, so that the incidence of digoxin toxicity increases significantly. Digitoxin and quinidine do not show any synergistic action.

10. Prevention of recurrent cardiac arrhythmia is another important aspect of anti-arrhythmic therapy.

11. Refractory arrhythmias often require a combination of two or more anti-arrhythmic agents.

12. Not uncommonly, some patients require DC shock and artificial pacemakers in addition to the anti-arrhythmic agents.

13. Anti-arrhythmic drug therapy alone is unsatisfactory in the treatment of sick sinus syndrome (SSS) in most cases. Thus, the use of an artificial pacemaker is the preferred treatment for sick sinus syndrome (SSS). In some cases with bradytachyarrhythmia syndrome (commonly a manifestation of

advanced SSS), one or more anti-arrhythmic agents are indicated even after pacing (Chapter 11).

14. For torsade de pointes (polymorphous ventricular tachycardia), the conventional anti-arrhythmic agents are not only ineffective but also more serious arrhythmias may be produced. Intravenous infusion of isoproterenol is the most effective agent under this circumstance. Artificial pacing with an over-driving rate (80 to 120 beats/min) is often a more effective and safer treatment for this ventricular tachycardia. Of course, a causative agent (commonly quinidine) should be discontinued immediately.

II. ELECTROPHYSIOLOGIC STUDY

Various anti-arrhythmic agents may alter the response of patients who have ventricular tachycardia to programmed ventricular stimuli or ventricular pacing. Many commonly used anti-arrhythmic drugs occasionally enhance the response to the stimuli. At times, the characteristics of ventricular tachycardia itself may be altered by certain agents. Most anti-arrhythmic agents are given IV, and less commonly by mouth during the acute phase of the electrophysiologic evaluation. In addition, long-term oral anti-arrhythmic drug therapy can be guided by the results of the electrophysiologic study. When an effective anti-arrhythmic agent is selected for a patient, after a review of the electrophysiologic test results, ventricular tachycardia can be effectively treated and prevented.

Because it is almost impossible to predict which anti-arrhythmic agent is effective in the suppression of ventricular tachycardia in a patient, various commonly used drugs are usually evaluated consecutively. In general, refractory ventricular tachycardia requires in-depth electrophysiologic study. During the electrophysiologic study, even when an effective anti-arrhythmic agent is selected, all other effective drugs are usually tested. The reason for this is that an alternative effective drug can be easily given if the patient develops serious untoward effects from the first drug chosen.

As a rule, it takes at least several days to complete the electrophysiologic evaluation of common anti-arrhythmic agents, because only one drug can be evaluated each day, except for lidocaine, which has a short half-life. It is essential to wait until the effects of each anti-arrhythmic agent are completely dissipated before the next drug is evaluated. For instance, lidocaine and procainamide may be evaluated during the initial complete electrophysiologic study, and the study may be followed by the evaluation of other drugs, including quinidine, propranolol, phenytoin, and disopyramide on consecutive days. When any new anti-arrhythmic agents under investigation are also tested, needless to say, additional days are necessary. During electrophysiologic study, a pervenous right ventricular electrode is often left in place, and continuous ECG monitoring is usually carried out for close observation of the patient.

The usual electrophysiologic study on various anti-arrhythmic drugs is conducted. Before any anti-arrhythmic agent is tested, of course, ventricular tachycardia is induced and is terminated by ventricular pacing in a patient. When procainamide is evaluated, a loading dose of the drug (1 to 2.5 g) is administered by IV infusion at a rate of about 50 mg/min. Then the programmed ventricular stimulation is repeated. When the ventricular tachycardia *cannot* be provoked by stimulation, blood is drawn to determine the concentration of procainamide, and oral drug (procainamide) therapy is initiated. The oral dosage of the drug is estimated by the IV doses required for the suppression of the ventricular tachycardia. By and large, the effective doses and the therapeutic blood concentrations are reported to be greater than those conventionally acceptable values. In one study, the effective doses of procainamide (Pronestyl) ranged from 6 to 12 g/day with the therapeutic blood concentrations ranging from 4.3 to 32.3 mg/L (average: 13.6 mg/L). The efficacy of procainamide has been repeatedly documented on follow-up electrophysiologic evaluation during oral drug therapy.

The usual IV doses or the electrophysiologic evaluation of other anti-arrhythmic agents are as follows: lidocaine (Xylocaine) is given with the dosage of 300 mg at a rate of 20 to 30 mg/min whereas the usual dosage of phenytoin (Dilantin) is 1000 mg at 20 mg/min. When propranolol (Inderal) is tested, 0.1 to 0.2 mg/kg of body weight is administered at 1 mg/min. The usual dosage of quinidine gluconate is 400 to 1600 mg at 20 mg/min. Disopyramide (Norpace) is administered orally for the study. The drug is given by mouth before the initiation of the electrophysiologic study in a loading dosage of 200 to 400 mg, followed by 100 to 300 mg every 6 hours for 36 hours. As a rule, relatively large amounts of each agent are given to obtain the therapeutic effect as long as no significant untoward effect is produced.

During short-term electrophysiologic evaluation of various anti-arrhythmic agents, the study is terminated when ventricular tachycardia is suppressed or significant side effects are observed. By and large, the evaluation should be discontinued immediately when the QRS duration or the Q-T interval is increased to more than 25 to 50% of the pre-existing values or when serious adverse effects such as hypotension are produced.

A good correlation exists between the results of the electrophysiologic study using various anti-arrhythmic agents and the efficacy of a drug to suppress ventricular tachycardia in clinical settings. In some patients, ventricular tachycardia is still inducible by programmed stimulation. Programmed stimulation, thus, may be more potent in the provocation of ventricular tachycardia than of spontaneous ventricular tachycardia during anti-arrhythmic drug therapy.

When dealing with patients who have recovered from cardiac arrest, cardiac arrhythmias (usually ventricular in origin), which were responsible for the production of the cardiac arrest, can be reproduced by the electrophysiologic study in many cases. Thus, an effective anti-arrhythmic drug program to prevent ventricular tachycardia or ventricular fibrillation can be established.

The rate of ventricular tachycardia is often decreased by various anti-arrhythmic drugs regardless of whether or not a drug is capable of reducing the ease of provoking the tachycardia by programmed stimulation. Occasionally, however, certain drugs may accelerate the rate of ventricular tachycardia. In general, the rate of ventricular tachycardia is nearly always reduced by quinidine, procainamide, and disopyramide when sufficient amounts are administered. The reason for this is that the conduction velocity of the re-entry cycle is slowed by a drug as a result of prolonged refractoriness in the involved ventricular myocardium.

The effect of procainamide on the tachycardiac zone varies considerably. The drug may cause narrowing or widening of the tachycardiac zone, and at times, no change may be evident. Although quinidine and disopyramide possess similar anti-arrhythmic effects on spontaneous or induced ventricular tachycardia, it is not possible to predict with certainty the true efficacy of these drugs in every case. Propranolol and verapamil have little effect on the rate of ventricular tachycardia or the tachycardiac zone.

One of the serious side effects of some anti-arrhythmic agents is the ability of these drugs to accelerate the rate of ventricular tachycardia in certain cases. This side effect is observed occasionally during the administration of lidocaine and phenytoin.

III. MANAGEMENT OF PREMATURE CONTRACTIONS (EXTRA-SYSTOLES)
1. The first step in management is the removal of any possible cause for the development of premature contractions regardless of the origin of the ectopic impulses. For example, digitalis-induced premature contractions, particularly ventricular in origin, are treated best by discontinuation of digitalis (Chapter 18).
2. Sedation is another important method to eliminate premature beats, especially in high-strung or nervous individuals.
3. Premature contractions are often eliminated by stopping heavy smoking or the excessive ingestion of coffee.
4. If the ventricular premature contractions are frequent (30 beats or more/hr), particularly in a diseased heart such as in acute MI, various anti-arrhythmic agents may be required.
5. Supraventricular (atrial or AV junctional) premature contractions are best treated with quinidine, if symptomatic (e.g., palpitations). Propranolol (Inderal) is almost equally effective in this case. By and large, supraventricular premature beats are self-limited and no active treatment is necessary as long as the arrhythmia does not cause any symptom.

6. Digitalis is particularly effective when premature contractions are associated with CHF.
7. Lidocaine (Xylocaine) is the drug of choice for the treatment of VPCs associated with acute MI, or during catheterization and cardiac surgery.
8. In the following situations, the treatment of VPCs is considered to be indicated:
   a. Frequent VPCs (30 or more beats/hour).
   b. R-on-T phenomenon (VPC superimposed on top of T wave of the preceding beat—vulnerable period).
   c. Multifocal VPCs.
   d. Grouped or paired VPCs.
   e. VPCs easily provoked by physical exercise or electrical stimulation in the electrophysiologic laboratory.
   f. Drug-induced VPCs (e.g., digitalis toxicity).
   g. VPCs in any active heart diseases (e.g. acute MI).
   h. VPCs after the termination of ventricular tachycardia or fibrillation.
9. For long-term therapy of VPCs, procainamide (Pronestyl) or quinidine is the preferred drug. Alternatively, disopyramide (Norpace) or phenytoin (Dilantin) may be used.
10. Phenytoin (Dilantin) is probably the best agent for the treatment of digitalis-induced premature beats (Chapter 18).
11. Beta-blocking agents (e.g., propranolol) are most effective in the treatment of various cardiac arrhythmias, particularly premature contractions associated with mitral valve prolapse syndrome.
12. Likewise, catecholamine-induced premature contractions are best treated with beta-blocking agents.
13. Calcium antagonists (e.g., verapamil or nifedipine) are the agents of choice for the treatment of VPCs associated with coronary artery spasm.
14. The most important factor to determine the indication vs. non-indication of anti-arrhythmic drug therapy for VPCs is the presence or absence of active underlying heart disease (e.g., acute MI).

IV. MANAGEMENT OF SUPRAVENTRICULAR TACHYARRHYTH-MIAS
   1. The first step in the management is the elimination of the cause if it is present. For instance, atrial fibrillation associated with thyrotoxicosis cannot be treated satisfactorily unless the thyroid function returns to euthyroid level.
   2. Carotid sinus stimulation (CSS) is often very effective in the termination of paroxysmal atrial or AV junctional tachycardia (Chapter 8).
   3. Digitalis is usually the drug of choice in the treatment of AF with rapid ventricular response.
   4. In digitalis-induced supraventricular tachyarrhythmias, digitalis must be discontinued immediately. In addition, phen-

ytoin (Dilantin) or potassium is found very effective in the termination of digitalis-induced supraventricular tachyarrhythmias (Chapter 18).

5. Quinidine is the best agent to prevent the recurrence of AF or flutter.
6. Propranolol (Inderal) is the most effective agent in the treatment of arrhythmias precipitated by exercise, emotional distress, or excessive sympathetic stimulation, and WPW syndrome or supraventricular tachyarrhythmias related to mitral valve prolapse syndrome.
7. Procainamide (Pronestyl) is less commonly used for the treatment of supraventricular tachyarrhythmias and lidocaine (Xylocaine) is rarely used in this case.
8. Verapamil is a useful drug for the treatment of various supraventricular tachyarrhythmias including those associated with the WPW syndrome.
9. Direct current (DC) shock is often very effective in the termination of various acute supraventricular tachyarrhythmias. In addition, elective cardioversion is another important therapy in the termination of chronic atrial fibrillation or flutter (Chapter 13).
10. In holiday heart syndrome, various tachyarrhythmias may be observed, but paroxysmal AF is the most common arrhythmia in this entity. Immediate discontinuation of alcohol consumption is the most important and the first therapeutic approach under this circumstance.
11. Artificial pacemakers (overdriving rate) are occasionally needed in the suppression of various supraventricular tachyarrhythmias that are refractory to various anti-arrhythmic agents or DC shock (Chapter 14).
12. Sedation is often beneficial for the treatment of supraventricular tachyarrhythmias in conjunction with other therapeutic measures.

V. MANAGEMENT OF VENTRICULAR TACHYARRHYTHMIAS

1. It is essential to eliminate any possible cause of ventricular tachyarrhythmias if it is present. Digitalis should be stopped immediately when ventricular tachyarrhythmias are due to digitalis toxicity (Chapter 18).
2. Quinidine or any other causative agents (procainamide or disopyramide) must be discontinued immediately in the treatment of torsade de pointes (a polymorphous or atypical ventricular tachycardia). In addition, artificial pacing with slight over-driving rate (80 to 120 beats/min) or IV infusion of isoproterenol is often indicated in this case. Quinidine-syncope or sudden death during quinidine therapy is often attributed to torsade de pointes (Chapter 12).
3. Direct current shock is the most effective way of terminating ventricular tachycardia, flutter, and fibrillation (Chapter 13). Defibrillation should be carried out immediately for the treat-

ment of ventricular fibrillation or flutter in addition to all the necessary cardiopulmonary resuscitation (CPR) as needed. Direct current (DC) shock, however, should be avoided as much as possible if ventricular tachycardia is induced by digitalis. The reason for this is that DC shock often produces new cardiac arrhythmias, particularly ventricular fibrillation, in this case.

4. Lidocaine (Xylocaine) is the drug of choice for the treatment of ventricular tachycardia associated with acute MI, or during anesthesia and cardiac catheterization. Procainamide (Pronestyl) and quinidine are the next commonly used drugs in this situation.

5. Bretylium (a new anti-arrhythmic agent) is a very effective drug for refractory ventricular tachyarrhythmias.

6. Disopyramide (Norpace) or propranolol (Inderal) is less commonly used for the treatment of ventricular tachyarrhythmias.

7. Phenytoin (Dilantin) is the best drug for the treatment of digitalis-induced ventricular tachycardia (Chapter 20).

8. Ventricular tachyarrhythmias associated with coronary artery spasm are best treated with calcium antagonists (e.g., nifedipine).

9. When ventricular tachyarrhythmias are refractory to anti-arrhythmic agents or DC shock, the use of an artifical pacemaker (overdriving pacing rate: 100 to 120 beats/min) is often a life-saving measure (Chapter 14).

10. For recurrent ventricular fibrillation, implantation of automatic mini-defibrillator should be strongly considered (see Chapter 13).

VI. MANAGEMENT OF SINUS BRADYCARDIA, SINUS ARREST, AND SA BLOCK

1. The therapeutic approaches vary markedly, depending upon the fundamental mechanism responsible for the production of bradyarrhythmias, the ventricular rate, the underlying cause, and the degree of symptoms.

2. Sinus bradycardia of mild degree (rate: 50 to 59 beats/min) is not uncommon in healthy individuals, especially in young athletes and elderly persons. When the sinus rate is between 40 and 50 beats/min, some symptoms may be present. Marked sinus bradycardia with a rate below 40 beats/min often produces significant hemodynamic alterations, especially when it is associated with acute MI.

3. The most common causes of sinus bradycardia include the therapeutic or toxic effects of various drugs including digitalis, propranolol, reserpine, guanethidine, methyldopa (Aldomet), and acute diaphragmatic MI. Drug-induced sinus bradycardia, sinus arrest or SA block is best treated by stopping that particular drug.

4. Active treatment is indicated when marked sinus bradycardia

persists and becomes symptomatic, and especially when it is associated with acute MI. The treatment of choice in this case is atropine and the next commonly used agent is isoproterenol (Isuprel).

5. Essentially the same therapeutic approach may be used in the treatment of symptomatic sinus arrest or SA block.

6. In drug-resistant sinus bradycardia, sinus arrest, or SA block, a temporary or even a permanent artificial pacemaker is the treatment of choice.

7. When dealing with persisting and drug-resistant sinus brady-arrhythmias, the underlying disorder is commonly sick sinus syndrome (SSS). For symptomatic or advanced SSS, permanent artificial pacemaker implantation is the treatment of choice (Chapter 11).

VII. MANAGEMENT OF AV BLOCK

1. AV block in itself does not require treatment. Therapeutic indication of AV block depends primarily on the degree, the site, and the etiology of the AV block, the ventricular rate, and the presence or absence of symptoms.

2. First-degree AV block does not usually require a particular treatment, except that the direct cause, such as digitalis intoxication, should be eliminated. Atropine is effective in abolishing digitalis-induced first and second-degree AV block. Isoproterenol (Isuprel) may be effective in this circumstance, but the drug often produces untoward reactions, such as an increase in ventricular irritability.

3. Wenckebach (Mobitz type I) AV block usually does not require active treatment unless significant symptoms are produced. Wenckebach AV block usually represents AV nodal block.

4. On the other hand, Mobitz type II AV block requires an artificial pacemaker because Mobitz type II AV block is considered to be an advanced form of bilateral bundle branch block. Mobitz type II AV block represents infranodal block.

5. In complete AV block, the therapeutic approach depends upon the ventricular rate, the exact site of the block, and the degree of the symptoms. Active treatment is usually not indicated when the ventricular rate is relatively rapid (40 to 60 min) in AV junctional escape rhythm due to complete AV block, such as in acute diaphragmatic MI, unless symptomatic. On the other hand, a permanent artificial pacemaker is indicated when the ventricular rate is slow (slower than 40/min) in ventricular escape (idioventricular) rhythm due to complete AV block such as seen in acute anterior MI, or in elderly individuals with degenerative changes in the conduction system.

6. Complete AV block in acute diaphragmatic MI represents AV nodal block whereas complete AV block in acute anterior MI

usually represents infranodal block—complete trifascicular block.

7. In general, AV nodal block is relatively benign and self-limited. Thus, active treatment is not indicated under this circumstance. On the other hand, the infra-nodal block is usually irreversible and a permanent pacemaker implantation is necessary in most cases.

8. Bilateral bundle branch block (bifascicular and trifascicular block) of varying degrees often requires a permanent artificial pacemaker, especially when it is symptomatic (Chapter 14).

9. In urgent situations before the insertion of an artificial pacemaker, various agents such as isoproterenol (Isuprel) or epinephrine (Adrenalin) may be tried.

SUGGESTED READINGS

Abdon, N., Johansson, B.W. and Lessem, J.: Predictive use of routine 24-hour elecrocardiography in suspected Adams-Stokes syndrome: Comparison with cardiac rhythm during symptoms. Br. Heart J. 47:553, 1982.

Akhtar, M., Tchou, P. and Jazayeri, M.: Use of calcium channel entry blockers in the treatment of cardiac arrhythmias. Circulation 80:IV-31, 1989.

Allen, B.J., Brodsky, M.A., Capparelli, E.V., et al.: Magnesium sulfate therapy for sustained monomorphic ventricular tachycardia. Am. J. Cardiol. 64:1202, 1989.

Anderson, J.L., Jolivette, M.D. and Fredell, P.A.: Efficacy and safety of flecainide for supraventricular arrhythmias. Prac. Cardiol. 15:35, 1989.

Brodsky, M.A. and Allen, B.J.: Stress, cardiac arrhythmias, and sudden cardiac death. Pract. Cardiol. 15:49, 1989.

Brodsky, M.A., Allen, B.J., Luckett, C.R., et al.: Antiarrhythmic efficacy of solitary beta-adrenergic blockade for patients with sustained ventricular tachyarrhythmias. Am. Heart J. 118:272, 1989.

Buxton, A.E., Marchlinski, F.E., Waxman, H.L., et al.: Prognostic factors in nonsustained ventricular tachycardia. Am. J. Cardiol. 53:1275, 1984.

Buxton, A.E., Waxman, H.L., Marchlinski, F.E., et al.: Role of triple extrastimuli during electrophysiologic study of patients with documented sustained ventricular tachyarrhythmias. Circulation 69:532, 1984.

Case, C.L., Crawford, F.A., Gillette, P.C., et al.: Management strategies for surgical treatment of dysrhythmias in infants and children. Am. J. Cardiol. 63:1069, 1989.

Crawford, W., Plumb, V.J., Epstein, A.E. and Kay, G.N.: Prospective evaluation of transesophageal pacing for interruption of atrial flutter. Am. J. Med. 86:663, 1989.

Chung, E.K.: Ambulatory Electrocardiography: Holter Monitor Electrocardiography. New York, Springer-Verlag, 1979.

Chung, E.K.: Artificial Cardiac Pacing, 2nd Ed. Baltimore, Williams & Wilkins, 1984.

Dobmeyer, D.J., Stine, R.A., Leier, C.V., et al.: The arrhythmogenic effects of caffeine in human beings. N. Engl. J. Med. 308:814, 1983.

Duffy, C.E., Swiryn, S., Bauernfeind, R.A., et al.: Inducible sustained ventricular tachycardia refractory to individual class I drugs: Effect of adding a second class I drug. Am. Heart J. 106:450, 1983.

El-Sherif, N., Mehra, R., Gough, W.B. and Zeiler, R.D.: Reentrant ventricular arrhythmias in the late myocardial infarction period: Interruption of reentrant circuits by cryothermal techniques. Circulation 68:644, 1983.

Ezri, M., Lerman, B.B., Marchlinski, F.E., et al.: Electrophysiologic evaluation of syncope in patients with bifascicular block. Am. Heart J. 106:693, 1983.

Funck-Brentano, C., Kroemer, H.K., Lee, J.T. and Roden, D.M.: Propafenone. N. Engl. J. Med. 322:518, 1990.

Gillette, P.C.: Advances in treatment of supraventricular tachyarrhythmias in children. Mod. Conc. Cardiovas. Dis. 58:37, 1989.

Hargrove, W.C. and Miller, J.M.: Risk stratification and management of patients with recurrent ventricular tachycardia and other malignant ventricular arrhythmias. Circulation 79:I-178, 1989.

Herre, J.M., Sauve, M.J., Malone, P., et al.: Long-term results of amiodarone therapy in patients with recurrent sustained ventricular tachycardia or ventricular fibrillation. J. Am. Coll. Cardiol. 13:442, 1989.

Hine, L.K., Gross, T.P. and Kennedy, D.L.: Outpatient antiarrhythmic drug use from 1970 through 1986. Arch. Intern. Med. 149:1524, 1989.

Huang, S.K.S.: Radio-frequency catheter ablation of cardiac arrhythmias: Appraisal of an evolving therapeutic modality. Am. Heart J. 118:1317, 1989.

Jazayeri, M.R., VanWyhe, G., Avitall, B., et al.: Isoproterenol reversal of antiarrhythmic effects in patients with inducible sustained ventricular tachyarrhythmias. J. Am. Coll. Cardiol. 14:705, 1989.

Josephson, M.E., Harken, A.H. and Horowitz, L.N.: Long-term results of endocardial resection for sustained ventricular tachycardia in coronary disease patients. Am. Heart J. 104:51, 1982.

Josephson, M.E., Horowitz, L.N., Spielman, S.R., et al.: Role of catheter mapping in the preoperative evaluation of ventricular tachycardia. Am. J. Cardiol. 49:207, 1982.

Josephson, M.E., Spear, J.E., Harken, A.H., et al.: Surgical excision of automatic atrial tachycardia: Anatomic and electrophysiologic correlates. Am. Heart J. 104:1076, 1982.

Kay, G.N., Epstein, A.E. and Plumb V.J.: Preferential effect of procainamide on the reentrant circuit of ventricular tachycardia. J. Am. Coll. Cardiol. 14:382, 1989.

Levine, J.H., Morganroth, J. and Kadish, A.H.: Mechanisms and risk factors for proarrhythmia with type Ia compared with Ic antiarrhythmic drug therapy. Circulation 80:1063, 1989.

McGovern, B.A., Garan, H. and Ruskin, J.N.: Treatment of ventricular arrhythmias. Curr. Probl. Cardiol. 13:787, 1988.

McGovern, B.A. and Ruskin, J.N.: Ventricular tachycardia: Initial assessment and approach to treatment. Mod. Conc. Cardiovas. Dis. 56:13, 1987.

Morady, F., Shen, E., Schwartz, A., et al.: Long-term follow-up of patients with recurrent unexplained syncope evaluated by electrophysiologic testing. J. Am. Coll. Cardiol. 2:1053, 1983.

Ochi, R.P., Goldenberg, I.F., Almquist, A., et al.: Intravenous amiodarone for the rapid treatment of life-threatening ventricular arrhythmias in critically ill patients with coronary artery disease. Am. J. Cardiol. 64:599, 1989.

Ohe, T.: Idiopathic sustained left ventricular tachycardia: Clinical characteristics and management. Pract. Cardiol. 15:47, 1989.

Peberdy, M.A. and Kowey, P.R.: Clinical guidelines for the use of amiodarone. Pract. Cardiol. 16:47, 1990.

Polikar, R., Geld, G.K., Dittrich, H.C., et al.: Effect of thyroid replacement therapy on the frequency of benign atrial and ventricular arrhythmias. J. Am. Coll. Cardiol. 4:999, 1989.

Salerno, D.M., Dias, V.C., Kleiger, R.E., et al.: Efficacy and safety of intravenous diltiazem for treatment of atrial fibrillation and atrial flutter. Am. J. Cardiol. 63:1046, 1989.

Salerno, D.M., Granrud, G., Sharkey, P., et al.: A controlled trial of propafenone for treatment of frequent and repetitive ventricular premature complexes. Am. J. Cardiol. 53:77, 1984.

Savage, D.D., Castelli, W.P., Anderson, S.J. and Kannel, W.B.: Sudden unexpected death during ambulatory electrocardiographic monitoring: The Framingham study. Am. J. Med. 74:148, 1983.

Scheinman, M.: Catheter and surgical treatment of cardiac arrhythmias. JAMA 263:79, 1990.

Singh, J.B., Rasul, A.M., Shah, A., et al.: Efficacy of mexiletine in chronic ventricular arrhythmias compared with quinidine: A single-blind, randomized trial. Am. J. Cardiol. 53:84, 1984.

Stanton, M.S., Prystowsky, E.N., Fineberg, N.S., et al.: Arrhythmogenic effects of antiarrhythmic drugs: A study of 506 patients treated for ventricular tachycardia or fibrillation. J. Am. Coll. Cardiol. 14:209, 1989.

Surawicz, B.: Ventricular arrhythmias: Why is it so difficult to find a pharmacologic cure? J. Am. Coll. Cardiol. 14:1401, 1989.

Surawicz, B.: Is hypomagnesemia or magnesium deficiency arrhythmogenic. J. Am. Coll. Cardiol. 14:1093, 1989.

Svenson, R.H., Littmann, L., Gallagher, J.J., et al.: Termination of ventricular tachycardia with epicardial laser photocoagulation: A clinical comparison with patients undergoing successful endocardial photocoagulation alone. J. Am. Coll. Cardiol. 15:163, 1990.

Uretz, E.F., Denes, P., Ruggie, N., et al.: Relation of ventricular premature beats to underlying heart disease. Am. J. Cardiol. 53:774, 1984.

Velebit, V., Podrid, P., Lown, B., et al.: Aggravation and provocation of ventricular arrhythmias by anti-arrhythmic drugs. Circulation 65:886, 1982.

Vrobel, T.R., Miller, P.E., Mostow, N.D. and Rakita, L.: A general overview of amiodarone toxicity: Its prevention, detection, and management. Prog. Cardiovas. Dis. 32:393, 1989.

Ware, J.A., Magro, S.A., Luck, J.C., et al.: Conduction system abnormalities in symptomatic mitral valve prolapse: An electrophysiologic analysis of 60 patients. Am. J. Cardiol. 53:1075, 1984.

Weaver, W.D., Cobb, L.A. and Hallstrom, A.P.: Ambulatory arrhythmias in resuscitated victims of cardiac arrest. Circulation 66:212, 1982.

Whitsett, T.L., Manion, C.V. and Christensen, H.D.: Cardiovascular effects of coffee and caffeine. Am. J. Cardiol. 53:918, 1984.

Zee-Cheng, C.S., Kouchoukos, N.T., Connors, J.P. and Ruffy, R.: Treatment of life-threatening ventricular arrhythmias with nonguided surgery supported by electrophysiologic testing and drug therapy. J. Am. Coll. Cardiol. 13:153, 1989.

c h a p t e r

11

THE SICK SINUS SYNDROME

Edward K. Chung

I. GENERAL CONSIDERATIONS

An increasing awareness of the clinical entity known as the sick sinus syndrome (SSS) has grown in the past 2 decades because the syndrome is found relatively commonly among our cardiac patients, particularly among elderly patients, and because in most cases it can be successfully treated with artificial cardiac pacing. The term SSS covers a broad spectrum of clinical manifestations (e.g., near syncope, syncope, dizziness, increased congestive heart failure, or angina pectoris and palpitations) that result from a dysfunctioning sinus node. The ECG manifestations of the SSS may include (1) persistent and marked sinus bradycardia, (2) sino-atrial (SA) block, (3) sinus arrest, (4) a long pause following an atrial premature contraction (APC), (5) chronic atrial fibrillation or flutter with a slow ventricular rate, (6) carotid sinus hypersensitivity, (7) lack of a stable sinus rhythm after cardioversion, (8) AV junctional escape rhythm with or without slow and unstable sinus activity, and (9) the brady-tachyarrhythmia syndrome (BTS). Those ECG findings in SSS are *not* drug induced.

Besides the sick sinus syndrome, other terms are used to describe those phenomena; the terms include sinoatrial syncope, sluggish sinus node syndrome, inadequate sinus mechanism, sick sinus node, and lazy sinus node. When tachyarrhythmia components are present intermittently or periodically during slow rhythm, various terms, such as brady-tachyarrhythmia syndrome, brady-tachy syndrome, and tachycardia-bradycardia syndrome have been used. Although some investigators use the terms SSS and BTS interchangeably, the BTS is one of the common manifestations of the SSS.

As can be expected, the degree of the sinus node dysfunction may be so minimal that the SSS may be manifested only by a slight sinus bradycardia. In such a case, the patient is usually asymptomatic. On the other hand, the sinus node may be severely diseased, leading to complete generator failure—prolonged sinus arrest or atrial fibrillation with a slow ventricular rate. The advanced SSS is nearly always symptomatic. Any symptoms in the SSS are usually related to the cardiac or the cerebral dysfunction. That is, the perfusion deficit in the heart or brain causes the production of various symptoms in the SSS. Near syncope or syncope is the most common clinical manifestation of the SSS.

II. ANATOMY AND ELECTROPHYSIOLOGY

The sinus node was discovered by Keith and Flack in 1907, and the electrophysiologic property of the sinus node as cardiac pacemaker was first described by Wybouw and by Lewis and his coworkers in 1910. The term sinus node is probably the most popular and appropriate one because embryologic studies have shown that the ultimate cardiac pacemaker is derived from the sinus venosus and not from the atria. Furthermore, the terms sinoatrial node and sinoauricular node are incorrect from a precise anatomic viewpoint because the node extends from the auriculocaval junction back to the atriocaval junction. Thus sinus node (Walmsley's term) is the most accurate one, and it is accepted as the standard name for the natural (primary) pacemaker of the heart.

The electrophysiologic event known as spontaneous phase 4 depolarization is the factor that distinguishes the pacemaker cells from the other cells. The sinus node is the dominant pacemaker because the sinus node cells possess the fastest spontaneous depolarization. The spontaneous sinus node depolarization can be altered by parasympathetic and sympathetic influences. For example, vagal stimulation of acetylcholine can slow the automaticity of the sinus node by reducing the slope of phase 4 depolarization as well as by hyperpolarizing the cells. On the other hand, sympathetic stimulation or catecholamine infusion enhances the spontaneous sinus node discharge rate, primarily as a result of an increase in the rate of phase 4 depolarization. The sinus node has both sympathetic and parasympathetic (vagal) innervation but the parasympathetic innervation is richer in the AV node.

Various investigative studies have confirmed that the sinus node is the primary pacemaker in the heart. Because the sinus node's inherent rate is faster than that of any other cardiac pacemaker, sinus rhythm is present in most healthy people. In the SSS, when the sinus node produces the cardiac impulses more slowly than usual (sinus bradycardia), or when it fails to produce any impulse (sinus arrest), or when the sinus impulse is not conducted to the atria because of SA block, the subsidiary pacemaker (commonly the AV junction) takes over the ventricular activity as an escape mechanism. On the other hand, the chronic generator failure (sinus arrest) not uncommonly leads to the establishment of chronic atrial fibrillation (often with a slow ventricular rate).

Considerable variation is present in the shape, size, and location of the sinus node. The exact location of the node depends on how the sinus artery encircles the base of the superior vena cava. In the human heart, the sinus node is generally located in the sulcus terminal near the junction of the superior vena cava and the right atrium. The node is somewhat elongated along the axis of the sulcus terminalis, and its anterior margin is a few millimeters posterior to a crest formed by the junction of the right atrial appendage with the superior vena cava. The sinus node is located more anteriorly when the caval encirclement by the node artery is clockwise (viewed from above) than when encirclement is counterclockwise. The size of the sinus node varies considerably, and it is not closely proportional to the size of the heart. In general, its size is approximately 15 mm in length, 5 to 7 mm in width, and 1.5 to 2 mm in thickness. The shape of the sinus node varies, but by and large it resembles an extended snail with its shell, which misleads one to think of the node as having a head, a body, and a tail. Since the sinus node is situated at a position that is less than 1 mm beneath the epicardial surface, the sinus node is vulnerable to many disease processes, including trauma (e.g., that of pericarditis). The superficial anatomical location of the sinus node may be directly or indirectly responsible for the development of the SSS in many patients.

In the human heart, the sinus node artery is commonly located near the center of the sinus node, but its location may be eccentric. In approximately 55 to 60% of human hearts, the sinus node artery arises from the proximal 2 to 3 cm of the right coronary artery, whereas in 40 to 45% of human hearts, it arises from the proximal 1 cm of the left circumflex coronary artery. Other origins of the sinus node artery are rare; they account for about 2% of the total. At times, there are two branches of the sinus node artery of equal size. The sinus node artery, regardless of whether it arises from the right or left coronary artery, courses along the anteromedial atrial wall of the base of the superior vena cava, which it encircles. The artery anastomoses with other atrial arteries of both ipsilateral and contralateral origin. Generally, the primary arterial supply of the sinus node is almost always unilateral in origin. Smaller branches of the artery are distributed throughout the sinus node.

Small veins are commonly found throughout the sinus node, whereas large veins are present infrequently.

Microscopically, the sinus node is composed of three types of cells, including P cells, transitional cells, and working cells. The term P cells is used because the cells are pale and thus resemble primitive myocardial cells. The P cells are thought to be responsible for sinus node pacemaker function.

The Purkinje-like fibers, the "internodal pathways" that connect from the sinus node to the specialized atrial conduction tissue have been described: the anterior, middle, and posterior internodal tracts. By electrophysiologic studies it has been demonstrated that the cardiac impulse from the sinus node reaches the AV node more rapidly than it would if it were conducted through the ordinary myocardium. Although any one of three internodal pathways may be responsible for intra-atrial conduction, in most normal hearts the conduction is thought to be carried out preferentially by way of the anterior tract. That theory is not universally accepted, however.

III. UNDERLYING DISORDERS

Although various drugs, such as digitalis, propranolol, and quinidine, frequently cause dysfunction of the sinus node, their functionally reversible effects on the sinus node are not considered part of the SSS. The basic underlying causes of the SSS are anatomic, with physiologic consequences that produce a long-standing and often irreversible process in the sinus node.

A. Coronary Artery Disease

Coronary heart disease, particularly myocardial infarction, has been reported as the most common underlying disease that produces the SSS. In one study, dysfunction of the sinus node was reported to occur in approximately 5% of patients with acute myocardial infarction. In addition, the sinus node dysfunction can be expected to be present in over 50% of patients who have diaphragmatic myocardial infarction. In one study, 31 out of 32 patients with diseased sinus node had diaphragmatic myocardial infarction. Dysfunction of the sinus node is usually observed during the first 4 days of diaphragmatic myocardial infarction. Commonly, the sinus node dysfunction is manifested by a progressive sinus bradycardia followed by various superventricular arrhythmias, including atrial fibrillation or flutter and AV junctional escape rhythm with a periodic restoration of sinus bradycardia and intermittent sinus arrest or SA block. Atrial myocardial infarction may cause the sinus node dysfunction on rare occasions. Atrial damage, including sinus node dysfunction, is common as a result of occlusions of the main right coronary artery (causing diaphragmatic myocardial infarction) and occlusions of the left circumflex artery (causing anterolateral myocardial infarction).

B. Idiopathic Disorders (Sclerotic-Degenerative Process)

When coronary heart disease is eliminated as a cause of the SSS, most of the remaining cases show no clear evidence of clinical heart disease as a cause of the SSS. In those latter cases, a sclerotic-degenerative process involving the sinus node is usually considered the cause of the SSS. Pathologic

Table 11–1.   The Sick Sinus Syndrome: Electrocardiographic Manifestations

Marked and persisting sinus bradycardia
Sinus arrest or SA block
Drug-resistant (e.g., to atropine or isoproterenol) sinus bradyarrhythmias
Long pause following an atrial premature contraction
Prolonged sinus node recovery time determined by atrial pacing
Chronic atrial fibrillation or the repetitive occurrence of atrial fibrillation (less
     commonly atrial flutter): (a) with slow ventricular rate (b) preceded or followed
     by sinus bradycardia, sinus arrest, or SA block
AV junctional escape rhythm (with or without slow and unstable sinus activity)
Carotid sinus syncope
Failure of restoration of sinus rhythm following cardioversion
Brady-tachyarrhythmia syndrome
Common coexisting AV block or intraventricular block
Any combination of the above

studies revealed that severe fibrosis involving the sinus node
and SA junction was the main feature of the SSS. In some
cases of the SSS, amyloid infiltration involving the sinus node
was demonstrated.

C. Miscellaneous Disorders

Other underlying causes of the SSS may be (1) rheumatic
heart disease, (2) cardiomyopathies, (3) congenital heart disease, (4) surgical trauma, (5) hypertension, (6) pericarditis or
myocarditis, (7) amyloidosis, (8) systemic lupus erythematosus, (9) muscular dystrophy, (10) Friedreich's ataxia, (11)
malignancy, (12) hemochromatosis, and (13) diphtheria.

Familial incidence of the SSS has been reported, and its
association with the long Q-T syndrome also has been
described. The SSS associated with systemic embolism and
the mitral valve prolapse syndrome has been reported.

In various congenital heart diseases, SSS seems to be relatively common among patients with atrial septal defect. This
observation may indicate that atrial septal defect may be associated with diffuse atrial disease including dysfunctioning
sinus node.

IV. ELECTROCARDIOGRAPHIC MANIFESTATIONS

Depending on the degree of the sinus node dysfunction, various
ECG abnormalities may be produced in the SSS (Table 11–1). Persistent and severe sinus bradycardia (not due to drugs) is the most
common (75 to 80% of all patients who had the SSS) and the earliest
manifestation of the SSS and it is followed by various other ECG
abnormalities as the syndrome progresses. In a long-standing SSS,
atrial fibrillation is the commonest underlying rhythm. When the
SSS is far advanced, it is manifested by the BTS, in which a variety
of cardiac rhythms are observed in many cases. In addition, AV
conduction disturbances as well as intraventricular blocks often
coexist in many persons with advanced SSS.

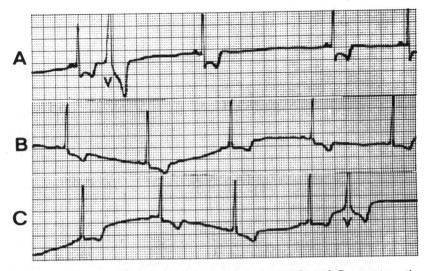

FIG. 11–1. The Holter monitor ECG rhythm strips A, B, and C are *not* continuous. The sick sinus syndrome is manifested by marked sinus bradycardia and arrhythmia (43 to 46 beats/min) with a ventricular premature contraction (VPC).

A. Sinus Bradycardia

Although some degree of sinus bradycardia is very common in healthy people, especially in athletes, a persistent and marked sinus bradycardia (one not due to drugs) deserves medical investigation. The SSS should be strongly suspected when chronic sinus bradycardia shows a rate slower than 45 beats/min (Fig. 11–1), with or without symptoms. Of course, marked sinus bradycardia frequently produces symptoms, such as light-headedness, near syncope, and syncope. It should be certain that the sinus bradycardia is not due to a drug, such as propranolol (Inderal), digitalis, reserpine (Serpasil), guanethidine (Ismelin), or methyldopa (Aldomet). On the other hand, the SSS may be "unmasked" by small amounts of drugs, particularly digitalis or propranolol. In other words, marked sinus bradycardia following the administration of small amounts of those drugs strongly suggests the SSS, especially in elderly people.

When sinus bradycardia is marked, one or more AV junctional or ventricular escape beats may occur, and incomplete AV dissociation is often produced (Fig. 11–2). At times, marked sinus bradycardia may lead to AV junctional escape bigeminy, in which sinus beats and AV junctional escape beats occur on every other beat. When the AV node as well as the sinus node is diseased—a common occurrence—the AV junctional escape rhythm also produces a markedly slow rate or

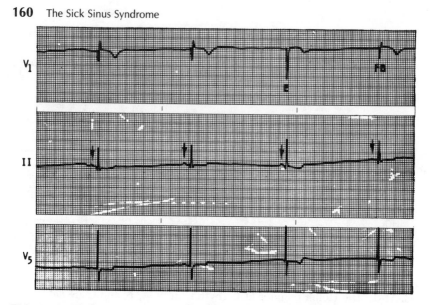

FIG. 11–2. These rhythm strips are those of an 85-year-old man who had had a diaphragmatic myocardial infarction 2 months previously. He complained of frequent dizzy spells. His slow heart rate failed to respond to atropine or isoproterenol. The rhythm is marked sinus bradycardia (28 beats/min) and a ventricular escape beat (in the third QRS complex). Note also the ventricular fusion beat (in the last QRS complex). That rhythm disorder is a manifestation of the sick sinus syndrome. In this tracing, the expected AV junctional escape beat failed to appear, and as a result, a ventricular escape beat occurred, a phenomenon that indicates coexisting AV node disease. A permanent-demand ventricular pacemaker was implanted in the patient.

ventricular escape beats appear because the AV node fails to produce any escape impulse (Fig. 11–2).

Marked sinus bradycardia is often irregular, and it may be followed by atrial or ventricular tachyarrhythmias (Figs. 11–1 and 11–3). First-degree AV block (in which the P-R interval is 0.28 sec or more) also commonly coexists (Fig. 11–3).

B. Sinus Arrest or Sinoatrial Block

When the SSS further progresses, the sinus node fails to produce any cardiac impulse, leading to sinus arrest (Fig. 11–4). The long P-P interval due to sinus arrest has no relationship to the basic P-P cycle. During sinus arrest, it is common to observe one or more AV junctional (less commonly ventricular) escape beats control the ventricular activity. In some other persons with SSS, SA block may be observed. In SA block, the sinus impulse is unable to conduct to the atria as a result of a block at the SA junction. SA block has two forms—Mobitz types I and II. Mobitz type II SA block is characterized by the intermittent absence of the expected P wave(s) in which the long P-P interval is a multiple of the

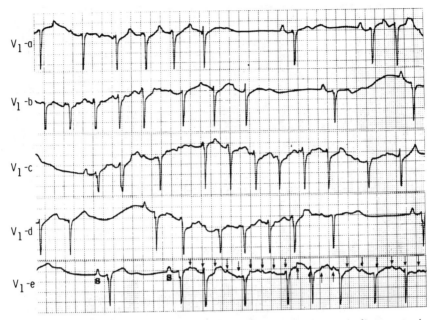

FIG. 11–3. Leads V_1-a, b, c, d, and e are continuous. The arrows indicate ectopic atrial activities. The sick sinus syndrome is manifested by marked sinus bradycardia (marked S) with first degree AV block and paroxysmal atrial fibrillation, flutter, and tachycardia. Digitalis is given to the patient, in addition to the implantation of a permanent-demand ventricular pacemaker.

basic P-P cycle (Fig. 11–5). On the other hand, Mobitz type I (Wenckebach) SA block produces a progressive shortening of the P-P cycles until a pause occurs. Mobitz type I (Wenckebach) SA block is analogous to Mobitz type I (Wenckebach) AV block, whereas Mobitz type II SA block is analogous to Mobitz type II AV block. In cases of far-advanced SA block or sinus arrest, the sinus activity is almost completely absent (at times, entirely absent), leading to atrial standstill. When

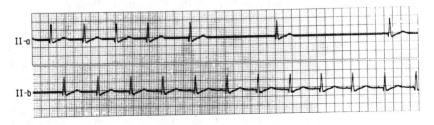

FIG. 11–4. Leads II-a and b are continuous. The sick sinus syndrome is manifested by sinus arrest.

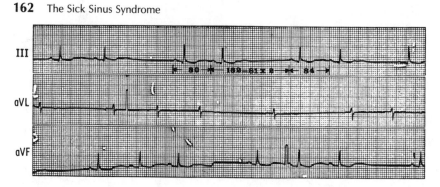

FIG. 11–5. The sick sinus syndrome is manifested by intermittent Mobitz type II and 2:1 SA block. (The numbers represent hundredths of a second.)

the basic sinus cycle is irregular, it is impossible to distinguish sinus arrest from SA block.

C. Drug-Resistant Sinus Bradyarrhythimas

When the sinus bradyarrhythmias fail to respond to atropine or isoproterenol, the presence of the SSS is almost certain (Figs. 11–1 and 11–2). The presence of the SSS is usually considered if the sinus rate is not accelerated beyond 90 beats/min by the IV injection of atropine sulfate (1 to 2 mg). For a similar reason, the SSS can be diagnosed when IV isoproterenol (1 to 2 mg/min) fails to enhance the sinus rate beyond 90 to 100 beats/min in sinus bradycardia. It should be noted that the administration of isoproterenol may provoke ventricular tachyarrhythmias.

D. Long Pause Following an Atrial Premature Contraction

In general, an atrial premature contraction (APC) is *not* followed by a full compensatory pause because the sinus node is passively activated by the ectopic atrial impulse. Thus the automaticity of the sinus node is momentarily disturbed by the ectopic atrial impulse. Occasionally, an APC is followed by a full compensatory pause when an APC occurs during late cardiac cycle so that the sinus node impulse formation is not disturbed. In such a case, the interference (collision) between the sinus impulse and the ectopic atrial impulse occurs at the SA junction, in the atria, or at the AV junction. Extremely rarely, an APC may be interpolated.

Although a postectopic pause following an APC is *not* fully compensatory, the returning cycle (the interval from the ectopic P wave to the first sinus P wave) is usually longer than the basic sinus P-P cycle because of a transient suppression of the sinus node by the ectopic atrial impulse—a physiologic phenomenon. When the returning cycle is longer than usual, however, an abnormally prolonged refractory period of the sinus node is suspected. In cases of a markedly prolonged sinus node recovery time due to the SSS, a single

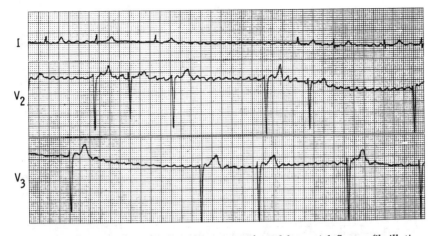

FIG. 11–6. The sick sinus syndrome is manifested by atrial flutter-fibrillation with a slow ventricular rate (15 to 30 beats/min) as a result of advanced AV block.

APC may be sufficient to produce sinus arrest, leading to absence of the sinus P waves for a long period of time. In such a case, AV junctional or ventricular escape rhythm frequently appears to activate the ventricles.

E. Prolonged Sinus Node Recovery Time Determined by Atrial Pacing

The prolonged sinus node recovery time determined by a rapid atrial pacing (120 to 150 beats/min) is a reliable indicator for the SSS. The rapid atrial pacing is particularly valuable when the ECG manifestations of the SSS are not obvious and when the clinical symptoms of the syndrome are vague. Detailed descriptions of the determination and usefulness of the sinus node recovery time are found elsewhere (see *Electrophysiologic Studies*).

F. Chronic Atrial Fibrillation or Repetitive Occurrence of Atrial Fibrillation (Less Commonly, of Atrial Flutter)

Chronic atrial fibrillation (AF) is the most common underlying rhythm in patients with far-advanced SSS, in which the sinus node is no longer capable of producing the cardiac impulse. In such a case, AF or flutter is often associated with a slow ventricular rate (30 to 50 beats/min) as a result of advanced AV block, and one or more AV junctional (less commonly, ventricular) escape beats may occur (Fig. 11–6). Until AF or flutter is well established as chronic, it is often preceded or followed by marked sinus bradycardia, sinus arrest, or SA block, with or without first-degree AV block, (a P-R interval of more than 0.28 sec; Figs. 11–3 and 11–7). In some people

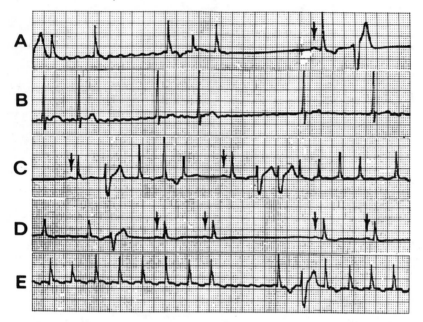

FIG. 11–7. Holter monitor ECG strips A, B, C, D, and E are *not* continuous. The arrows indicate sinus P waves. The sick sinus syndrome is manifested by sinus bradycardia and areas of atrial fibrillation, atrial flutter with a 2:1 AV response, and occasional ventricular premature contractions, as well as by aberrant ventricular conduction, producing the brady-tachyarrhythmia syndrome.

with the SSS, however, the ventricular rate is relatively fast in AF or flutter, leading to the BTS (Fig. 11–7).

G. AV Junctional Escape Rhythm (with or without Slow and Unstable Sinus Activity)

When marked sinus bradycardia becomes worse, it is often followed by sinus arrest, and AV junctional escape rhythm may become the underlying rhythm with or without unstable sinus activity (Fig. 11–8). The AV junctional escape rhythm is commonly irregular until it becomes well established as chronic. In chronic AV junctional escape rhythm, the cycle is usually regular (Fig. 11–8). In such a case, retrograde P waves may be preceded or followed by the QRS complexes (Fig. 11–8), and at times no P wave is discernible.

H. Carotid Sinus Syncope

It has been reported that the sudden development of sinus arrest by carotid sinus stimulation lasting more than 3 sec is highly suggestive of inappropriate sinus responsiveness—the SSS (Fig. 11–9). Similarly, the appearance of a long ventricular standstill in chronic AF or flutter induced by carotid sinus stimulation probably has the same clinical significance.

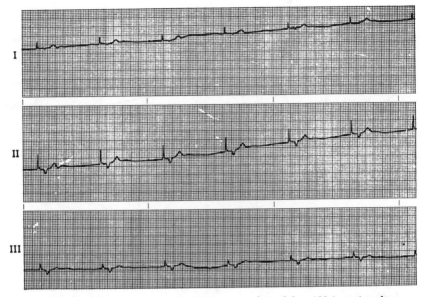

FIG. 11–8. The sick sinus syndrome is manifested by AV junctional escape rhythm (40 beats/min). Note the retrograde P waves following each QRS complex.

I. Failure to Restore Sinus Rhythm Following Cardioversion

The SSS is strongly suspected when the heart is unable to restore a stable sinus rhythm for a long period of time following the termination of any ectopic tachyarrhythmias by direct current shock (Fig. 11–10), particularly following the termination of AF or flutter. In that circumstance, the AV

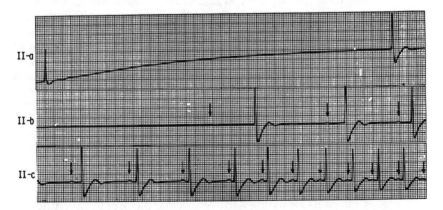

FIG. 11–9. Leads II-a, b, and c are continuous. The arrows indicate sinus P waves. A long period of sinus arrest with a long ventricular standstill (7.86 sec) is produced as a result of a hypersensitive reaction to carotid sinus stimulation (CSS).

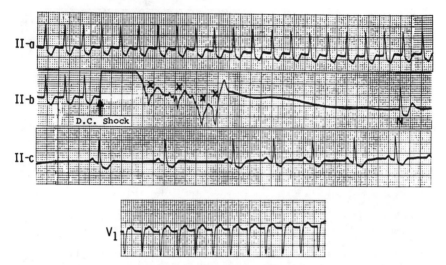

FIG. 11–10. Leads II-a, b, and c are continuous. Direct current (DC) shock was applied for supraventricular tachycardia (arrow). Note the long ventricular standstill and frequent ventricular premature contractions (marked X) with group beats and an AV junctional escape beat (marked N) until sinus rhythm is restored.

junctional escape rhythm often becomes the dominant rhythm, with or without unstable sinus P waves In far-advanced SSS, AF may persist, with unstable AV junctional or ventricular escape rhythm following the termination of ventricular tachyarrhythmias by direct current shock.

J. The Brady-Tachyarrhythmia Syndrome

Although some investigators use the terms BTS and SSS interchangeably, the conditions are by no means identical. As mentioned, the BTS is one of the common manifestations of advanced SSS. In the BTS, the bradyarrhythmia component is commonly marked sinus bradycardia (Figs. 11–1, 11–3, and 11–7) and less commonly chronic atrial fibrillation with a slow ventricular rate (Fig. 11–11). The tachyarrhythmia component in the BTS is most commonly AF or flutter-fibrillation with rapid ventricular response (Fig. 11–3) and less commonly atrial flutter with rapid (often 2:1) ventricular response (Fig. 11–7). Paroxysmal atrial tachycardia (PAT) or AV junctional tachycardia as a tachyarrhythmia component in the BTS is not too common. The incidence of ventricular tachyarrhythmia in the BTS (Figs. 11–11 and 11–12) has been reported by different authors to be 8 to 10%.

K. Common Coexisting Atrioventricular Block or Intraventricular Block

Although AV block or intraventicular block per se is *not* a part of the SSS, either condition often coexists with the SSS

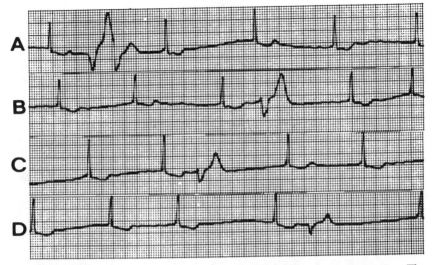

FIG. 11–11. Holter monitor ECG strips A, B, C, and D are *not* continuous. The sick sinus syndrome is manifested by atrial fibrillation with advanced AV block causing slow ventricular rate (30 to 42 beats/min) and frequent ventricular premature contractions with group beats—the brady-tachyarrhythmia syndrome.

because the same underlying disease process—degenerative-sclerotic change—may diffusely involve the entire conduction system. That is why advanced or even complete AV block often occurs in chronic AF or flutter, leading to a very slow ventricular rate in advanced SSS (Figs. 11–6, 11–7, 11–11 and 11–12). In addition, first-degree AV block (a P-R interval greater than 0.24 sec) is extremely common in the BTS (Fig. 11–3), and it is often preceded or followed by AF with a slow ventricular rate (Fig. 11–3). Furthermore, various forms of intraventricular block frequently coexist with the SSS (Fig. 11–13).

L. Any Combination of the above Electrocardiographic Manifestations

As can be expected, various ECG manifestations of the SSS itself may be present, or common ECG abnormalities (e.g., AV block, intraventricular block, and AV junctional or ventricular escape rhythm) may coexist with the SSS. For example, an ECG tracing in advanced SSS may show marked sinus bradycardia, sinus arrest, AV junctional and ventricular escape beats, paroxysmal AF, and ventricular premature contractions. Another ECG may show sinus bradycardia, intermittent SA block, marked first-degree AV block, and AV junctional escape beats. When the expected AV junctional escape beats fail to appear (e.g., marked sinus bradycardia, sinus

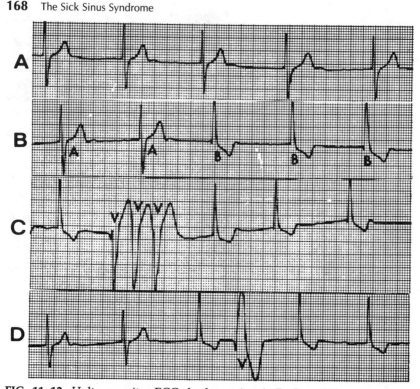

FIG. 11–12. Holter monitor ECG rhythm strips A, B, C, and D are *not* continuous. The rhythm is atrial fibrillation with escape rhythms from two foci (marked A and B) due to advanced AV block and frequent multifocal ventricular premature contractions (marked V) with ventricular group beats. Those ECG findings represent the brady-tachyarrhythmia syndrome as a manifestation of the sick sinus syndrome.

arrest, etc.) the finding often indicates the diseased AV node, which frequently coexists with dysfunctioning sinus node.

V. CLINICAL CONSIDERATIONS

Laslett made the original report on the syncopal attacks associated with bradycardia (in 1909). There has been increasing interest and awareness of the therapeutic problems regarding the SSS and the BTS among physicians since Short described the therapeutic dilemma in patients presenting with sinus bradycardia and tachyarrhythmia associated with syncope. The clinical manifestations in patients with the SSS are fundamentally due to hypoperfusion of the vital organs, particularly the brain, heart, and kidney as a result of a markedly slow ventricular rate that may or may not be associated with tachyarrhythmias.

A. Sex and Age

There is no particular sexual preponderance in the SSS, but the syndrome has been reported more frequently among eld-

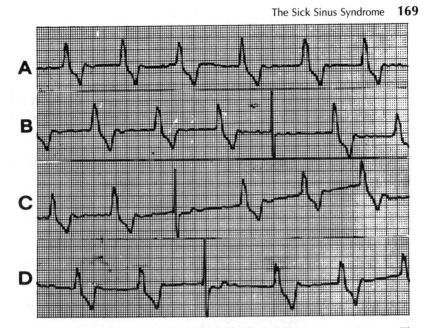

FIG. 11–13. Holter monitor ECG strips A, B, C, and D are *not* continuous. The sick sinus syndrome is manifested by atrial fibrillation with advanced AV block causing slow ventricular rate. Broad QRS complexes in the tracing probably represent coexisting left bundle branch block. Alternative diagnosis is intermittent ventricular escape rhythm.

erly women than among men. The SSS may involve any age group although it is reported to reach a peak in people in their 60s and 70s. It has been suggested that the SSS may be the cause of sudden death in some young athletes. Another report described eight Africans with the SSS; all of them were 32 years of age or younger. The life expectancy in the different parts of the world seems to greatly affect the peak incidence of the SSS.

B. Underlying Heart Diseases

As described earlier, the most common underlying heart disease in the SSS has been reported to be coronary heart disease (the incidence is about 50%). The next most common underlying disease process seems to be idiopathic, namely, sclerotic-degenerative changes in the sinus node and other conduction systems (the incidence is about 30 to 35%). Of course, many patients with the SSS may have more than one underlying cardiac disease. The less common underlying diseases of the SSS are rheumatic heart disease, congenital heart disease, hypertension, cardiomyopathy, amyloidosis, hemochromatosis, surgical injury, myocarditis, pericarditis, Friedreich's ataxia, progressive muscular dystrophy, collagen disease, and metastatic disease.

C. Clinical Manifestations

The clinical manifestations of the SSS may be multifaceted, and they may occur only intermittently. The most common manifestations of the advanced SSS are lightheadedness and near syncope or syncope. But in mild cases, the patient may be totally asymptomatic, and in the early stage, the condition may be extremely difficult to recognize or evaluate.

1. Cerebral Manifestations

In mild cases or in the early stage of the SSS, diminished cerebral arterial blood flow may be manifested by generalized fatigue, muscle ache, or slight personality changes, including irritability, intermittent memory loss, and insomnia. When the SSS progresses, the cerebral manifestations may be slurred speech, pareses, erroneous judgment, lightheadedness, and near syncope followed by syncope. Several of the cerebral manifestations, such as near syncope and syncope, are almost always due to a marked slowing of the heart rate or to cardiac arrest; the tachycardia component seldom produces significant cerebral symptoms.

Because the SSS is primarily a disease of the elderly, the various cerebral manifestations are frequently misinterpreted as cerebrovascular accidents or simply as "senility." Near syncope or syncope is reported in 40 to 70% of patients with the SSS. Dizziness was reported in 6 to 7% of patients with the SSS.

2. Cardiac Manifestations

As can be expected, the various cardiac manifestations are the second most common finding in the SSS. In the early stage of mild SSS, the cardiac manifestations may be completely absent except for a slow heart rate or a mixture of slow and rapid cardiac rhythms. The three most common cardiac manifestations in the SSS are palpitations, increased signs of congestive heart failure, and increased angina pectoris. In some instances, a sudden occurrence of acute pulmonary edema or episodic acute pulmonary edema may be the first sign of the SSS because the patient may not seek medical attention during the mild stage of the syndrome. The feeling of palpitations may be due to an extremely slow rhythm itself (e.g., sinus bradycardia or AF with advanced AV block), irregular rhythm, or a mixture of slow and rapid rhythms (the BTS). Most patients experience palpitations when the cardiac rhythm suddenly changes—from slow rhythm to rapid rhythm, or vice versa. The three most common cardiac manifestations (palpitations, increased signs of congestive heart failure, and angina pectoris) of the SSS are closely interrelated, and one symptom frequently aggravates the others. In my experience, palpitations have been the most

Table 11–2. The Sick Sinus Syndrome: Diagnostic Approach

Clinical manifestations
Routine 12-lead ECG
Ambulatory (Holter monitor) ECG
Carotid sinus stimulation and Valsalva maneuver
Cardioversion
Exercise (stress) ECG test
Drugs (e.g., atropine, isoproterenol)
Electrophysiologic studies
    Determination of sinus node recovery time by atrial pacing
    Determination of SA conduction time by atrial extrastimulus technique
    His bundle electrocardiography

common cardiac manifestation of the SSS although Moss and Davis found that increased signs of congestive heart failure were the most common cardiac manifestation (occurring in 22% of cases). Moss and Davis found also that the incidence of palpitations or an increase in angina pectoris was about equal (each symptom occurring in 15% of cases).

In far-advanced cases of the SSS, the patients may develop prolonged cardiac arrest or ventricular fibrillation leading to death.

3. Other Manifestations

Various nonspecific manifestations, such as oliguria and gastrointestinal distress, are not uncommon in the SSS, but those manifestations are usually secondary to hypoperfusion of the heart itself.

VI. DIAGNOSTIC APPROACH (See also Table 11–2)

In mild cases of the SSS, it is not always easy to make a definitive diagnosis. The physician often needs a high index of suspicion to arrive at the diagnosis during the early stage of the SSS. The presence of a marked and persistent sinus bradycardia (that is not due to drugs) should always raise the possibility of the SSS, even in totally asymptomatic young people, including athletes.

A. Clinical Manifestations

The diagnosis of the SSS cannot be made definitively on the basis of the clinical manifestations alone. The SSS, however, must be included in the differential diagnosis when the patient has a history of near syncope or syncope. Similarly, the SSS should be considered as an underlying disorder in any person with unexplainable pulmonary edema, palpitations, or angina pectoris, particularly when those manifestations (singly or together) are associated with a slow heart rate that is not due to drugs (e.g., digitalis and propranolol).

B. Routine 12-Lead ECG

The diagnosis of the advanced SSS can be confirmed by the

typical ECG findings shown on a routine 12-lead ECG or long rhythm strips (Figs. 11–2 to 11–6; 11–8).

C. Ambulatory (Holter Monitor) ECG

When the typical ECG findings of the SSS are not documented on the routine 12-lead ECG because the findings occur intermittently, the Holter monitor ECG is the best diagnostic tool (Figs. 11–1, 11–7, 11–11 to 11–13).

D. Carotid Sinus Stimulation and the Valsalva Maneuver

Sinus arrest lasting more than 3 seconds with carotid sinus stimulation strongly suggests inappropriate sinus node responsiveness—the SSS (Fig. 11–9). The response to the Valsalva maneuver may also be useful in demonstrating the sinus node dysfunction. The Valsalva maneuver produces the expected changes in the aortic pulse pressure but causes little or no change in the pulse rate. In contrast, the physiologic bradycardia of the elderly demonstrates the expected acceleration of the heart rate during the strain phase (phase 2) and the subsequent slowing of the heart rate during the blood pressure overshoot (phase 4). Carotid sinus stimulation and the Valsalva maneuver, however, do not provide direct diagnostic evidence of the sinus node disease; they give a clue to the functional status of the sinus node. Further investigation is indicated in many cases.

E. Cardioversion

Needless to say, cardioversion is *not* a diagnostic method for the SSS. Failure, however, to restore sinus rhythm following the termination of any ectopic tachyarrhythmia by cardioversion strongly suggests the SSS (Fig. 11–10).

F. The Exercise ECG Test

When the sinus rate is not increased significantly by the standard exercise ECG (e.g., the treadmill) protocol, the SSS may be suspected provided that the inappropriate sinus rate change is *not* related to a drug (e.g., propranolol). Of course, people in good physical condition (e.g., runners and other athletes) may not show a significant increase in the heart rate with the exercise ECG protocol simply because the exercise load is insufficient, not because they have a sinus node dysfunction.

G. Drugs

The SSS is often suspected when anyone, particularly an elderly person, develops marked sinus bradycardia following the administration of a small amount of digitalis or propranolol; the SSS may be "unmasked" by the drug. That finding, however, is not always reliable in the diagnosis of the SSS. Atropine has been used frequently to evaluate the response of the sinus node. Physiologic sinus bradycardia responds to the IV administration of atropine by a normal or exaggerated acceleration of the sinus rate. On the other hand, no significant increment of the sinus rate is observed in the SSS following the administration of atropine. It has been suggested that when IV atropine sulfate (1 to 2 mg) fails to increase the sinus rate beyond 90 beats/min in sinus bradycardia and when the sinus node recovery time remains prolonged by rapid (120 to 140 beats/min for 2 to 4 min) atrial pacing after atropine injection, the diagnosis of the SSS can be made. Similarly the presence of the SSS may be considered when the sinus rate does not increase beyond 90 to 100 beats/min in sinus bradycardia following the IV administration of isoproterenol (1 to 2 mg/min).

H. Electrophysiologic Studies

1. Determination of Sinus Node Recovery Time by Atrial Pacing

Of the various electrophysiologic studies, the determination of the sinus node recovery time (post-pacing pause) by rapid atrial pacing is the most reliable provocative test to uncover indirect evidence of the SSS. The determination can be made by the use of a pervenous right atrial pacing catheter and the conventional ECG recordings. The artificial pacing can be performed by placing the pacing catheter either within the coronary sinus or at the junction of the superior vena cava and right atrium, whichever location permits the most effective and consecutive atrial capture. The initial pacing rate is usually 90 beats/min, and it is progressively increased by 10 beats every 2 to 4 min, up to 150 beats/min. The pacing is terminated suddenly at the end of each period, and the post-pacing pause (the interval from the last pacing spike to the onset of the next sinus P wave) is measured. When a complete absence of sinus P wave (atrial standstill) follows the termination of pacing, the first AV junctional escape interval (the interval from the last pacing spike to the first AV junctional escape beat) is measured. To avoid syncope, however, atrial pacing must be restarted immediately when there has been complete cardiac arrest for 4 seconds.

The post-pacing pause is expected to occur in people with normal sinus nodes as well as in those with diseased sinus nodes; it is comparable to the post-tachyarrhythmia pause. The diseased sinus node, however, requires an abnormally long recovery time until its automaticity as the primary pacemaker is re-established. Thus clear distinction is documented between normal and abnormal responses.

It has been reported that the actual sinus node recovery time following the termination of atrial pacing is closely related to the resting sinus rate—the slower the resting sinus rate, the longer the maximum post-pacing pause. When the resting sinus rate is between 75 and 85 beats/min, the maximum post-pacing pause is estimated to be

115 and 128%, respectively, of the resting cycle length (the post-pacing pause is 800 to 900 msec). In sinus bradycardia (45 to 60 beats/min), the maximum post-pacing pause is expected to be much longer, and an abnormally long sinus node suppression can be easily recognized. In sinus rhythm with a rate of 60 beats/min (the cycle length is 1000 msec), a post-pacing pause showing 125% of the resting value (1250 msec) strongly suggests the SSS; and the presence of the SSS is almost certain when the post-pacing pause is longer than 1250 msec. When the resting sinus rate is 45 beats/min (the cycle length is 1420 msec), the post-pacing pause of 1700 msec or greater is diagnostic of the SSS although the percentage increase is only 120%. In severe SSS the post-pacing pause may reach 2000 to 6000 msec. Extremely prolonged sinus node recovery times (13,680 msec following atrial pacing of 120 beats/min and 19,400 msec following atrial pacing of 140 beats/min) have been demonstrated in a patient with far-advanced SSS due to cardiac amyloidosis.

Narula and co-workers proposed the concept of corrected sinus node recovery time (CSRT)—the difference between the post-pacing pause and the resting sinus P/P cycle. The normal maximum CSRT is calculated to be 525 msec or less, whereas the abnormal CSRT is calculated to be 1880 ± 1079 msec.

It should be noted that although the determination of the sinus node recovery time by atrial pacing is still the best indirect diagnostic approach for the SSS, the test may still have false negative results in some instances.

2. Determination of SA Conduction Time by the Atrial Extrastimulus Technique

In other kinds of electrophysiologic studies, the SA conduction times (SACTs) were measured indirectly by the atrial extrastimulus technique. In one study, a prolonged (more than 152 msec) calculated SACT was associated with a high incidence of sinus node or atrial disease. But in another study, the SACT in the control group was not significantly different from the SACT in the patients with the SSS.

3. His Bundle Electrocardiography

Because the SSS is often associated with various abnormalities in the impulse formation and conduction elsewhere in the heart, His bundle electrocardiographic studies can provide useful information. For example, the presence of abnormal electrophysiologic properties in the AV junction may indirectly support the diagnosis of SSS. In addition, by recognizing the coexisting conduction disturbance, a specific type of artificial pacing may be selected for a patient who has the SSS.

VII. THERAPEUTIC APPROACH
   The fact that anti-arrhythmic drug therapy alone has been unsatisfactory in the treatment of the SSS has been repeatedly emphasized. The use of a permanent artificial pacemaker is the treatment of choice for all patients with the SSS. Drug therapy alone for the SSS is unsuccessful because:
   1. The drug used to treat the tachyarrhythmia component is harmful for or aggravates the bradyarrhythmia component and vice versa.
   2. The drugs used to treat bradyarrhythmia (e.g., atropine sulfate and isoproterenol) are not effective enough.
   3. Many patients experience significant and intolerable side effects from the drugs.
   For those reasons it is generally agreed that artificial pacemaker therapy is mandatory in almost every case of advanced SSS even if the patent is asymptomatic. In fact, at present the most common indication for the artificial pacemaker is the SSS.
   A. Artificial Packmaker Therapy
   Permanent artificial pacing is indicated for all patients who have symptomatic or advanced SSS. The ideal artificial pacemaker in the treatment of SSS is programmable AV sequential (bifocal) pacing so that various pacemaker parameters can be adjusted noninvasively after pacemaker implantation according to the individual patient's need. The ordinary demand ventricular pacemaker, however, is satisfactory for many patients who have SSS (Fig. 11–14). AV sequential pacing is recommended in patients who have SSS when the atrial contribution (kick) is essential and when coexisting advanced or complete AV block is present.
   Coexisting AV conduction disturbances in the SSS can be identified readily by the His bundle ECG. When the His bundle recording is not available, the atrial pacing can provide valuable information. Thus significant AV block is reasonably excluded when the P-R interval remains less than 0.22 sec during atrial pacing (120 to 140 beats/min). But when AV block of any degree (commonly, the Wenckebach AV block) is produced by the atrial pacing, the presence of AV conduction disturbances is certain.
   When the possibility of a coexisting AV block is reasonably excluded, atrial pacing may be considered. An important advantage of the atrial pacing (80 to 120 beats/min) is that the atrial tachyarrhythmia component in the BTS can be suppressed (in up to 50% of cases) by pacing without the use of an anti-arrhythmic drug. For that purpose, coronary-sinus pacing is the preferred atrial pacemaker therapy. One of the disadvantages of coronary sinus pacing is that one cannot always be sure that the pacing may remain stable and constant.
   When the atrial kick is considered to be definitely needed

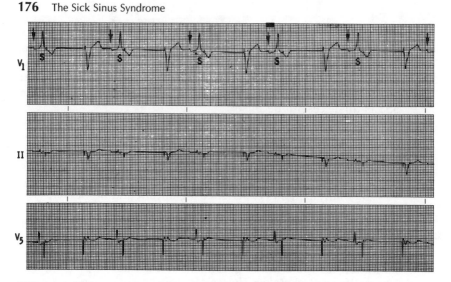

FIG. 11–14. The arrows indicate sinus P waves. The tracing shows marked sinus bradycardia (30 beats/min) with demand ventricular pacemaker rhythm. Note that the patient's sinus beats and the pacing beats alternate throughout the tracing.

in patients who have coexisting AV block, the use of a bifocal (AV sequential) demand pacemaker should be considered. The bifocal demand pacemaker, like the ventricular demand pacemaker, monitors ventricular electrical activity but it programs both atrial and ventricular stimulation. It consists of two demand pacemaker units—a conventional QRS-inhibited demand pacemaker and a QRS-inhibited atrial demand pacemaker. The pacing escape interval of the atrial pacemaker is shorter than that of the ventricular pacemaker. The difference between those two escape intervals determines the AV sequential interval—the P-R interval. The ventricular electrodes have a dual function. They sense the ventricular signal and they stimulate the ventricles as required. The atrial electrode stimulates the atria but it does not have a sensing function. Thus the signal detected by the ventricular electrode is responsible for both atrial and ventricular pacing. The bifocal demand pacemaker can stimulate both atria and ventricles in sequence, or it may stimulate the atria alone, or it may remain totally dormant. Thus the pacemaker functions automatically according to the individual patient's needs.

It should be noted that AV sequential or atrial pacing mode is useless in terms of the atrial kicking when there is chronic AF as a result of SSS. In this case, ventricular demand pacing has to be used.

A programmable pacemaker has been introduced in clinical

medicine, particularly for the treatment of the sick sinus syndrome. The programmable pacemaker is often ideal for many patients who have sick sinus syndrome, particularly the brady-tachyarrhythmia syndrome, because the ideal pacing rate can be achieved noninvasively after implantation. In many patients who have the BTS, a slightly overdriving pacing rate (80 to 100 beats/min) is required.

B. Anti-arrhythmic Drug Therapy

As mentioned previously, anti-arrhythmic drug therapy alone is unsatisfactory (and often hazardous) for the patient who has the SSS. Anti-arrhythmic drug therapy, however, can be instituted with relative safety following the implantation of a permanent pacemaker. Anti-arrhythmic drugs are often required for the SSS because the tachyarrhythmia component is usually not suppressed by the pacing alone although atrial pacing may be capable of eliminating atrial tachyarrhythmias.

The indications for specific anti-arrhythmic drugs are similar to those for various tachyarrhythmias that are not associated with the SSS (Chapter 12). Digitalis is the drug of choice for AF, flutter, or tachycardia with rapid ventricular response (Figs. 11–3 and 11–7). Digitalis and diuretics may improve myocardial function and indirectly suppress the atrial tachyarrhythmias in patients who have the SSS associated with congestive heart failure. At times, propranolol may be added when an atrial tachyarrhythmia with rapid ventricular response is not well controlled by digitalis alone. Quinidine is useful for the prevention of atrial tachyarrhythmias. When a ventricular tachyarrhythmia is not controlled by artificial pacing, various drugs, such as procainamide, quinidine, phenytoin, or propranolol may be tried either one at a time or combined (Figs. 11–11 and 11–12). Every physician should be clearly aware of the fact that no patient is immune to any drug intoxication, particularly digitalis intoxication, even after artificial pacing (Chapter 14).

VIII. PROGNOSIS

The natural course of disease of the sinus node seems to be that it is chronic, progressive, and long-standing, but it is difficult to determine the long-term prognosis. At present, the diseased sinus node cannot be cured, and in most cases only symptomatic treatment with hemodynamic improvement—artificial pacing to replace the natural pacemaker—can permit the patient with the SSS to lead a normal life. The exact length of time from the first manifestation of the SSS until death is unknown, but in most cases it seems to be from many months to 5 to 10 years. At present, it is more difficult to evaluate the natural course of the SSS because of the ready availability of artificial pacemakers to treat the SSS in the early stage. The danger of sudden death is always possible in people who have untreated SSS.

The initial stage of the SSS is marked by chronic sinus brady-cardia that is progressively followed by development of sinus arrest or SA block. Advanced SSS is manifested by chronic AF or flutter with slow ventricular rate due to advanced AV block or the BTS. Although chronic AF is considered the end stage of the SSS, it is difficult to predict when it may appear in a person with the SSS. In addition, it is also difficult to predict the life expectancy of people with the SSS who develop chronic AF. Careful clinical observations and more in-depth investigations may give more precise information about the long-term prognosis of the SSS.

In a study of 39 patients who have the SSS, after pacemaker implantation, the long-term (6 to 59-month follow-up period) prognosis was reported poor. In that study, 15 patients (42%) died during the follow-up period. Eleven of the 15 deaths (73%) were related to cardiac problems, but none were associated with either cardiac arrhythmias or pacemaker failure. Symptoms recurred or persisted after pacemaker implantation in 14 patients, and 9 of those 14 died. Twenty-two patients became asymptomatic after pacing, and 6 of those 22 died.

IX. SUMMARY

1. The SSS may be manifested by a variety of ECG abnormalities, including marked and persistent sinus bradycardia (that is not due to drugs), sinus arrest, SA block, chronic AF or flutter with slow ventricular rate, AV junctional escape rhythm with or without unstable sinus activity, a hypersensitive response to carotid sinus stimulation or the Valsalva maneuver, a failure to restore sinus rhythm following cardioversion, and the BTS.

2. Sinus bradycardia is the earliest finding in the SSS.

3. Chronic AF is considered the end stage of the SSS.

4. The BTS is one of the common manifestations of advanced SSS.

5. Direct documentation of the typical ECG manifestations of the SSS by the 12-lead ECG or the Holter monitor ECG is the best diagnostic approach.

6. Many provocative diagnostic tests are available for the diagnosis of the SSS but none of them are perfect. The determination of the sinus node recovery time by atrial pacing is the best test, but it may have a false negative result.

7. The various clinical manifestations of the SSS are due to hypoperfusion of the vital organs, particularly the brain and the heart itself.

8. The most common clinical manifestations of the SSS are cerebral symptoms, including lightheadedness, near syncope, and syncope.

9. The next most common clinical manifestations of the SSS are cardiac symptoms, including palpitations, increased

signs of congestive heart failure, and angina pectoris. Acute pulmonary edema may occur.

10. Anti-arrhythmic drug therapy alone is unsatisfactory for the SSS, and all patients who have symptomatic and/or advanced SSS should be treated with permanent artificial pacemakers.

11. The ideal artificial pacemaker in the treatment of SSS is programmable AV sequential (bifocal) pacing so that various pacemaker functions can be adjusted according to the individual patient's need. Ordinary demand ventricular pacing, however, is satisfactory for many patients who have SSS.

12. After artificial pacing, some patients require one or more anti-arrhythmic drugs (e.g., digitalis, propranolol, quinidine, procainamide) for the treatment of the tachyarrhythmia component of the BTS.

13. It is important to re-emphasize that no one is immune to any drug intoxication, particularly digitalis intoxication, even after artificial pacing.

14. The long-term prognosis in the SSS is uncertain, but it appears to take many months to 5 to 10 years after the onset of the first manifestations of the SSS to the patient's death. In one study, the long-term (6 to 59-month follow-up period) prognosis, following pacemaker implantation for 39 patients with the SSS, was poor. Nevertheless, the immediate prognosis after pacing seems favorable in many cases of SSS.

15. The incidence of the SSS is reported to reach a peak in people in their 60s and 70s, but a person of any age may have the SSS.

16. These is no sex preponderance.

17. The SSS is always a possibility in anyone, especially an elderly person who has marked and chronic sinus bradycardia (that is not due to drugs) with or without symptoms.

18. For a similar reason, the possibility of the SSS should always be considered in any person who experiences near syncope or syncope.

19. Sudden death is always a possibility in anyone who has advanced, untreated SSS.

SUGGESTED READINGS

Alboni, P., Malcarne, C., Pedroni, P., et al.: Electrophysiology of normal sinus node with and without autonomic blockage. Circulation 65:1236, 1982.

Arguss, N.S., Rosin, E.V. and Adolph R.J.: Significance of chronic sinus bradycardia in elderly people. Circulation 46:924, 1972.

Asseman, P., Berzin, B., Desry, D., et al.: Persistent sinus nodal electrograms during abnormally prolonged postpacing atrial pauses in sick sinus syndrome in humans: sinoatrial block vs overdrive suppression. Circulation 68:33, 1983.

Beder, S.D., Gillette, P.C., Garson, A., Jr., et al.: Symptomatic sick sinus syndrome in children and adolescents as the only manifestation of cardiac abnormality or associated with unoperated congenital heart disease. Am. J. Cardiol. 51:1133, 1983.

Benditt, D.G., Strauss, H.C., Scheinman, M.M., et al.: analysis of secondary pauses following termination of rapid atrial pacing in man. Circulation 54:436, 1976.

Blanc, J.J., Gestin, E., Guillerm, D., et al.: Response of normal and abnormal sinus node to right ventricular stimulation. Am. J. Cardiol. 48:429, 1981.

Bolognesi, R., Benedini, G., Affatato, A., et al.: Electrophysiological evaluation of the sinus node in patients with atrioventricular and/or intraventricular conduction defects. J. Electrocardiol. 22:297, 1989.

Breithardt, G., Seipel, L. and Loogen, F.: Sinus node recovery time and calculated sinoatrial conduction time in normal subjects and patients with sinus node dysfunction. Circulation 56:43, 1977.

Brooks, C.M. and Lu, H.H.: The Sinoatrial Pacemaker of the Heart. Springfield, IL, Charles C Thomas, 1972.

Caralis, D.G. and Varghese, P.J.: Familial sinoatrial node dysfunction. Increased vagal tone a possible aetiology. Br. Heart J. 38:951, 1976.

Chughtai, A.L., Yans, J. and Kwatra, M.: Carotid sinus syncope. Report of 2 cases. JAMA 237:2320, 1977.

Chung, E.K.: Artificial Cardiac Pacing: Practical Approach, 2nd Ed. Baltimore, Williams & Wilkins, 1984.

Chung, E.K.: Sick sinus syndrome: Current views (Part I), Mod. Conc. Cardiovas. Dis. 49:61, 1980.

Chung, E.K.: Sick sinus syndrome: Current views (Part II), Mod. Conc. Cardiovas. Dis. 49:67, 1980.

Chung, E.K.: Principles of Cardiac Arrhythmias, 4th Ed., Baltimore, Williams & Wilkins, 1989.

Clark, E.B. and Kugler, J.D.: Preoperative secundum atrial septal defect with coexisting sinus node and atrioventricular node dysfunction. Circulation 65:976, 1982.

Crook, B., Kitson, D., McComish, M. and Jewitt, D.: Indirect measurement of sinoatrial conduction time in patients with sinoatrial disease and in controls. Br. Heart J. 39:771, 1977.

DeSilva, R.A. and Shubrooks, S.J.: Mitral valve prolapse with atrioventricular and sinoatrial node abnormalities of long duration. Am. Heart J. 93:772, 1977.

Dhingra, R.C., Amat-Y-Leon, F., Wyndham, C., et al.: Clinical significance of prolonged sinoatrial conduction time. Circulation 55:8, 1977.

Dhingra, R.C., Amat-Y-Leon, F., Wyndham, C., et al.: Electrophysiologic effects of atropine on sinus node and atrium in patients with sinus nodal dysfunction. Am. J. Cardiol. 38:848, 1976.

Easley, R. and Goldstein, S.: Sino-atrial syncope. Am. J. Med. 50:166, 1971.

Ector, H. and Van Der Hauwaert, L.G.: Sick sinus syndrome in childhood. Br. Heart J. 44:684, 1980.

Evans, R. and Shaw, D.B.: Pathological studies in sinoatrial disorder (sick sinus syndrome). Br. Heart J. 39:778, 1977.

Fairfax, A.J., Lambert, C.D. and Leatham, A.: Systemic embolism in chronic sinoatrial disorder. N. Engl. J. Med. 295:190, 1976.

Ferrer, M.I.: The natural history of the sick sinus syndrome. J. Chronic Dis. 25:313, 1972.

Ferrer, M.I.: The sick sinus syndrome. Circulation 47:635, 1973.

Fowler, N.O., Fenton, J.C. and Conway, G.F.: Syncope and cerebral dysfunction caused by bradycardia without atrioventricular block. Am. Heart J. 80:303, 1970.

Gang, E.S., Reiffel, J.A., Livelli, F.D., Jr., and Bigger, J.T., Jr.: Sinus node recovery times following the spontaneous termination of supraventricular tachycardia and following atrial overdrive pacing: a comparison. Am. Heart J. *105*:210, 1983.

Gillette, P.C., Shannon, C., Garson, A., Jr., et al.: Pacemaker treatment of sick sinus syndrome in children. J. Am. Coll. Cardiol. *1*:1325, 1983.

Gomes, J.A.C., Kang, P.S. and El-Sherif, N.: The sinus node electrogram in patients with and without sick sinus syndrome: techniques and correlation between directly measured and indirectly estimated sinoatrial conduction time. Circulation *66*:864, 1982.

Gray, L.W., Duca, P. and Chung, E.K.: Sick sinus syndrome due to cardiac amyloidosis. Cardiology *63*:212, 1978.

Greenwood, R.D., Rosenthal A., Sloss, L.J., et al.: Sick sinus syndrome after surgery for congenital heart disease. Circulation *52*:208, 1975.

Guntheroth, W.G.: Sudden infant death syndrome (crib death). Am. Heart J. *93*:784, 1977.

Gupta, P.K., Lichstein, E., Chadda, K.D. and Badui, E.: Appraisal of sinus nodal recovery time in patients with sick sinus syndrome. Am. J. Cardiol. *34*:265, 1974.

Hanne-Paparo, N., Drory, Y., Schoenfeld, Y., et al.: Common ECG changes in athletes. Cardiology *61*:267, 1976.

Hatle, L., Bathen, J. and Rokseth, R.: Sinoatrial disease in acute myocardial infarction: Long-term prognosis. Br. Heart J. *38*:410, 1976.

Hattori, M., Toyama, J., Ito, A., et al.: Comparative evaluation of depressed automaticity in sick sinus syndrome by Holter monitoring and overdrive suppression test. Am. Heart J. *105*:587, 1983.

Hoffman, B.F. and Cranefield, P.F.: Electrophysiology of the Heart. New York, McGraw-Hill, 1961.

Ikeme, A.C., D'Arbela, P.G. and Somers, K.: The sick sinus syndrome in Africans. Am. Heart J. *89*:295, 1975.

James, T.N.: Anatomy of the human sinus node. Anat. Rec. *141*:109, 1961.

James, T.N.: The specialized conducting tissue of the atria. *In* L.S. Dreifus and W. Likoff (eds.): Mechanisms and Therapy of Cardiac Arrhythmias. New York, Grune & Stratton, 1966.

James, T.N.: Pericarditis and the sinus node. Arch. Intern. Med. *110*:305, 1962.

James, T.N.: Anatomy of the Coronary Arteries. New York, Hoeber, Medical Division of Harper & Row, 1961.

James, T.N.: The coronary circulation and conduction system in acute myocardial infarction. Prog. Cardiovasc. Dis. *10*:410, 1968.

Jordan, J., Yamaguchi, I. and Mandel, W.J.: Characteristics of sinoatrial conduction in patients with coronary artery disease. Circulation *55*:569, 1977.

Jordan, J.L., Yamaguchi, I., and Mandel, W.J.: The sick sinus syndrome. JAMA *237*:682, 1977.

Juillard, A., Guillerm, F., Chuong, H.V., et al.: Sinus node electrogram recording in 59 patients: comparison with simultaneous estimation of sinoatrial conduction using premature atrial stimulation. Br. Heart J. *50*:75, 1983.

Kang, P.S., Gomes, J.A.C., Kelen, G. an El-Sherif, N.: Role of autonomic regulatory mechanisms in sinoatrial conduction and sinus node automaticity in sick sinus syndrome. Circulation *64*:832, 1981.

Kaplan, B., Langendorf, R., Lev, M. and Pick, A.: Tachycardia-bradycardia syndrome (so-called "sick sinus syndrome"). Am. J. Cardiol. *31*:497, 1973.

Kay, R., Estioke, M., Wiener, I., et al.: Primary sick sinus syndrome as an indication for chronic pacemaker therapy in young adults: incidence, clinical features, and long-term evaluation. Am. Heart J. *103*:338, 1982.

Keith, A. and Flack, M.: Form and nature of muscular connection between the primary division of the vertebrate heart. J. Anat. Physiol. *41*:172, 1907.

Kerr, C.R. and Strauss, H.C.: The measurement of sinus node refractoriness in man. Circulation *68*:1231, 1983.

Kozakewich, H.P.W., McManus, B.M. and Vawter, G.F.: The sinus node in sudden infant death syndrome. Circulation 65:1242, 1982.

Kulbertus, H.E., De Leval-Rutten, F., Mary, L. and Casters, P.: Sinus node recovery time in the elderly. Br. Heart J. 37:420, 1975.

Langslet, A., and Sorlord, S.J.: Surdocardiac syndrome of Jervell and Lange-Nielsen, with prolonged QT interval present at birth, and severe anaemia and syncopal attacks in childhood. Br. Heart J. 37:830, 1975.

Leichtman, D., Nelson, R., Gobel, F.L., et al.: Bradycardia with mitral valve prolapse. A potential mechanism of sudden death. Ann. Intern. Med. 85:453, 1976.

Lown, B.: Electrical version of cardiac arrhythmias. Br. Heart J. 29:469, 1967.

Lu, H.H., Lange, G. and Brookes, C.M.: Factors controlling pacemaker action in cells of the sinoatrial node. Circ. Res. 17:460, 1965.

Macieira-Coelho, E., Silva, E., Alves, M.G. and Machado, H.B.: Postexercise electrocardiographic and clinical changes in patients with sick sinus syndrome. J. Electrocardiol. 22:139, 1989.

Mandel, W., Hayakawa, H., Danzig, R. and Marcus, H.S.: Evaluation of sino-atrial node function in man by overdrive suppression. Circulation 44:59, 1971.

Mandel, W., Hayakawa, H., Allen, H.H., et al.: Assessment of sinus node function in patients with sick sinus syndrome. Circulation 46:761, 1972.

Mazuz, M. and Friedman, H.S.: Significance of prolonged electrocardiographic pauses in sinoatrial disease: Sick sinus syndrome. Am. J. Cardiol. 52:485, 1983.

Metzger, A.L., Goldberg, A.N. and Hunter, R.L.: Sick sinus node syndrome as the presenting manifestation of reticulum cell sarcoma. Chest 60:602, 1971.

Morley, C.A., Perrins, E.J., Grant, P., et al.: Carotid sinus syncope treated by pacing: analysis of persistent symptoms and role of atrioventricular sequential pacing. Br. Heart J. 47:411, 1982.

Moss, A.J. and Davis, R.F.: Brady-tachy syndrome. Prog. Cardiovasc. Dis. 16:439, 1974.

Narula, O.S., Samet, P. and Javier, R.P.: Significance of the sinus-node recovery time. Circulation 45:140, 1972.

Nordenberg, A., Varghese, P.J. and Nugent, E.W.: Spectrum of sinus node dysfunction in two siblings. Am. Heart J. 91:507, 1976.

Parameswaran, R., Ohe, T. and Goldberg, H.: Sinus node dysfunction in acute myocardial infarction. Br. Heart J. 38:93, 1976.

Probst, P., Muhlberger, V., Lederbauer, M., et al.: Electrophysiologic findings in carotid sinus massage. PACE 6:689, 1983.

Rakovec, P., Jakopin, J., Rode, P., et al.: Clinical comparison of indirectly and directly determined sinoatrial conduction time. Am. Heart J. 102:292, 1981.

Rasmussen, K.: Chronic sino-atrial heart block. Am. Heart J. 81:38, 1971.

Reiffel, J.A., Bigger, J.T., Jr. and Giardina, E.G.V.: "Paradoxical" prolongation of sinus nodal recovery time after atropine in the sick sinus syndrome. Am. J. Cardiol. 36:98, 1975.

Reiffel, J.A., Bigger, J.T., Jr., Cramer, M. and Reid, D.S.: Ability of Holter electrocardiographic recording and atrial stimulation to detect sinus nodal dysfunction in symptomatic and asymptomatic patients with sinus bradycardia. Am. J. Cardiol. 40:189, 1977.

Reifel, J.A., Gang, E., Bigger, J.T., et al.: Sinus node recovery time related to paced cycle length in normals and patients with sinoatrial dysfunction. Am. Heart J. 104:746, 1982.

Rosen, K.M., Loeb, H.S., Sinno, M.Z., et al.: Cardiac conduction in patients with symptomatic sinus node disease. Circulation 43:836, 1971.

Rosenqvist, M.: Atrial pacing for sick sinus syndrome. Clin. Cardiol. 13:43, 1990.

Rokseth, R. and Hatle, L.: Sinus arrest in acute myocardial infarction. Br. Heart J. 33:639, 1971.

Rubinstein, J.J., Schulman, C.L. and Yurchak, P.M.: Clinical spectrum of the sick sinus syndrome. Circulation 46:5, 1972.

Scarpa, W.J.: The sick sinus syndrome. Am. Heart J. 92:648, 1976.

Schwartz, P.J., Periti, M. and Malliani, A.: The long Q-T syndrome, Am. Heart J. 89:378, 1975.

Shaw, D.B.: The etiology of sino-atrial disorder (sick sinus syndrome). Am. Heart J. 92:539, 1976.

Spellberg, R.D.: Familial sinus node disease. Chest 60:246, 1971.

Steinbeck, G. and Luderitz, B.: Comparative study of sinoatrial conduction time and sinus node recovery time. Br. Heart J. 37:956, 1975.

Strasberg, B., Sagie, A., Erdman, S., et al.: Carotid sinus hypersensitivity and the carotid sinus syndrome. Prog. Cardiovas. Dis. 31:379, 1989.

Swartz, M.H., Teichholz, L.E. and Donoso, E.: Mitral valve prolapse. A review of associated arrhythmias. Am. J. Med. 62:377, 1977.

Tabatznik, B., Mower, M.M., Somson, E.B. and Prempree, A.: Syncope in the "sluggish sinus node syndrome." Circulation 40:200, 1969.

Tan, A.T.H., Ee, B.K.H., Mah, P.K., et al.: Diffuse conduction abnormalities in an adolescent with familial sinus node disease. PACE 4:645, 1981.

Toyama, J., Ito, A, Sawada, K., et al.: Overdrive suppression in diagnosis of sick sinus syndrome. J. Electrocardiol. 8:209, 1975.

Thery, C., Gosselin, B., Lekieffre, J. and Warembourg, H.: Pathlogy of sinoatrial node. Correlations with electrocardiographic findings in 111 patients. Am. Heart J. 93:735, 1977.

Van Mechelen, R., Hagemeijer, F., De Boer, H., and Schelling, A.: Atrioventricular and ventriculoatrial conduction in patients with symptomatic sinus node dysfunction. PACE 6:13, 1983.

Vincent, G.M., Abildskov, J.A. and Burgess, M.J.: Q-T interval syndrome. Prog. Cardiovasc. Dis. 16:523, 1974.

Wohl, A.J., Laborde, J., Atkins, J.M., et al.: Prognosis of patients permanently paced for sick sinus syndrome. Arch. Intern. Med. 136:406, 1976.

Woolliscroft, J. and Tuna, N.: Permanent atrial standstill: The clinical spectrum. Am. J. Cardiol. 49:2037, 1982.

chapter

ANTIARRHYTHMIC DRUG THERAPY

Edward K. Chung

I. GENERAL CONSIDERATIONS

Since direct current (DC) cardioverters and artificial pacemakers have become readily available, the therapeutic results of the management of various arrhythmias have improved markedly in the past two decades. The best therapeutic results can be obtained when a precise diagnosis of the arrhythmia is entertained because some drugs are more effective, or almost specific, for certain arrhythmias. For instance, digitalis is usually the drug of choice for atrial fibrillation (AF) with rapid ventricular response. Conversely, digitalis is ineffective, or even contraindicated, in the treatment of ventricular tachyarrhythmias.

It is essential to eliminate the cause if it is still present. For instance, the most important and the first step in treating digitalis-induced arrhythmias is immediate discontinuation of digitalis. In addition, underlying etiological factors also significantly influence the therapeutic result. For example, ventricular tachycardia (VT) associated with acute myocardial infarction (MI) is best treated with lidocaine (Xylocaine), whereas digitalis-induced VT responds best to phenytoin (Dilantin) or potassium.

Prevention of the recurrence of tachyarrhythmias is another important aspect of management. For this reason, maintenance therapy with digitalis and many other antiarrhythmic drugs (see Table 12–1) is often necessary for long periods of time or even indefinitely. Quinidine is known to be the best agent for the pre-

Table 12–1.   Anti-tachyarrhythmic Agents, Including Dosage, Action, Indications, Adverse Effects, and Toxicity*

Dosage	Full Dosage	Maintenance Dosage	Onset of Action	Maximum Effect	Therapeutic Plasma Levels	Duration of Action	Indications	Adverse Effects and Toxicity
Digoxin (Lanoxin)	0.5–1 mg IV initially, then 0.25–0.5 mg q. 2 h as needed (total: 1–2.5 mg)	0.125–0.75 mg (average: 0.25 mg) daily (PO)	10–30 min	2–3 h	0.5–2.5 ng/ml	3–6 days	SV tachyarrhythmias (especially for AF and AFl)	Almost every known arrhythmia aggravation of CHF, anorexia, nausea, vomiting, color vision, blurring vision, headache, dizziness, confusion, allergic manifestations (urticaria, eosinophilia); idiosyncrasy, thrombocytopenia, GI hemorrhage, necrosis
Deslanoside (Cedilanid-D)	0.8–1.6 mg IV initially, then 0.4 mg q. 2 h as needed (total: 1.2–2 mg)	—	10–30 min	2–3 h	—	3–6 days		
Ouabain (G-Strophantin)	0.25–0.5 mg IV initially, then 0.1 mg q. ½ h as needed (total: 0.5–1.2 mg)	—	3–10 min	½–1 h	—	12 h–3 days		
Lidocaine (Xylocaine)	75–100 mg direct IV q. 10–20 min as needed (total: 750 mg) or 200–250 mg IM	1–5 mg/min IV infusion	At once	At once	2–5 µg/ml	Minutes	Primary: V tachyarrhythmias Secondary: SV tachyarrhythmias with anomalous conduction in WPW syndrome	Dizziness, drowsiness, confusion, muscle twitching, disorientation, euphoria, cardiac and respiratory depression, convulsion, hypotension, AV and I-V block
Procainamide (Pronestyl)	1–2 g/200 ml 5% D/W IV drip. 100 mg q. 2–4 min (1 g in ½–1 h) (total 2 g) or 1 g PO initially, then 0.5 g q. 2–3 h (total: 3.5 g)	0.25–0.5 g q. 3 h PO	At once Rapid	Minutes 1–2 h	3–10 µg/ml	6 h 6–8 h	Primary: V tachyarrhythmias Secondary: SV tachyarrhythmias including those with anomalous conduction in WPW syndrome	AV and I-V block, ventricular arrhythmias, LE, nausea, vomiting, lymphadenopathy, hypotension, convulsion, allergic manifestations (eosinophilia, urticaria), agranulocytosis

Table 12–1. Anti-tachyarrhythmic Agents, Including Dosage, Action, Indications, Adverse Effects, and Toxicity* *Continued*

Dosage	Full Dosage	Maintenance Dosage	Onset of Action	Maximum Effect	Therapeutic Plasma Levels	Duration of Action	Indications	Adverse Effects and Toxicity
Quinidine gluconate	0.8 g/200 ml 5% D/W IV drip 25 mg/min or 0.4–0.6 g IM initially then 0.4 g q. 2–4 h (total: 2.6 g)		10–15 min 10–15 mn	Not immediately 30–90 min	—	6–8 h 6–8 h	Primary: SV tachyarrhythmias including those with anomalous conduction in WPW syndrome Secondary: V tachyarrhythmias	AV and I-V block, nausea, vomiting, headache, photophobia, diplopia, headache, tinnitus, diarrhea, ventricular arrhythmias, respiratory depression, hypotension, convulsion, rashes (macular or papular), thrombocytopenic purpura, thrombocytopenia, hemolytic anemia
Quinidine sulfate	Oral route (see text)	0.3–0.4 g q. 6 h PO	—	2–3 h	2–6 mg/ml	6–8 h		
Phenytoin (Dilantin)	125–250 mg IV q. 10–20 min as needed (total: 750 mg/h)	100–200 mg q. 6 h PO	At once	Minutes		4–8 h	Primary: Digitalis-induced arrhythmias Secondary: Nondigitalis-induced V tachyarrhythmias	Cardiac depression, hypotension, AV, S-A block, sinus bradycardia, ataxia, tremor, gingival hyperplasia, allergic manifestations (urticaria, purpura, and eosinophilia)
Propranolol (Inderal)	1–3 mg IV initially, then second dose may be repeated after 2 min; additional medication should not be given less than 4 h (total: 10 mg)	10–40 mg q. 6 h PO	At once	Minutes	50–100 ng/ml	3–6 h	Various tachyarrhythmias (very effective for those in WPW syndrome and MVPS)	Marked SB, S-A, and AV block. CHF, nausea, vomiting, diarrhea, asthma, hypotension, shock, erythematous rashes, paresthesias of hands, and fever
Disopyramide (Norpace)	300 mg PO initially, followed by 100–200 mg q. 6 h	100–200 mg q. 6 h PO	1 h	2–3 h	3–8 µg/ml	6–9 h	Primary: V tachyarrhythmias Secondary: SV tachyarrhythmias including those with anomalous conduction in WPW syndrome	Dry mouth, urinary hesitancy or retention, blurred vision, constipation, precipitation of glaucoma, prolonged Q-T interval, V tachycardia or fibrillation, syncope, CHF, hypotension, AV block, I-V block, aggravation of SSS, skin rash, jaundice, psychosis, hypoglycemia, agranulocytosis

Drug	Dosage		Onset of Action		Therapeutic Serum Level	Half-Life	Indications	Side Effects/Adverse Reactions
Bretylium	5–10 mg/kg direct IV (slow) q. 15–20 min as needed (total: 30 mg/kg)	5–10 mg/kg (slow) IV or IM q. 6–8 h or IV infusion at 1–2 mg/min	5–10 min for antifibrillatory effect and 20 min–2 h for prevention of V arrhythmias	—	1.33 µg/ml	5–10 h	Life-threatening or recurrent refractory V tachycardia or fibrillation	Hypotension (especially postural), dizziness, vertigo, syncope, nausea, vomiting, parotid pain, new V arrhythmias, worsening of preexisting V arrhythmias
Verapamil	0.075–0.15 mg/kg direct IV (slow) followed by 5–10 mg IV, repeated at 30 min or IV infusion at 0.005 mg/kg/min	IV infusion at 0.005 mg/kg/min or 40–80 mg PO q. 8 h (maximum: 720 mg/day)	5 min (IV) 2 hr (PO)	2–5 h	—	3–7 h	SV tachyarrhythmias (AF, AFl, AT, AV JT) including those in WPW syndrome	Nausea, headache, dizziness, rash, flushing, urinary retention, constipation, ankle edema, hypotension. AV block, SB sinus arrest
Amiodarone	800–1600 mg/day for 1–2 weeks PO for 7–10 days 5–10 mg/kg IV, over 20–30 min, followed by IV infusion of 10–12 mg/kg/24 h for 3–5 days	200–600 mg/day	—	Days to weeks	1.0–3.5 µg/ml	20–60 days	Various supraventricular and ventricular tachyarrhythmias	Pulmonary pneumonitis and fibrosis, photodermatitis and bluish-gray skin discoloration, corneal microdeposits of brownish crystals, hypothyroidism, hyperthyroidism, GI disorders, liver function abnormalities, neuromuscular disorders, SB, aggravation of CHF, nausea, headache
Tocainide	400–800 mg t.i.d. PO	400–800 mg t.i.d. PO	—	2 h	4–12 µg/ml	12–14 h	V tachyarrhythmias	Nausea, vomiting, rash, dizziness, tremor, paresthesias, leukopenia, blurred vision, ataxia, convulsions, personality changes, inability to concentrate, insomnia, nightmares, cervical muscle spasm

Table 12–1. Anti-tachyarrhythmic Agents, Including Dosage, Action, Indications, Adverse Effects, and Toxicity* *Continued*

Dosage	Full Dosage	Maintenance Dosage	Onset of Action	Maximum Effect	Therapeutic Plasma Levels	Duration of Action	Indications	Adverse Effects and Toxicity
Mexiletine	200–400 mg t.i.d. PO	200–400 mg t.i.d. PO	—	2–4 h	0.75–2 µg/ml	8–12 h	V tachyarrhythmias	Nausea, vomiting, indigestion, hepatitis, dizziness, vertigo, tremor, confusion, dysarthria, drowsiness, paresthesia, nystagmus, diplopia, ataxia, hypotension, sinus bradycardia, worsening of arrhythmias, skin rash, thrombocytopenia, positive antinuclear factor
Flecainide	100–400 mg q. 12 h PO 1–2 mg/kg IV injection over 10 min, followed by IV infusion of 0.15–0.25 mg/kg/h	100–400 mg q. 12 h PO	—	2–4 h	0.2–1.0 µg/ml	7–22 h	Various supraventricular and ventricular tachyarrhythmias	Blurred vision, nausea, dry mouth, headache, dizziness, paresthesia, fatigue, tremor, nervousness, aggravation of ventricular arrhythmias, aggravation of CHF, AV block, worsening of SSS, interference of artificial pacing, rash, abdominal pain, diarrhea, impotence

*Abbreviations: AF = atrial fibrillation; AFl = atrial flutter; AT = atrial tachycardia; AVJT = AV junctional tachycardia; CHF = congestive heart failure; D/W = dextrose in water; GI = gastrointestinal; h = hours; IM = intramuscular injection; IV = intravenous injection; I-V = intraventricular; LE = lupus erythematosus; MVPS = mitral valve prolapse syndrome; PO = orally; q. = every; S-A = sinoatria; SB = sinus bradycardia; SSS = sick sinus syndrome; SV = supraventricular; t.i.d. = 3 times a day; V = ventricular; WPW = Wolff-Parkinson-White

Table 12–2. Antiarrhythmic Agents: Classification

Class I: Membrane-stabilizing Agents
Inhibit fast sodium channels leading to reduction in rate of depolarization phase of cardiac action potential and slow conduction.
    A. *Quinidine-like drugs:* Quinidine, procainamide, disopyramide
        Reduce rate of depolarization and conduction velocity
        Lengthen the effective refractory period
    B. *Lidocaine-like drugs:* Lidocaine, tocainide, phenytoin, mexiletine, aprindine
        Shorten action potential duration
        Increase relative refractory period
    C. *Other membrane-stabilizing agents:* Encainide, lorcainide, flecainide, cibenzoline, propafenone, indecainide

Class II: Beta-adrenergic Blocking Agents
    Propranolol and other beta-blocking agents
        Inhibit electrophysiologic action of adrenergic stimulation

Class III: Agents Which Widen Action Potential Duration by Prolongation of Repolarization
    Amiodarone, bretylium, sotalol

Class IV: Calcium-Channel Blocking Agents
    Verapamil, diltiazem and other calcium-channel blockers
        Inhibit slow inward calcium current
        Decrease rate of sinus node diastolic depolarization
        Depress conduction and increase refractoriness in AV node

vention of recurrence of atrial fibrillation (AF) or flutter, whereas procainamide (Pronestyl) is known to be the best agent for the prevention of ventricular tachyarrhythmias in long-term therapy. Propranolol (Inderal) or other beta-blocking agents are shown to be the most effective agents in the treatment of catecholamine-induced arrhythmias and arrhythmias related to Wolff-Parkinson-White (WPW) syndrome. Many new antiarrhythmic agents have been introduced in clinical medicine recently, and some of them are still under investigation. These new antiarrhythmic agents will be discussed later in this chapter. Various antiarrhythmic agents have been classified into four major categories according to their electrophysiologic properties and pharmacologic actions (see Table 12–2).

Antibradyarrhythmic agents (see Table 12–3) have recently become much less frequently used because of the ready availability of artificial pacemakers. Commonly used antibradyarrhythmic agents include atropine and isoproterenol (Isuprel), especially during acute MI.

It is not uncommon to use various antiarrhythmic drugs in conjunction with DC cardioverters and artificial pacemakers when dealing with refractory cardiac arrhythmias.

Since electrophysiologic studies (EPS) have been carried out extensively, it has been possible to use a specific antiarrhythmic agent for a specific cardiac arrhythmia (see Table 12–4). For exam-

Table 12-3. Antibradyarrhythmic Agents*

Drugs	Dosage	Onset of Action	Maximum Effect	Duration of Action	Indications	Side Effects and Toxicity
Atropine sulfate	0.3–2 mg q. 4–6 h IV as needed or the same dose may be given SC (total: 4 mg) or 0.4–0.8 mg q. 4–6 h PO for mild form	1–5 min	Few minutes–30 min	4–6 hr	Primary: Sinus bradycardia, sinus arrest, S-A block Secondary: First degree and, occasionally, second degree AV block	Dry mouth, urinary retention, exacerbation of glaucoma, hallucinations, hyperpyrexia, postural hypotension, sinus tachycardia, VPC, ventricular tachycardia
Isoproterenol (Isuprel)	0.02–0.05 mg (up to 0.1 mg) IC or IV or 0.1–0.4 mg SC or IM q. 2–6 h as needed or 1 mg/200 ml 5% D/W IV infusion, 1–4 µg/min initially and may increase to 5–10 µg/min as needed; 10–30 mg sublingually q. 1–6 h (for mild cases)	At once / Irregular	At once / Irregular	Minutes / Minutes	Ventricular standstill, severe A-S syndrome Primary: High degree or complete AV block Secondary: Sinus bradycardia, sinus arrest and S-A block	Tremor, nausea, nervousness, sweating, weakness, dizziness, headache, palpitation, VPC, ventricular tachycardia and fibrillation, hypotension
Epinephrine hydrochloride (Adrenalin)	0.3–0.6 ml of 1:1000 solution IV, IM, SC or IC or 0.5–1 mg/250 ml 5% D/W IV infusion, 1–4 µg/min initially and may increase to 4–8 µg/min as needed	At once	At once	Very short	High degree or complete AV block and ventricular standstill	Trembling, pallor, nervousness, hypertension, VPC, ventricular tachycardia and fibrillation
Ephedrine	30–60 mg PO q. 2–4 h	—	—	—	High degree or complete AV block	Urinary retention, nervousness, vertigo, insomnia, hypertension, ventricular tachyarrhythmias

*Abbreviations: A-S = Adams-Stokes; AV = atrioventricular; CHF = congestive heart failure; D/W = dextrose in water; h = hour; IC = intracardiac; IM = intramuscular, IV = intravenous; q. = every; PO = by mouth; S-A = sinoatrial; SC = subcutaneous; TB = tuberculosis; VPC = ventricular premature contraction.

Table 12–4. Effects of Cardiac Drugs on Conduction Time

Drug	A-H Interval (AV Nodal Conduction Time)	H-V Interval (His-Purkinje Conduction Time)
Digitalis	Increasing (slowing)	No change
Propranolol (Inderal)	Increasing (slowing)	No change
Quinidine	Decreasing (accelerating)	Increasing (slowing)
Procainamide (Pronestyl)	No change or increase (slowing)	Increasing (slowing)
Phenytoin (Dilantin)	Decreasing (accelerating) or no change	No change
Lidocaine (Xylocaine)	No change	No change
Disopyramide (Norpace)	No change	Increasing (slowing)
Tocainide	No change	No change
Bretylium	No change	No change
Amiodarone	Increasing (slowing)	No change or increase (slowing)
Flecainide	Increasing (slowing)	Increasing (slowing)
Mexiletine	No change or increase (slowing)	No change or increase (slowing)
Encainide	Increasing (slowing)	Increasing (slowing)
Verapamil	Increasing (slowing)	No change
Atropine	Decreasing (accelerating)	No change
Isoproterenol (Isuprel)	Decreasing (accelerating)	No change or decrease

ple, supraventricular (reciprocating) tachycardia with normal QRS complexes in WPW syndrome is best treated with either propranolol or digitalis because these drugs block the normal atrioventricular (AV) conduction. On the other hand, quinidine or a quinidine-like drug is found to be extremely effective in terminating AF with anomalous AV conduction in WPW syndrome (see Table 12–5).

Recent electrophysiologic investigative studies using extrastimulation technique have shown that the best antiarrhythmic agent for a specific tachyarrhythmia can be chosen according to its efficacy. For example, when VT under a given clinical circumstance cannot be induced by extrastimulation (arrhythmia-induction) technique following administration of a certain antiarrhythmic agent (e.g., quinidine) in an electrophysiologic laboratory, that drug will be the agent of choice for that clinical circumstance. This extrastimulation technique is very useful when dealing with refractory VT, and the technique is also extremely beneficial for a long-term prophylactic antiarrhythmic therapy.

II. GUIDE TO ANTIARRHYTHMIC THERAPY
   A. The purpose of the drug therapy for cardiac arrhythmias is the prevention of various untoward sequelae of the arrhythmias.
   B. The common untoward sequelae of arrhythmias include congestive heart failure (CHF), angina pectoris, fainting, dizziness, weakness, palpitations, skipped heart beats, convulsion, feel-

Table 12–5. Effect of Drugs on the Refractory Periods of the Normal AV and Anomalous Pathways

	Effective Refractory Period	
Drug	AV Node	Accessory Pathway
Propranolol (Inderal)	Lengthened	No change
Digitalis	Lengthened	Shortened
Lidocaine (Xylocaine)	No change	Lengthened
Quinidine	Shortened	Lengthened
Disopyramide (Norpace)	Variable	Lengthened
Procainamide (Pronestyl)	No change	Lengthened
Phenytoin (Dilantin)	Shortened	Variable
Verapamil	Lengthened	Variable
Amiodarone	Lengthened	Lengthened
Flecainide	Lengthened	Lengthened
Sotalol	Lengthened	Lengthened
Propafenone	Lengthened	Lengthened
Encainide	Lengthened	Lengthened
Aprindine	Lengthened	Lengthened
Ajmaline	Lengthened	Lengthened

ing of impending death, cerebral ischemia, and even actual death.

C. Correct diagnosis of a given arrhythmia is essential. There are three major categories:
   1. Tachyarrhythmias, including premature contractions (extrasystoles) of various origins
   2. Bradyarrhythmias
   3. Bradytachyarrhythmias

D. Careful consideration must be given to indications and contraindications for various agents from electrophysiologic approaches (see Tables 12–4 and 12–5).

E. All physicians should be familiar with the recommended dosages of various antiarrhythmic agents (see Tables 12–1 and 12–3).

F. Prevention of side-effects and toxicity of various agents is essential.

G. The direct or indirect cause of a given arrhythmia should be eliminated if possible before any antiarrhythmic agent is used.

H. When dealing with any unexplainable tachyarrhythmia, especially in young patients, common underlying problems should be considered before initiating any antiarrhythmic agent. Common underlying factors or disorders that frequently cause various cardiac arrhythmias include:
   1. Use of cocaine or similar drugs
   2. Vigorous exercise, excessive use of coffee, tea, or cola drinks, cigarette smoking, and emotional stress
   3. Hyperthyroidism (thyrotoxicosis)

4. Mitral valve prolapse syndrome
5. WPW syndrome
I. Various antiarrhythmic agents may show synergistic or antagonistic actions. For example, the serum digoxin level often rises excessively when digoxin and quinidine are administered together, so that the incidence of digoxin toxicity increases significantly. However, digitoxin and quinidine do not seem to show any synergistic action.
J. Prevention of recurrent cardiac arrhythmia is another important aspect of antiarrhythmic therapy.
K. Refractory arrhythmias often require a combination of 2 or more antiarrhythmic agents.
L. Not uncommonly, patients require DC shocks and artificial pacemakers in addition to the antiarrhythmic agents.
III. MANAGEMENT OF PREMATURE CONTRACTIONS (EXTRA-SYSTOLES)
A. The first management step is to remove any possible cause for the development of premature contractions regardless of the origin of the ectopic impulses. For example, digitalis-induced premature contractions, particularly those of ventricular origin, are treated best by discontinuation of digitalis.
B. Sedation is another important method of eliminating premature beats, especially when dealing with high strung or nervous patients.
C. Premature contractions are often eliminated by stopping heavy smoking or excessive ingestion of coffee.
D. If the premature contractions are frequent (30 beats or more per hour) particularly in a diseased heart, such as in acute MI, various antiarrhythmic agents may be required.
E. Supraventricular (atrial or AV junctional) premature contractions are best treated with quinidine, if symptomatic (e.g., palpitations). Propranolol is almost equally effective in this situation. By and large, supraventricular premature beats are self-limited, and no active treatment is necessary as long as the arrhythmia does not cause any symptoms.
F. Digitalis is particularly effective when premature contractions are associated with CHF.
G. Lidocaine is the drug of choice for the treatment of ventricular premature contractions (VPCs) associated with acute MI, or during catheterization and cardiac surgery.
H. In the following situations, treatment of VPCs is indicated
1. Frequent VPCs (30 or more beats per hour)
2. R-on-T phenomenon (a VPC superimposed on top of the T-wave of preceding beat) in some cases
3. Multifocal VPCs
4. Grouped or paired VPCs
5. VPCs after the termination of VT or ventricular fibrillation (VF)

6. VPCs associated with any active or acute cardiac disease (e.g., acute MI).
I. For long-term therapy of the VPCs, procainamide or quinidine is the drug of choice. Alternatively, tocainide, amiodarone, mexiletine, disopyramide (Norpace), or phenytoin may be used.
J. Phenytoin is probably the best agent for the treatment of digitalis-induced premature beats.
K. Calcium antagonists (e.g., verapamil or nifedipine) are the agents of choice for the treatment of VPCs associated with coronary artery spasm.
IV. MANAGEMENT OF SUPRAVENTRICULAR TACHYARRHYTH-MIAS

The first step of management is elimination of the cause if present. For instance, AF associated with thyrotoxicosis cannot be treated satisfactorily unless thyroid function returns to euthyroid level. Carotid sinus stimulation is often effective in terminating paroxysmal atrial or AV junctional tachycardia.

Digitalis is usually the drug of choice in the treatment of AF with rapid ventricular response. In digitalis-induced supraventricular tachyarrhythmias, digitalis must be discontinued immediately. In addition, phenytoin or potassium is found to be effective in terminating digitalis-induced supraventricular tachyarrhythmias. Quinidine is the best agent to prevent the recurrence of atrial fibrillation or flutter. Propranolol has been shown to be the most effective agent in the treatment of arrhythmias precipitated by exercise, emotional distress, excessive sympathetic stimulation, and supraventricular tachyarrhythmias related to WPW syndrome or mitral valve prolapse syndrome. Procainamide is less commonly used for the treatment of supraventricular tachyarrhythmias, and lidocaine is rarely used in this situation except in WPW syndrome. Verapamil is found to be useful for the treatment of various supraventricular tachyarrhythmias.

DC shock is often effective in terminating various acute supraventricular tachyarrhythmias. In addition, elective cardioversion is another important therapy of terminating chronic AF or flutter. Artificial pacemakers (overdriving rate) are occasionally needed in the suppression of various supraventricular tachyarrhythmias that are refractory to various antiarrhythmic agents and/or DC shock. Sedation is often beneficial for the treatment of supraventricular tachyarrhythmias in conjunction with other therapeutic measures.
V. MANAGEMENT OF VENTRICULAR TACHYARRHYTHMIAS

It is essential to eliminate any possible cause of ventricular tachyarrhythmias if present. Digitalis should be stopped immediately when ventricular tachyarrhythmias are due to digitalis toxicity. DC shock is the most effective way of terminating ventricular tachycardia, flutter, and fibrillation. Defibrillation should be carried out immediately in addition to all necessary cardiopulmonary resuscitation (CPR). However, DC shock should be avoided as much as possible if VT is induced by digitalis. The reason for this is that DC shock often produces new cardiac arrhythmias, particular VF, in this situation.

Lidocaine is the drug of choice for the treatment of VT associated with acute MI, or during anesthesia and cardiac catheterization. Procainamide and quinidine are the next most commonly used drugs in this situation. Bretylium (a new antiarrhythmic agent) has been found to be an effective drug for refractory ventricular tachyarrhythmias. Amiodarone is becoming a popular drug in the treatment of refractory ventricular tachyarrhythmias. Disopyramide or propranolol is less commonly used for the treatment of ventricular tachyarrhythmias. Phenytoin is the best drug for the treatment of digitalis-induced VT. Ventricular tachyarrhythmias associated with coronary artery spasm are best treated with calcium antagonists (e.g., nifedipine).

When ventricular tachyarrhythmias are refractory to antiarrhythmic agents and/or DC shock, the use of an artificial pacemaker (over-driving pacing rate: 100 to 120 bpm) is often a life-saving measure. For recurrent and drug-resistant ventricular tachyarrhythmias, implantation of an automatic mini defibrillator should be strongly considered.

VI. MANAGEMENT OF SINUS BRADYCARDIA, SINUS ARREST, AND SINOATRIAL BLOCK

Therapeutic approaches vary markedly depending upon the fundamental mechanism responsible for the production of bradyarrhythmias, the ventricular rate, and the degree and underlying cause of symptoms.

Sinus bradycardia of mild degree (rate: 50 to 59 bpm) is not uncommon in healthy persons especially in young athletes and elderly persons. Marked sinus bradycardia with a rate below 40 bpm may produce some hemodynamic alterations, especially when it is associated with acute MI. The most common causes of sinus bradycardia include the therapeutic or toxic effects of various drugs including digitalis, propranolol, reserpine, guanethidine, and methyldopa (Aldomet), as well as acute diaphragmatic MI. Drug-induced sinus bradycardia, sinus arrest, or sinoatrial (SA) block is best treated by stopping the particular drug. Active treatment is indicated when marked sinus bradycardia persists and becomes symptomatic and especially when it is associated with acute MI. The treatment of choice in this case is atropine, and the next commonly used agent is isoproterenol.

Essentially the same therapeutic approach may be used in the treatment of symptomatic sinus arrest or SA block. In drug-resistant sinus bradycardia, sinus arrest, or SA block, a temporary or even a permanent artificial pacemaker is the treatment of choice. When dealing with persisting and drug resistant sinus bradyarrhythmias, the underlying disorder is commonly sick sinus syndrome (SSS). For symptomatic or advanced SSS, permanent artificial pacemaker implantation is the treatment of choice.

VII. MANAGEMENT OF ATRIOVENTRICULAR BLOCK

AV block per se does not require treatment. Therapeutic indication for AV block depends primarily on the degree, site, etiology, ventricular rate, and the presence or lack of symptoms.

First-degree AV block usually requires no particular treatment except that the direct cause, such as digitalis intoxication, should be eliminated. It has been reported that atropine is effective in abolishing digitalis-induced first and second-degree AV block. Isoproterenol may be effective in this circumstance, but often produces untoward reactions, such as increasing ventricular irritability.

Wenckebach (Mobitz type I) AV block usually does *not* require active treatment unless significant symptoms are produced. Wenckebach AV block usually represents AV nodal block.

On the other hand, Mobitz type II AV block requires an artificial pacemaker because this disorder is considered to be a precursor of complete bilateral bundle branch block (BBBB). Mobitz type II AV block represents infranodal block.

In complete AV block, the therapeutic approach depends upon the ventricular rate, the exact site of the block, and the degree of symptoms. Active treatment is usually *not* indicated when the ventricular rate is relatively rapid (40 to 60 bpm) in AV junctional escape rhythm, as in acute diaphragmatic MI, unless it is symptomatic. On the other hand, a permanent artificial pacemaker is indicated when the ventricular rate is slow (less than 40 bpm) in ventricular escape (idioventricular) rhythm due to complete AV block, as seen in acute anterior MI or in elderly patients with degenerative changes in the conduction system.

Complete AV block in acute diaphragmatic MI represents AV nodal block, whereas complete AV block in acute anterior MI usually represents infranodal block—complete trifascicular block.

In general, AV nodal block is relatively benign and self-limited. Thus active treatment is not indicated under this circumstance. On the other hand, infranodal block is usually irreversible and permanent pacemaker implantation is necessary in most cases.

Bilateral bundle branch block (bifascicular and trifascicular block) of varying degrees often requires a permanent artificial pacemaker especially when symptomatic.

In urgent situations before the insertion of an artificial pacemaker, various agents such as isoproterenol or epinephrine (Adrenalin) may be tried.

VIII. ANTITACHYARRHYTHMIC AGENTS

As emphasized previously, the best therapeutic results can be obtained when a precise diagnosis of the arrhythmia is entertained, because some drugs are more effective and almost specific for certain arrhythmias. In addition, indications of various antitachyarrhythmic agents (see Table 12–1) vary markedly depending upon the underlying cause for the tachycardia. Most commonly used antitachyarrhythmic agents include cardiac glycosides, quinidine, lidocaine, procainamide, phenytoin, and propranolol. New antitachyarrhythmic agents include bretylium, disopyramide, verapamil, amiodarone aprindine, tocainide, encainide, flecainide, ethmozine, acecainide mexiletine, metoprolol, sotalol, pirmenol, cibenzoline lorcainide, propafenone, and acebutolol. Some of these agents are still under investigation and they are not available for routine clinical use.

A. QUINIDINE

Quinidine has been probably the most valuable antiarrhythmic agent available for more than 50 years. Quinidine has 2 major effects—direct and indirect. The direct effect of the drug is on the cell membrane, whereas the indirect effect is anticholinergic. As a result of the net clinical effect of combined anticholinergic and direct actions, a marked prolongation of the refractory period in the atria and a lesser prolongation of the ventricles are produced. In addition, a shortening of the refractory period in the AV junction is induced by quinidine. The sinus rate tends to be slowed by the direct effect of quinidine, but the indirect (vagolytic) effect tends to reverse this. As a result, the sinus rate may not be altered significantly by quinidine, or it may be accelerated. It should be emphasized that the serum digoxin level rises significantly when digoxin and quinidine are given together so that digoxin toxicity may easily be produced.

1. Indications
   a) Quinidine has been an indispensable drug primarily to convert atrial fibrillation or flutter to sinus rhythm. Before DC cardioverters were available, large amounts of quinidine sulfate had to be used to restore sinus rhythm, but it is no longer necessary to do so except when a DC cardioverter is not available.
   b) At present, the role of quinidine is primarily to prevent the recurrence of atrial fibrillation (AF) or flutter following a restoration of sinus rhythm by either digitalization or DC shock.
   c) Quinidine is also useful in the treatment of various acute supraventricular, as well as ventricular, tachyarrhythmias. With respect to acute tachyarrhythmias, quinidine is found to be more effective for the treatment of supraventricular than ventricular ones.
   d) Quinidine is also useful for the suppression of premature beats of various origin, including VPCs.
   e) Quinidine is effective in the treatment of supraventricular tachyarrhythmias with anomalous conduction in WPW syndrome.

2. Full Dosage
   a) For the treatment of acute tachyarrhythmias, quinidine gluconate 0.8 g diluted in 200 ml of 5% dextrose in water may be given intravenously at a rate of about 25 mg per

minute under continuous electrocardiographic monitoring.

b) Intramuscular administration of quinidine gluconate may be carried out by giving 0.4 to 0.6 g initially, followed by 0.4 g every 2 to 4 hours as needed. Total intramuscular dosage should not exceed 2 to 2.4 g.

3. Maintenance Dosage

   The usual maintenance dosage of quinidine sulfate for the prevention of recurrence of various arrhythmias is 0.3 to 0.4 g every 6 hours.

4. Side Effects and Toxicity

   a) Side effects or mild toxic manifestations include nausea, vomiting, diarrhea, tinnitus, slight impairment of hearing and vision, and slight widening of the QRS complex or Q-T interval.

   b) When quinidine toxicity is advanced, the above manifestations become more severe. Thus, the patient may develop blurring vision, disturbed color perception, photophobia, diplopia, abdominal pain, headache, confusion, and ventricular tachyarrhythmias.

   c) When the patient has an unusual sensitivity or idiosyncracy to quinidine, respiratory depression, hypotension, convulsion, urticaria, macular or papular rashes, fever, thrombocytopenia, hemolytic anemia, and even sudden death may occur.

   d) The most serious side effect and toxicity of quinidine is the production of multiformed and irregular VT, which is usually initiated by VPCs with the R-on-T phenomenon as a result of a markedly prolonged Q-T interval with a broad T wave induced by quinidine. This multiformed VT has been termed torsade de pointes (Figure 12–1). This serious arrhythmia often transforms into VF leading to death.

   e) It has been shown that so-called quinidine syncope or sudden death from quinidine is attributed to VF as a result of R-on-T phenomenon initiated by multiformed VT.

B. LIDOCAINE

The discovery of antiarrhythmic properties of lidocaine is probably the most important addition to the therapeutic approach to cardiac arrhythmias. Lidocaine has a structure similar to quinidine or procainamide, but its electrophysiologic properties are quite different. Because lidocaine has little effect on the atria, it is of little use in the treatment of atrial tachyarrhythmias except for those associated with WPW syndrome. Lidocaine depresses diastolic depolarization and automaticity in the ventricles. Lidocaine, in standard doses, has no effect on conduction velocity and generally shortens both the action potential and the refractory period. Approximately 90% of an

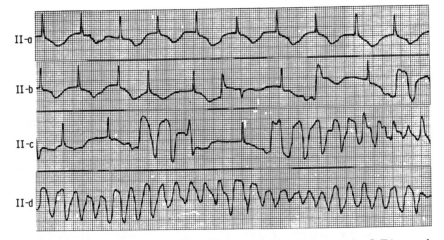

FIG. 12–1. Torsade de pointes induced by quinidine. Note that the Q-T interval is extremely prolonged as a result of a broad T wave. Leads II-a, b, c and d are continuous.

administered dose of the drug is metabolized in the liver, and the remaining 10% is excreted unchanged by the kidneys. The action of lidocaine is more transient than that of procainamide, and the former penetrates the cardiac tissues more rapidly than the latter.

1. Indications
    a) Lidocaine has been widely used, primarily for the treatment of ventricular tachyarrhythmias and VPCs associated with acute MI and cardiac surgery or cardiac catheterization.
    b) In the past decade, lidocaine has gradually replaced procainamide because the former is more effective and seldom produces hypotension when given properly.
2. Administration
    a) For the initiation of therapy, direct injection of 75 to 100 mg of lidocaine (1 to 1.5 mg/kg) is given slowly and the dose may be repeated 5 minutes later.
    b) In general, total doses should not exceed 750 mg, and it is advisable that no more than 300 mg be administered during a 1 hour period.
    c) When intravenous injection is not immediately feasible, 200 to 300 mg of lidocaine may be given intramuscularly into the deltoid muscle. An additional intramuscular injection may be given 60 to 90 minutes later as needed.
    d) It is recommended that lidocaine be administered under continuous electrocardiographic monitoring.
    e) Following the termination of ventricular tachyarrhythmia, continuous intravenous infusion with a rate of 1 to

5 mg per minute is needed for 24 to 72 hours, in most cases, to prevent recurrence of the arrhythmia.

f) When ventricular tachyarrhythmias do not recur, lidocaine may be replaced gradually with oral procainamide or quinidine (or a similar antiarrhythmic agent).

3. Side Effects and Toxicity

a) Toxicity is relatively uncommon.

b) It may produce dizziness, drowsiness, confusion, muscle twitching, disorientation, euphoria, cardiac and respiratory depression, convulsion, and hypotension.

c) Caution should be employed in the repeated use of lidocaine in patients with severe liver or renal disease because accumulation may led to toxicity.

C. PROPRANOLOL

Propranolol is a beta-adrenergic receptor-blocking agent that has been widely used for management of various tachyarrhythmias, including those induced by digitalis and those resistant to digitalis. Antiarrhythmic actions of propranolol are produced by two effects: 1) inhibition of adrenergic stimulation of the heart, and 2) direct action on the electrophysiologic properties of cardiac tissue. The inhibition of adrenergic stimulation of the heart is needed for the treatment of catecholamine-induced arrhythmias. Direct membrane action on the electrophysiologic property is essential in the treatment of digitalis-induced arrhythmias. Thus, the overall effects of propranolol usually result in reduction of automaticity, including reduction of sinus rate, and prolongation of atrial and AV conduction time.

Other beta-blocking agents may be used in place of propranolol.

1. Indications

a) Tachyarrhythmias associated with WPW syndrome: Propranolol is considered to be the drug of choice in the treatment of regular supraventricular (reciprocating) tachycardia with normal QRS complexes.

b) Catecholamine-induced tachyarrhythmias: Propranolol is effective in the treatment of tachyarrhythmias (of any origin) precipitated by physical exercise, emotional distress, or any other excessive sympathetic stimulation.

c) Arrhythmias associated with mitral valve prolapse syndrome (Barlow's syndrome).

d) Digitalis-induced tachyarrhythmias: Propranolol is used when potassium or phenytoin is found to be ineffective or contraindicated.

e) Atrial fibrillation or flutter: Propranolol is useful to reduce the ventricular rate in atrial fibrillation or flutter when the rapid ventricular response is difficult to control by digitalis.

f) Miscellaneous indications: Propranolol is found to be effective in terminating some cases of multifocal atrial tachycardia (MAT). Propranolol is also useful when the arrhythmias are associated with idiopathic hypertrophic subaortic stenosis (IHSS), angina pectoris, or anesthesia.

2. Contraindications

   a) Bradyarrhythmias

   Marked sinus bradycardia, sinus arrest, SA block, second or third-degree AV block, bradytachyarrhythmia syndrome (BTS)

   b) CHF

   c) Hypotension, cardiogenic shock

   d) Bronchial asthma, bronchitis, and other chronic lung diseases

   e) History of hypersensitive reaction to beta-blockers

3. Administration and Dosage

   a) Intravenous injection: Propranolol should be administered slowly under the ECG monitoring. The usual dosage is 1 to 2 mg; the second dose can be repeated 5 to 10 minutes later. Total dosage should not exceed 10 mg.

   b) Oral administration when the clinical situation is not urgent. Propranolol may be given orally in doses ranging between 10 and 40 mg, 3 to 4 times daily. Up to 240 mg 4 times daily have been tried by some investigators. The same dosage is recommended for long-term use or for prophylactic purposes.

4. Side Effects or Toxicity

   Various side effects or toxicity of propranolol can be divided into three major categories: cardiovascular manifestation, respiratory manifestations, and miscellaneous manifestations.

   a) Cardiovascular Manifestations

   (1) Marked slowing of the heart rate. This may include sinus bradycardia, sinus arrest, SA block, AV junctional escape rhythm, ventricular escape rhythm, and ventricular standstill. Note that atropine should be used to counteract propranolol action.

   (2) Development or worsening of CHF. Proper digitalization and diuretic therapy are essential.

   (3) Development of hypotension. Isoproterenol should be used.

   (4) Development of acute MI. This has been reported upon sudden discontinuation of propranolol. Thus, gradual reduction of dosage is preferable whenever feasible.

   (5) Difficulty of cardiac resuscitation. When the patient on propranolol therapy develops cardiac arrest, especially during cardiac surgery, it is often difficult to resuscitate him. Thus, it is recommended that pro-

pranolol be discontinued for 24 to 48 hours before cardiac surgery, if possible.

b) Respiratory Manifestations

Asthmatic attacks have been reported in susceptible persons, particularly in patients with history of asthma or bronchitis. The reason is that propranolol increases airway resistance.

c) Miscellaneous Manifestations

(1) Hypoglycemia has been reported in patients under insulin therapy or recovering from anesthesia, and in infants and children during periods of restricted food intake.

(2) Neurologic manifestations: These may include light-headedness, fatigue, lethargy, hallucination, mental depression, insomnia, and peripheral neuropathy.

(3) Nonspecific or allergic manifestations include nausea, vomiting, diarrhea, constipation, fever, erythematous rashes, thrombocytopenia, granulocytosis, and alopecia.

D. PROCAINAMIDE

Procainamide had been the traditional drug of choice in the treatment of VT until lidocaine was proven in the past decade to be safer and more effective. Large amounts of procainamide were often used in the treatment of VT, especially until DC cardioverters became readily available.

Procainamide has electrophysiologic effects very similar to quinidine. Procainamide slows electrical conduction, increases the refractory period, and depresses diastolic depolarization and automaticity. It has an indirect vagolytic action, and AV conduction may be facilitated when low doses are used. However, the direct effect of procainamide is depression of AV conduction with higher doses. Therapeutic levels are easily achieved by oral administration since this drug is almost completely absorbed from the gastrointestinal tract. Procainamide should be administered with caution to patients with significant renal disease because it is excreted primarily by the kidneys in unchanged form.

1. Indications

a) Although procainamide has electrophysiologic actions very similar to those of quinidine, the former drug has been used primarily in the treatment of ventricular tachyarrhythmias.

b) At present, the primary indication for procainamide is to prevent the recurrence of ventricular tachyarrhythmias following their termination by DC shock and/or intravenous lidocaine.

c) Procainamide is also effective for the treatment of supraventricular tachyarrhythmias, although it is not the primary drug of choice. Procainamide has been used in place of quinidine when the patient is unable to take the latter drug.

    d) At present, large doses of parenteral procainamide are used only when a DC cardioverter is not available and lidocaine is found to be ineffective.

    e) Procainamide is effective for suppression of ventricular premature beats.

2. Full Dosage

    a) Intravenous Administration:

When intravenous procainamide has to be used, 1 to 2 g of the drug diluted in 200 ml of 5% dextrose in water are administered by continuous intravenous drip at a rate of 100 mg every 2 to 4 minutes under continuous ECG monitor. A total intravenous dose should not exceed 2 g.

    b) Oral Administration:

When the clinical situation is not urgent, procainamide may be given orally. Initially, 1 g of procainamide may be given by mouth and followed by 0.5 g every 2 to 3 hours as needed. A total oral dose should not exceed 3.5 g.

3. Maintenance Dose

The usual maintenance dose of procainamide is 0.25 to 0.5 g every 3 hours by mouth. Some investigators have tried up to 1000 mg 4 times daily.

4. Side Effects and Toxicity

    a) Side effects and toxic manifestations of procainamide include nausea, vomiting, fever, leukopenia, lymphadenopathy, a lupus erythematosus-like syndrome, convulsion, AV block, intraventricular block of varying degrees, ventricular tachyarrhythmias, and hypotension.

    b) In some patients who are sensitive to procainamide, allergic manifestations such as eosinophilia, urticaria, and agranulocytosis may be observed.

    c) The major disadvantage of procainamide is that it has to be given every 3 hours (by mouth) in order to maintain the therapeutic blood level. However, a long-acting procainamide is available in the market at the present time.

    d) Torsade de pointes is occasionally produced by procainamide.

E. PHENYTOIN

The discovery of the antiarrhythmic properties of phenytoin is another important addition to the management of various cardiac arrhythmias, particularly those induced by digitalis. Phenytoin has a structure similar to that of barbiturates, but its electrophysiologic properties are quite different from other antiarrhythmic agents. Conduction velocity in the atria is accelerated by phenytoin, resulting from a faster depolarization of the atria, although the sinus rate is usually uninfluenced by this drug. Although phenytoin may not influence AV conduction, it may accelerate it. It does not alter intraventricular conduction significantly. One of the most important actions of phenytoin is to counteract the depressant effect of the AV conduction induced by digitalis or procainamide. In addition, it depresses diastolic depolarization and automaticity, and shortens the duration of the action potential and the effective refractory period.

1. Indications

 a) Phenytoin is considered to be the drug of choice in the treatment of various tachyarrhythmias induced by digitalis. This is especially true in the management of digitalis-induced VT.

 b) As a secondary indication, it is also useful in place of procainamide or lidocaine when these drugs are found to be ineffective.

2. Full Dosage

 a) Intravenous Administration

 The initial dose of phenytoin is between 125 and 250 mg intravenously for 1 to 3 minutes under ECG monitoring. Most patients respond within 3 seconds to 5 minutes. The same dose may be repeated every 10 to 20 minutes as needed, but a total dose should not exceed 750 mg per hour. Continuous intravenous drip of phenytoin is not practical because the drug easily precipitates with various commonly-used intravenous solutions.

 b) Oral Administration

 When the situation is not urgent, 200 mg of phenytoin may be given orally as an initial dose, followed by 100 mg every 4 to 6 hours as needed.

3. Maintenance Dosage

 Following the termination of the tachyarrhythmias, a maintenance dose of phenytoin 100 mg 3 to 4 times daily is often needed for varying periods depending upon the clinical situation. Oral phenytoin is often useful in place of procainamide or quinidine for a long-term therapy.

4. Side Effects and Toxicity

 Side effects and toxic manifestations of phenytoin include respiratory and cardiac depression, skin reactions such as urticaria and purpura, eosinophilia, drowsiness, ataxia, tremor, depression, nervousness, arthralgia, gingival hyperplasia, hypotension, and AV block of varying degree. Fortunately these manifestations are rare.

F. DISOPYRAMIDE

Disopyramide is an antiarrhythmic oral agent similar to quinidine. Disopyramide is a local anesthetic that possesses a direct electrophysiologic effect on the heart similar to that of quinidine and procainamide. It also possesses intense anticholinergic effects that may alter some of the drug's direct electrophysiologic properties.

It is important to remember that among all antiarrhythmic

drugs, disopyramide is considered one of the most potent negative inotropic agents available in the market. Thus it should not be administered in the presence of CHF or cardiogenic shock.

Approximately 85 to 90% of orally administered disopyramide is absorbed from the gastrointestinal tract, and peak plasma levels are reached within 2 to 3 hours. Renal excretion is the primary route of elimination, and about 50% of the drug is excreted unchanged in the urine. This is the reason why special caution must be taken in the presence of renal impairment when using disopyramide; a smaller dosage than usual is recommended in this circumstance.

In the normal heart, disopyramide has little or no effect on sinus node recovery time, or on the sinus rate. In SSS, however, the abnormally prolonged sinus node recovery time is often further prolonged by disopyramide. Likewise, it can further prolong the H-V interval when there is preexisting conduction disturbance, although it has little or no effect on the P-R, QRS, Q-T, A-H, or H-V intervals in normal hearts. The effective refractory period of the anomalous pathway in WPW syndrome is prolonged by disopyramide, but the drug possesses varible effects on the effective refractory period of the AV node. It usually prolongs the effective refractory period of the atria.

It is interesting to note that disopyramide does not seem to affect the serum digoxin level although the drug is very similar to quinidine in many other respects.

1. Indications
   a) Indications are essentially the same as those of quinidine and procainamide.
   b) Primary indications are for the prevention and treatment of ventricular tachyarrhythmias (e.g., frequent VPCs).
   c) Secondary indications include the prevention of various supraventricular tachyarrhythmias, such as AF or flutter.
   d) Disopyramide may be used in the prevention and treatment of various tachyarrhythmias with anomalous AV conduction in WPW syndrome because the drug prolongs the effective refractory period of the accessory pathway.
   e) The capability of disopyramide to reduce the slope of phase-4 depolarization is important in the treatment of cardiac arrhythmias by means of enhanced automaticity.
2. Contraindications
   a) CHF
   b) Cardiogenic shock
   c) SSS
   d) Renal insufficiency
   e) Hypersensitivity to disopyramide

3. Administration and Dosage
   a) The usual recommended loading dosage (by mouth) is 300 mg.
   b) The usual maintenance dosage is 100 to 200 mg every 6 hours following the loading dosage.
   c) In some reports, 400 mg every 6 hours have been administered with varying degrees of success.
   d) The therapeutic plasma levels of disopyramide are 3 to 8 μg/ml, and the maximum effect is reached within 2 to 3 hours after oral administration.
4. Side Effects and Toxicity
   a) Cardiovascular effects:
      (1) Disopyramide may cause multiformed ventricular tachycardia (torsade de pointes) initiated by VPCs with the R-on-T phenomenon as a result of prolonged Q-T interval, and it may lead to VF, syncope, and sudden death.
      (2) Negative inotropic effect may cause heart failure, aggravate pre-existing CHF, and/or cardiogenic shock.
      (3) Sinus node recovery time is further prolonged by disopyramide in SSS.
      (4) The H-V interval is further prolonged when there is pre-existing conduction abnormality, so that various intraventricular blocks may occur.
      (5) The drug may cause AV block of varying degrees.
   b) Anticholinergic effects:
      (1) Dry mouth, nausea or vomiting
      (2) Urinary hesitancy or retention
      (3) Blurred vision and precipitation of glaucoma
      (4) Constipation
   c) Other effects:
      Skin rash, jaundice, psychosis, hypoglycemia, and agranulocytosis have been reported in medical literature.
G. BRETYLIUM
   Bretylium tosylate (Bretylol) has been approved recently only for parenteral use for the treatment of life-threatening, drug-resistant, and/or DC shock-resistant VT and fibrillation in the United States. The oral form of bretylium is still under investigation primarily because it is poorly and erratically absorbed from the gastrointestinal tract.
   The onset of antiarrhythmic effect occurs within a few minutes to 10 minutes following intravenous injection, and 20 minutes following intramuscular injection. The primary route of elimination of bretylium is the kidneys and about 80 to 90% is excreted unchanged in the urine. Thus, the dosage should be reduced in patients with renal insufficiency.
   The electrophysiologic effects of bretylium on the heart result directly from direct membrane effects on the myocardium and indirectly from the sympathetic innervation of the heart. The

direct membrane effects on cardiac tissue prolong the action potential duration and effective refractory period of the Purkinje fibers and ventricular myocardium.

Bretylium possesses dual adrenergic effects. Its initial sympathomimetic effect is to release norepinephrine from adrenergic nerve endings. During this early stage, a new ventricular arrhythmia may be provoked or the preexisting ventricular arrhythmia may be aggravated by bretylium, leading to more serious clinical outcome—undesirable effects. When the transient sympathomimetic effect subsides, bretylium inhibits the release of norepinephrine from adrenergic nerve endings. These antiadrenergic effects of the drug are the important antiarrhythmic properties.

1. Indications
    a) Bretylium is used primarily for life-threatening VT or fibrillation when these arrhythmias are refractory to more commonly used drugs such as lidocaine or procainamide and DC shock.
    b) Bretylium may be capable of terminating VF (chemical defibrillation).
    c) DC shock is often effective in terminating VF following administration of bretylium even when the initial DC shock was ineffective.
    d) Bretylium may be effective to prevent VF by raising the ventricular fibrillatory threshold.
2. Administration and Dosage
    a) Bretylium is given either by intravenous injection, intravenous infusion, or intramuscular injection.
    b) Oral use is not approved for clinical use.
    c) The initial dose of intravenous injection is 5 to 10 mg/kg (i.e., 350 to 500 mg), slowly over 10 to 20 minutes.
    d) When VF or life-threatening VT continues or recurs, the same dosage may be repeated and DC shock may be repeated every 15 minutes until the total dose of 30 mg/kg is reached.
    e) For maintenance dose, 5 to 10 mg/kg may be given slowly by intravenous injection every 6 to 8 hours or, alternatively, the drug can be given by continuous intravenous infusion at 1 to 2 mg/minute.
    f) When use of the intravenous route is not immediately feasible, bretylium may be given intramuscularly, 5 to 10 mg/kg every 6 to 8 hours.
    g) The onset of the antifibrillatory effect occurs within a few minutes to 10 minutes following intravenous injection, and the therapeutic plasma levels are found to be 1.33 μg/ml.
3. Side Effects and Toxicity
    a) Hypotension, particularly postural hypotension, is a serious side-effect.

  b) Vertigo, dizziness, and syncope may occur.
  c) During acute therapy, nausea and vomiting are common.
  d) During long-term therapy, severe parotid pain may be observed.
  e) The most undesirable effect of bretylium is its transient sympathomimetic effect soon after administration. During this stage, bretylium may provoke a new ventricular arrhythmia or aggravate the preexisting ventricular arrhythmia.

H. VERAPAMIL

Verapamil is a papaverine derivative with unique electro-pharmacologic properties. Initially, verapamil was introduced during the 1960s as an antianginal agent, but the drug is now considered to be one of the most important antiarrhythmic agents in the treatment of various supraventricular tachyarrhythmias.

Verapamil is a calcium blocking agent; it blocks the influx of calcium and possibly sodium ions through the slow channels of cardiac tissue. Verapamil slows the sinus rate, and prolongs A-H interval and the functional, as well as effective, refractory periods of the AV node. The H-V interval and the QRS duration are not altered by the drug.

Orally administered verapamil is almost completely (90% to 100%) absorbed from the gastrointestinal tract, but bioavailability is not more than 10 to 20% as a result of extensive first-pass metabolism through the liver. Thus, the hepatic metabolism is the major route of elimination and only 7% of the drug is excreted in the urine unchanged. Oral doses of verapamil are about 8 to 10 times larger than intravenous doses because of the first-pass hepatic effect. By and large, orally administered verapamil is not as effective as intravenous verapamil either in terminating a variety of supraventricular tachyarrhythmias or in reducing the ventricular rate in AF or flutter.

1. Indications
   a) For termination of various supraventricular tachyarrhythmias, particularly those generated by re-entry mechanism.
   b) Conversion of AF or flutter to sinus rhythm by verapamil has been reported, but the primary role of the drug is to reduce the ventricular rate in these atrial arrhythmias.
   c) Verapamil is found to be *not* effective for ventricular arrhythmias.
2. Contraindications
   a) Advanced or complete AV block.
   b) Tachyarrhythmias with anomalous conduction in WPW syndrome.
   c) SSS and brady-tachyarrhythmia.
3. Administration and Dosage
   a) Recommended dosage for intravenous injection is 0.075

to 0.15 mg/kg (5 to 10 mg bolus) slowly over 1 to 3 minutes followed by intravenous infusion of 0.005 mg/kg per minute or 5 to 10 mg over 1 to 3 minutes, repeated at 30 minutes.

b) For children, the same dosage regimen (0.075 to 0.15 mg/kg) has been recommended.

c) For oral administration, the usual recommended dosage is 40 to 120 mg every 6 to 8 hours, and the maximum doses should be not more than 480 mg/day.

4. Side Effects and Toxicity
   a) Verapamil may cause hypotension, AV block of varying degrees, marked sinus bradycardia, and sinus arrest.
   b) SSS and pre-existing AV block are often worsened by verapamil.
   c) It is extremely important to remember that the ventricular rate may be enhanced by verapamil when the drug is given in the treatment of various tachyarrhythmias with anomalous conduction in WPW syndrome. The reason for this is that the conduction via an accessory pathway is enhanced by verapamil. Under this circumstance, ventricular fibrillation or even sudden death may occur.
   d) The noncardiac adverse effects of verapamil may include nausea, headache, constipation, dizziness, rash, flushing, urinary retention, and ankle edema.

I. AMIODARONE

Amiodarone, an iodinated benzofuran derivative, is a class III antiarrhythmic agent (see Table 12–2) found to be effective in the prevention and treatment of a variety of supraventricular, as well as ventricular, tachyarrhythmias, including those associated with WPW syndrome. Amiodarone was initially introduced in 1967 as a vasodilating drug to treat angina pectoris, but was later found to possess potent antiarrhythmic properties.

Amiodarone hydrochloride is available for clinical use in both oral and intravenous forms, and recently the drug has been approved by the FDA in the United States. When amiodarone is given by mouth, it is absorbed slowly with a bioavailability of approximately 35% (range from 22 to 46%). The drug is 95% protein-bound and has a large volume of distribution (about 5000 liters). The main locations of deposition include liver, fat, lungs, myocardium, kidneys, thyroid, and skeletal muscles in descending order. Amiodarone is a lipid-soluble agent, and it has a high affinity for adipose tissue. A large loading dose is necessary because of large volume of distribution. Since amiodarone has a long terminal elimination half-life (mean 24.8 ± 11.7 days), the duration of antiarrhythmic effects as well as adverse effects is long, even when the drug is discontinued.

For the same reason, it takes days to weeks to achieve the full antiarrhythmic effect of amiodarone. There is a linear relationship between the dose and the plasma concentration of the drug during chronic oral administration. The therapeutic plasma concentration of amiodarone ranges from 0.75 to 3.5 μg/ml, but it should be maintained below 2.5 μg/ml in order to minimize or avoid side effects.

In isolated tissue preparations, amiodarone significantly prolongs the action potential duration and increases the refractory period of the atria, ventricles, and Purkinje fibers. The drug possesses little effect on the maximum rate of depolarization (Phase 0) and resting membrane potential. Clinical electrophysiologic studies have demonstrated that amiodarone causes slowing of sinus node automaticity, slowing of the AV nodal conduction time, and the lengthening of the refractory periods in the atria and the ventricles. The H-V interval may increase slightly or may not be changed by the drug. In addition, the refractory period of the antegrade conduction of the accessory pathway in WPW syndrome is usually increased by amiodarone.

1. Indications
    a) Amiodarone is effective in the prevention and treatment of various supraventricular as well as ventricular tachyarrhythmias.
    b) The drug has been shown to be effective in suppressing VPCs and nonsustained ventricular tachycardia (VT) even when the arrhythmias are refractory to other conventional antiarrhythmic drugs.
    c) The drug is shown to be effective in the prevention of recurrent AF or flutter and supraventricular tachycardia with or without anomalous AV conduction.
    d) Induction of VT by programmed electrical stimulation following 2 to 4 weeks of amiodarone therapy does not necessarily preclude a favorable long-term therapeutic result. When VT cannot be induced after amiodarone therapy, the clinical arrhythmia will definitely remain suppressed.
    e) Amiodarone is highly recommended for almost all types of tachyarrhythmias which have not responded to other conventional antiarrhythmic agents.
2. Administration and Dosage
    a) The most common oral dosages range from 800 to 1600 mg/day (in a single or divided dose) for 1 to 2 weeks, followed by a maintenance dose of 200 to 600 mg/day.
    b) Amiodarone may be given intravenously with oral administration concomitantly when more rapid control of serious ventricular tachyarrhythmia is desired.
    c) The usual intravenous dosage of amiodarone is 5 to 10 mg/kg over 20 to 30 minutes, followed by a continuous infusion of 10 to 12 mg/kg per 24 hours for 3 to 5 days.
    d) The rapid intravenous infusion may be repeated within 30 minutes.

e) Amiodarone should be diluted with dextrose in water and *not* in saline solution because the drug often precipitates in saline solution.

f) The usual maintenance oral dose is 200 to 600 mg per day.

3. Side Effects and Toxicity

a) The most common side effects include photodermatitis, bluish-gray skin discoloration, hypothyroidism and hyperthyroidism, pulmonary pneumonitis and fibrosis, corneal micro-deposits of brownish crystals, asymptomatic liver function abnormalities, gastrointestinal disorders, neuromuscular disorders, and marked sinus bradycardia.

b) Pulmonary toxicity, abnormal liver functions, neurological and ocular problems seem to be dose-related adverse effects.

c) When the plasma level exceeds 2.5 μg/ml, the risk of developing various side effects is much greater.

d) Pulmonary toxicity is one of the most serious side effects and may lead to death in some cases.

e) Serial chest x-ray films should be obtained during long-term amiodarone therapy, especially in patients with the pre-existing pulmonary interstitial abnormalities.

f) If pulmonary toxicity is suspected, tests for diffusion capacity, and possibly bronchoscopy with bronchial lavage for cytologic examination may be valuable in the diagnosis.

g) Corticosteroids are often beneficial in patients with respiratory failure due to amiodarone toxicity; it may be life saving in some cases.

h) Worsening of the pre-existing ventricular arrhythmias has been reported, and torsade de pointes may be induced by amiodarone. Amiodarone should be given with caution when the drug is administered concomitantly with quinidine or quinidine-like drugs because of a danger of provoking torsade de pointes.

i) The plasma concentrations of quinidine and procainamide are often raised by concomitant administration of amiodarone. Amiodarone is known to interact with other drugs including digoxin, phenytoin, warfarin, and, possibly, propafenone and mexiletine.

j) When beta-blockers or calcium channel-blockers are administered together with amiodarone, AV block, marked sinus bradycardia, and significant hypotension may be produced. In some cases, temporary artificial pacing may be required.

k) From these observations, the dosage of these drugs should be reduced considerably (one-third to one-half), and the plasma concentrations of these agents should be

closely monitored during concomitant amiodarone therapy.
J. TOCAINIDE

Tocainide, an analog of lidocaine, has recently been approved by the FDA in the United States in the treatment of ventricular arrhythmias. The antiarrhythmic effects of tocainide were demonstrated in man for the first time in 1976.

The bioavailability of the drug is essentially complete, and its peak plasma levels are observed within 2 hours following oral administration. Approximately 50% of tocainide is bound to plasma protein at the therapeutic concentrations.

Tocainide is primarily excreted by the kidneys, and 40% of an orally-given dose is recovered unchanged in the urine within 48 hours. The drug has no active metabolites, and the elimination half-life ranges from 12 to 14 hours. Since the kidneys are the primary route of excretion, the dosage should be reduced in elderly individuals and in patients with renal failure.

Tocainide is classified as a type I-B antiarrhythmic agent. Its electrophysiologic properties are very similar to those of lidocaine. The drug depresses membrane responsiveness and shortens the effective refractory period and action potential duration. The effects on the AV conduction time, P-R interval, QRS interval, or Q-T interval are insignificant.

1. Indications
    a) Tocainide is found to be effective in the treatment of various ventricular tachyarrhythmias including VPCs and VT even when other conventional antiarrhythmic drugs have been unsuccessful.
    b) The success rates of tocainide in the treatment of various ventricular arrhythmias have been reported to be 46 to 95%.
    c) The lack of a response to lidocaine predicts failure of the efficacy of tocainide, but a response to lidocaine correlates less with the efficacy of tocainide.
    d) Podrid and Lown reported that 87% of patients who failed to respond to lidocaine also failed to respond to tocainide. On the other hand, only 63% of patient who responded to lidocaine also responded to tocainide.
    e) In general, the efficacy of tocainide for suppression of VPCs is favorable, but the drug is less effective than quinidine or procainamide in the prevention of recurrent VT or VF.
2. Administration and Dosage
    a) The recommended oral doses of tocainide are 400 to 800 mg 3 times daily. The maximum dose is often necessary for the treatment of malignant ventricular arrhythmias.
    b) The drug may be given only twice daily when the total doses are relatively small amounts.

c) The therapeutic plasma concentrations range from 4 to 12 μg/ml.

d) The maintenance doses range from 400 to 800 mg 3 times daily.

3. Side Effects and Toxicity

   a) The side effects are gastrointestinal (e.g., nausea, vomiting) or neurological, and discontinuation of the drug may be necessary in about 11%.

   b) The neurological side effects may include dizziness, tremor, ataxia, convulsions, blurred vision, personality changes, insomnia, nightmares, parasthesias, inability to concentrate, and cervical muscle spasm. These side effects of tocainide are dose related in many cases.

   c) Many patients develop a skin rash, but this problem is not serious.

K. MEXILETINE

Mexiletine, a class I-B antiarrhythmic agent, is structurally and pharmacologically similar to lidocaine, and is recently approved by the FDA to treat ventricular arrhythmias. Mexiletine is effective in suppressing VPCs in patients with acute MI and chronic coronary artery disease (CAD). However, the drug is less effective in the treatment of refractory sustained VT or VF. Mexiletine is a local anesthetic and an anticonvulsant; its antiarrhythmic action was first observed in 1972.

Mexiletine is well absorbed, with a bioavailability of 80 to 90% in healthy people. The peak plasma levels are observed within 2 to 4 hours, and 70% is protein bound. The drug is mostly metabolized in the liver, and less than 10% is excreted unchanged in the urine. The elimination half-life of the drug is 8 to 12 hours in healthy individuals, and is significantly delayed in patients with acute MI, heptic disease, or renal failure.

Mexiletine possesses electrophysiologic properties similar to those of lidocaine. The drug has little effect on sinus node function in healthy people, so that the sinus rate, sinus node recovery time, sinoatrial conduction time, or atrial refractory period are *not* significantly altered by intravenous injection of mexiletine. However, marked sinus bradycardia and prolonged sinus node recovery time have been reported in patients with sick sinus syndrome. The effective refractory period of the atria as well as ventricles is not altered by mexiletine. When there is any pre-existing intraventricular conduction disturbance, however, mexiletine often causes lengthening of the H-V interval and refractory period of His-Purkinje system. The P-R interval, QRS interval or Q-T interval are *not* significantly altered by intravenous or oral administration of mexiletine.

1. Indications:

   a) Mexiletine is found to be effective to suppress VPCs associated with various clinical circumstances including acute

MI, chronic CAD, cardiac surgery, and digitalis intoxication.
   b) The drug is effective in some cases even when VPCs are refractory to lidocaine, procainamide, or beta-blockers.
   c) However, mexiletine is effective only in a minority of patients with chronic sustained VT or VF.
2. Administration and Dosage
   a) The usual recommended oral doses range from 200 to 400 mg 3 times daily (10 to 15 mg/kg/day).
   b) The therapeutic plasma concentrations are 0.75 to 2.0 μg/ml.
   c) The maintenance oral doses are 200 to 400 mg 3 times daily.
3. Side Effects and Toxicity
   a) The most common side effects of mexiletine are neurological and gastrointestinal disorders.
   b) Gastrointestinal side effects include nausea, vomiting, and indigestion.
   c) Neurological side effects are drowsiness, dizziness, vertigo, confusion, tremor, paresthesia, diplopia, and nystagmus.
   d) Cardiac side effects may include marked sinus bradycardia, worsening of the pre-existing ventricular arrhythmias, and hypotension.
   e) Other less common adverse effects are skin rash, thrombocytopenia, hepatitis and positive anti-nuclear factor.
   f) Side effects are mostly dose-related, and toxic effects are observed when the plasma concentrations are above 1.5–3.0 μg/ml in the majority of cases.
   g) Mexiletine should be given with caution to patients with SSS, intraventricular conduction disturbances and renal or hepatic disorders.
L. FLECAINIDE

Flecainide, a fluorinated benzamide derivative, was recently approved by the FDA in the United States in the treatment of supraventricular as well as ventricular tachyarrhythmias. The drug has been used primarily in the management of ventricular arrhythmias by mouth. Flecainide is a class I-C antiarrhythmic agent that was synthesized in 1972, and its antiarrhythmic effect in animals was first reported in 1975.

Flecainide is a potent local anesthetic, and is well absorbed on oral administration. Approximately, 50% of a dose is metabolized in the liver, 30% is excreted unchanged in the urine, and only 5% excreted in the feces. The bioavailability of flecainide is as high as 95%, and the peak plasma levels are achieved within 2 to 4 hours following a single oral dose. The plasma half-life varies from 7 to 22 hours (mean 13 hours) in man after a single intravenous or oral dose, and even longer (mean 16 hours) after repeated doses in healthy people, in elderly individuals, and in patients with renal or cardiac disease. The therapeutic plasma levels range from 0.2 to 1.0 μg/ml.

The sinus rate, sinoatrial conduction time, and sinus node recovery time are *not* significantly altered by flecainide. However, this drug often causes a significant increase in corrected sinus node recovery time in patients with SSS. The drug produces a significant lengthening of the P-A interval, A-H interval, H-V interval, and the QRS interval: the Q-T interval is not altered by this drug. Likewise, effective refractory periods of the atria, AV node, and ventricles are *not* altered by flecainide. In patients with WPW syndrome, the drug causes lengthening of both antegrade and retrograde refractory periods of the accessory pathway, and this effect is more pronounced in the retrograde conduction.

1. Indications
   a) Flecainide is effective in the treatment of various supraventricular as well as ventricular tachyarrhythmias including those associated with WPW syndrome.
   b) The drug is more frequently used for ventricular arrhythmias, and is effective to suppress VPCs in 80 to 100% of cases according to different reports.
   c) In a multicenter double-blind trial, the efficacy of oral flecainide was compared with oral quinidine in 280 cases with chronic VPCs. At least 80% suppression of VPCs was observed in 85% of the flecainide-treated group as compared with only 57% suppression among the quinidine-treated group.
   d) In this study, 68% of the flecainide-treated group had complete suppression of ventricular group beats (couplets) and VT as compared with only 33% suppression among the quinidine-treated group.
   e) Flecainide may also prevent induction of sustained or nonsustained VT by programmed ventricular stimulations even when those arrhythmias are refractory to other conventional antiarrhythmic agents (60% success rate in some studies).
   f) Flecainide is also effective for prevention of recurrent VT or VF in some cases.

2. Administration and Dosage
   a) The usual recommended oral dosages are 100 to 400 mg every 12 hours; twice-daily oral doses seem to be most ideal.
   b) In patients with poor left ventricular function, low dosage regimen (100 mg every 12 hours) should be the initial treatment, and the dosage may be increased at 4-day intervals to a maximum of 200 mg every 12 hours as needed. The plasma levels should be monitored closely.
   c) For intravenous injection, 1 to 2 mg/kg are administered over 10 minutes, followed by an infusion of 0.15 to 0.25

mg/kg/hour. Lower doses are recommended for patients with left ventricular dysfunction or with renal failure. Flecainide has a negative inotropic action when the drug is administered intravenously.

    d) The maintenance oral doses of flecainide are 100-400 mg every 12 hours.

3. Side Effects and Toxicity

    a) In a multicenter trial with oral flecainide, about 60% of the patients developed at least one side effect: the drug had to be discontinued in 13% because of various side effects.

    b) The most common side effects are related to central nervous system disorders including nausea, headache, fatigue, nervousness, dizziness, blurred vision, paresthesia, and tremor.

    c) Cardiac side effects include aggravation of ventricular arrhythmias, CHF, and SSS. Flecainide may produce AV block and may interfere with the function of artificial cardiac pacing by increasing pacing thresholds.

    d) Less common side effects are skin rash, abdominal pain, diarrhea, and impotence.

M. SOTALOL

Sotalol, a class III antiarrhythmic drug, is a noncardioselective beta-adrenergic blocking agent, and is still under investigation. Initially sotalol was tried in the treatment of supraventricular, as well as ventricular arrhythmias, but recently the drug has been used to suppress VPCs.

Sotalol is absorbed rapidly and completely, and the peak plasma level is reached within 2 to 3 hours. Approximately 75% is excreted in the urine, and the remaining fraction is eliminated in bile. The serum half-life is 14 to 20 hours during chronic oral administration. When the drug is given intravenously, the serum half-life is 6 to 8 hours after a single dose. The therapeutic plasma concentrations range from 1.0 to 3.0 μg/ml.

Sotalol increases the action potential duration as a result of prolongation of repolarization. The drug increases the effective refractory periods in the AV node, atria, ventricles, and accessory pathways. The Q-T interval is often prolonged significantly by sotalol.

1. Indications

    a) Sotalol is primarily used to suppress VPCs, although the drug had been tried initially in the treatment of various supraventricular and ventricular tachyarrhythmias.

    b) In some studies, sotalol was effective to suppress or reduce VPCs in patients with CAD in 88.5% using 320 mg per day by mouth.

    c) Some reports indicate that sotalol may also be useful in the treatment of recurrent sustained VT or VF. In one study dealing with 18 patients assessed by programmed electrical stimulation, intravenous sotalol (1.5 mg/kg) was effective in preventing induction of sustained VT in 12 patients (67%).

2. Administration and Dosage

   a) The therapeutic plasma concentrations of sotalol range from 1 to 3 μg/ml.

   b) The recommended maintenance oral dosage is 80 to 240 mg every 12 hours.

   c) Intravenously, sotalol 1.5 mg/kg has been administered for the treatment of sustained VT or VF.

3. Side Effects and Toxicity

   a) Major side effects include hypotension and prolonged Q-T interval, that may lead to torsade de pointes.

   b) The drug may cause gastrointestinal or neurological side effects which are commonly observed with class I antiarrhythmic agents.

   c) Marked sinus bradycardia may be observed, especially in patients with SSS.

   d) AV block may easily be produced when there is any pre-existing AV conduction disturbance.

   e) CHF may be aggravated by intravenous injection or during a few days of oral administration.

   f) Sotalol should be used with extreme caution when the drug is administered concomitantly with other drugs which cause prolonged Q-T interval.

N. ETHMOZINE

Ethmozine (Moricizine), a phenothiazine derivative, was synthesized in the Soviet Union in 1964 as an antiarrhythmic agent in the treatment of supraventricular as well as ventricular tachyarrhythmias. Ethmozine is still an investigational drug in the USA. This drug is well absorbed and extensively metabolized. Less than 1% of the compound is found in feces and urine. The peak plasma concentration is reached within 1 to 1½ hours after oral administration, and the elimination half-life is about 2 to 5 hours following a single oral dose. When dealing with patients with advanced cardiac disease or renal failure, the elimination half-life is significantly prolonged.

Intravenous injection of ethmozine produces significant prolongation of P-A interval, A-H interval, and P-R interval, but sinus rate, Q-T interval, or H-V interval are *not* altered significantly. Likewise, the effective refractory periods in the AV node, atria and ventricles are *not* significantly changed. On the other hand, the drug may produce significant increase in the refractory periods of the antegrade as well as retrograde conduction of the accessory pathways.

1. Indications

   a) Ethmozine is shown to be effective in the treatment of supraventricular as well as ventricular tachyarrhythmias.

   b) The drug is fairly effective in the suppression of VPCs,

but less effective in preventing inducible sustained VT or VF.

c) Further investigations will be necessary in order to determine the efficacy of ethmozine in the prevention and treatment of recurrent VT or VF.

2. Administration and Dosage

a) The therapeutic plasma concentrations of ethmozine range from 0.5 to 0.9 μg/ml.

b) The usual recommended oral doses are 10 to 15 mg/kg/24 hours in divided doses every 8 hours.

c) Although the precise therapeutic dosage schedule has *not* been fully established, intravenous injection of ethmozine in doses of 1 to 3 mg/kg was reported to produce the onset of therapeutic effect within 5 minutes.

3. Side Effects and Toxicity

a) Major side effects are gastrointestinal and neurological disorders.

b) Gastrointestinal side effects are nausea, vomiting, diarrhea and indigestion.

c) Neurological side effects include dizziness, vertigo, fatigue, confusion, nervousness, euphoria, and perioral numbness.

d) Other side effects may include headache, insomnia, blurred vision, and dry mouth.

e) Hypotension and aggravation of ventricular arrhythmias may be produced.

O. PROPAFENONE

Propafenone hydrochloride *cannot* be classified according to conventional classification criteria. The drug was synthesized in 1970 and has been used extensively in Germany since then. Propafenone was found to be effective in the treatment of ventricular as well as supraventricular tachyarrhythmias, including those associated with WPW syndrome. The drug was just recently approved by the FDA.

Propafenone is rapidly and almost completely absorbed after oral administration. The biovailability of this agent is approximately 50%, and the peak blood levels are observed within 2 hours. The elimination half-life is about 3 to 6 hours, but an antiarrhythmic effect may last up to 10 hours following a single dose. Propafenone is rapidly metabolized in the liver, and only 1% is excreted unchanged in the urine. The therapeutic plasma concentrations are reported to be 0.2 to 3.0 μg/ml. The drug possesses local anesthetic action, weak beta-adrenergic blocking, and calcium channel-blocking actions. This agent may cause a negative inotropic effect with higher plasma concentrations.

Propafenone has a potent membrane-stabilizing activity, but does not have a significant effect on the action potential duration or duration of repolarization. Significant lengthening of

A-H interval, H-V interval, and refractory periods of the atria as well as the ventricles is observed after intravenous injection of propafenone (2 mg/kg) followed by intravenous infusion (2 mg/min), but sinus node recovery time or sinoatrial conduction time was not altered. Oral administration of the drug produced similar electrophysiologic effects. In patients with WPW syndrome, the effective refractory periods of antegrade as well as retrograde accessory pathways are significantly prolonged by propafenone. The P-R interval and the QRS interval are prolonged by the drug, but the Q-T interval is unchanged.

1. Indications
    a) Propafenone is shown to be effective in the treatment of supraventricular as well as ventricular tachyarrhythmias.
    b) The drug is useful in the prevention and treatment of various tachyarrhythmias associated with WPW syndrome.
    c) Propafenone is reported to be effective to suppress VPCs in 80 to 85%.
    d) When this drug is administered with quinidine or procainamide together, VPCs may easily be suppressed at reduced doses of all drugs, so that side effects may be prevented.
    e) The efficacy of propafenone for sustained VT or VF is much less favorable (53% success rate in some series).
    f) In the electrophysiologic studies, various investigators reported that this drug failed to prevent the induction of VT in most patients during the initial treatment periods, as assessed by programmed electrical stimulation technique. However, the induction of VT under this circumstance does not necessarily preclude the efficacy of propafenone in the clinical settings. Propafenone often causes significant reduction of the heart rate, even though VT may persist.
2. Administration and Dosage
    a) Intravenous loading dose is 2 mg/kg followed by an infusion of 2 mg/min.
    b) The therapeutic plasma concentrations are 0.2 to 3.0 μg/ml.
    c) The recommended oral dose is 150 to 300 mg every 8 hours.
3. Side Effects and Toxicity
    a) The incidence of side effects is generally low, and the drug is well tolerated by most patients.
    b) The most common side effects are gastrointestinal disorders including nausea, vomiting, and alteration in taste or smell.
    c) Cardiac side effects are uncommon, but may include AV block, sinus arrest, intraventricular conduction disturbances, aggravation of ventricular arrhythmias, and wors-

ening of CHF in patients with pre-existing left ventricular dysfunction.

d) This drug may also cause dry mouth, headache, fatigue, dizziness and blurred vision in some cases.

P. OTHER NEW ANTIARRHYTHMIC AGENTS
1. Aprindine
   a) Aprindine, which was originally developed in Belgium, has been relatively popular in many European countries in the treatment and prevention of various supraventricular as well as ventricular tachyarrhythmias. The drug is available for oral as well as parenteral use.
   b) The initial enthusiasm regarding its clinical use has been tempered by an extremely narrow toxic-therapeutic ratio with serious adverse effects such as agranulocytosis, which may be fatal unless detected early. The drug has been under clinical investigation in the United States.
   c) Aprindine has a potent local anesthetic effect and has a terminal amine structure similar to lidocaine. By and large, the electrophysiologic properties of aprindine are similar to those of quinidine and procainamide.
   d) The effect of aprindine on the sinus rate is variable, but it slows the conduction diffusely at almost all levels in the heart. Specifically, it prolongs the A-H, P-R, QRS, and H-V intervals. The effective refractory period of the atria, AV node, and His-Purkinje system is prolonged by aprindine.
   e) Aprindine has been widely used in Europe in the prevention and treatment of various tachyarrhythmias associated with WPW syndrome because it slows the conduction in the anomalous pathway. Aprindine has been found to be especially useful in the treatment of various arrhythmias associated with mitral valve prolapse syndrome.
   f) Aprindine is easily absorbed from the gastrointestinal tract, and about 65% of the drug and its metabolites are excreted in the urine.
   g) The onset of action following intravenous injection and oral administration occurs after 5 to 10 minutes and 2 hours, respectively. The maximum antiarrhythmic effect following oral administration is usually observed within several days because the half-life is long (20 to 30 hours).
   h) The recommended intravenous dose is 200 mg at a rate of 2 mg/min, followed by 100 mg over 30 minutes, and then 100 mg over 6 hours. The oral loading dose is 200 to 300 mg, and is followed by 100 to 150 mg daily in 2 to 3 doses. The therapeutic plasma levels of aprindine are reported to be 1 to 2 μg/ml.
   i) Common side-effects are dose-related neurologic symp-

toms including ataxia, dizziness, nervousness, tremors, seizures, and impairment of memory. The most serious adverse effects of aprindine are agranulocytosis and cholestatic jaundice. Because it possesses a moderate negative inotropic effect, it may cause slight ventricular dysfunction even with therapeutic doses.

2. Encainide
   a) Encainide was developed in the United States and recently approved by the FDA as a new antiarrhythmic agent for ventricular arrhythmias, particularly VPCs.
   b) Encainide possesses local anesthetic properties, and the chemical structure resembles that of procainamide. The drug is reported to be extremely active at low blood concentrations.
   c) The usual oral dose of encainide is 100 to 300 mg per day in 4 to 6 divided doses. The therapeutic plasma half-life is reported to be 3 to 4 hours.
   d) Orally administered encainide is reported to significantly prolong the atrial and ventricular effective refractory periods, AV nodal conduction, conduction through anomalous pathways in WPW syndrome, and conduction through the His-Purkinje system. Thus, it commonly prolongs the P-R interval, QRS duration, and Q-T interval on the ECG. These ECG changes do not appear to indicate toxicity of encainide, however.
   e) Adverse effects of encainide are reported to be mild and infrequent. They include leg cramps, metallic taste in the mouth, dizziness, vertigo, paresthesia, and diplopia.

3. Acebutolol
   a) Acebutolol is a cardioselective beta-adrenergic blocking agent, and was recently approved by the FDA. It possesses the usual beta-blocking effects, including prolongation of AV nodal as well as S-A conduction. In addition, His-Purkinje conduction may be slowed at high plasma concentration.
   b) Acebutolol is reported to reduce the ventricular response in atrial fibrillation or flutter, and it may convert these atrial arrhythmias to sinus rhythm. It has been shown that acebutolol is effective in treating VPCs in various clinical circumstances, including MI. The potential role of acebutolol in treating a variety of cardiac arrhythmias associated with chronic obstructive pulmonary disease including multifocal atrial tachycardia, has been reported.
   c) The recommended intravenous dose of acebutolol is 1 to 20 mg every 4 hours, whereas the oral dosage is 300 mg every 8 hours.
   d) Side effects include marked sinus bradycardia, AV block

of varying degrees, and depression of myocardial contractility.

4. Lorcainide

   a) Lorcainide, an acetanilide derivative with a potent class I-C antiarrhythmic drug, is under investigation in the treatment of ventricular arrhythmias.

   b) Lorcainide is a potent local anesthetic antiarrhythmic agent.

   c) The major electrophysiologic effects of lorcainide include prolongation of intra-atrial, His-Purkinje, and intraventricular conduction times.

   d) Atrial and ventricular effective refractory periods are usually *not* affected or slightly prolonged by this agent. However, the effects on AV nodal effective refractory periods are variable. The conduction time via an accessory pathway may be prolonged by lorcainide.

   e) Lorcainide is available both orally and intravenously, and the drug is found to be effective in controlling various ventricular arrhythmias.

   f) The efficacy of lorcainide by intravenous administration was found to be comparable to that of intravenous lidocaine when 30 patients with frequent and complex VPCs (unassociated with acute MI) were treated. Side effects were also similar in both groups.

   g) In healthy individuals, the half-life of lorcainide ranges from 5 to 7.5 hours, but it may be markedly prolonged in patients with cardiac disease.

   h) Common neurologic side effects include nervousness, headache, sleep disturbance, dizziness, and confusion as well as nausea and vomiting. Transient flushing may be observed frequently following bolus injections of the drug.

   i) The usual dosage schedule has not been fully established.

5. Pirmenol

   a) Antiarrhythmic, electrophysiologic, and electrocardiographic effects of pirmenol are comparable to those of quinidine. Pirmenol is still being investigated in the United States.

   b) Pirmenol is easily and safely administered orally or intravenously (bolus or infusion).

   c) The antiarrhythmic effects and its relatively long plasma half-life (7 to 9 hours) correlate well with the therapeutic plasma concentrations.

   d) The direct negative inotropic action of pirmenol appears to be less than that of other antiarrhythmic drugs.

   e) The drug does not possess alpha or beta-adrenergic blocking effect.

   f) Anticholinergic effect of pirmenol is less than that of quinidine or disopyramide.

g) Suppression or marked reduction of VPCs (often refractory to other drugs) is usually accomplished with pirmenol in 60 to 80% of cases.

h) Mean therapeutic oral dose was reported to be 100 mg per day, and mean plasma concentration during chronic oral therapy was 2.3 μg/ml.

i) The P-R interval is *not* altered by pirmenol, but QRS interval may be prolonged slightly. Significant lengthening of the Q-T interval has *not* been observed during pirmenol therapy, and consequently, torsade de pointes has *not* been reported.

j) During chronic pirmenol therapy, the side effects are metallic or bitter taste in about 15% of cases. Dry mouth or constipation may also occur.

6. Cibenzoline

a) Cibenzoline, an imidazoline derivative, has antiarrhythmic properties and electrophysiologic characteristics of class I-C antiarrhythmic drug.

b) Cibenzoline is still under investigation in the United States, and has been shown to be effective in suppressing experimental, as well as clinical, ventricular arrhythmias.

c) The drug produces significant lengthening of P-R interval as well as QRS duration, but Q-T interval is *not* significantly altered by the drug.

d) In a study dealing with 49 patients with ventricular arrhythmias, acute therapy with 260 to 330 mg/day of cibenzoline resulted in more than 75% suppression of VPCs in 29 of 49 patients, more than 90% suppression of paired VPCs in 31 of 42 patients, and complete suppression of ventricular group beats (3 or more VPCs in a row) or VT in 21 of 27 patients.

e) From available data, the efficacy of cibenzoline in the treatment of ventricular arrhythmias appears to be comparable (even superior in some studies) to that of quinidine, procainamide, disopyramide, and tocainide.

f) The incidence of side effects of cibenzoline also seems to be similar to that of other commonly used antiarrhythmic drugs. The most common side effects include nervousness and tremulousness, but gastrointestinal disorders are uncommon.

g) Aggravation of CHF or ventricular arrhythmias by cibenzoline is probably less common compared with many other antiarrhythmic agents.

IX. ANTI-BRADYARRHYTHMIC AGENTS

Because of ready availability of artificial pacemakers, various anti-bradyarrhythmic agents (see Table 12–3) have been less commonly used in the past decade. Nevertheless, these agents are valuable for the management of such milder forms of slow rhythms as marked but transient sinus bradycardia. In addition, anti-bradyarrhythmic agents are extremely useful for urgent situations, such as Adams-Stokes syndrome, when artificial pacemakers are not immediately available. Atropine sulfate and isoproterenol are probably the most commonly used drugs.

A. ATROPINE SULFATE
  1. Indications
      a) Atropine is primarily used to accelerate the sinus rate by vagal inhibition. Thus, this is the drug of choice for marked symptomatic sinus bradycardia, sinus arrest, or SA block, usually associated with acute diaphragmatic MI or digitalis toxicity.
      b) Secondary indication of atropine is for Wenckebach AV block due to digitalis toxicity or acute diaphragmatic MI when the patient is symptomatic from the arrhythmia itself. However, in most cases, Wenckebach AV block does not require treatment.
  2. Administration and Dosage
      a) Atropine is best administered intravenously in a dosage between 0.3 and 1 mg (up to 2.0 mg); a similar dosage may be repeated every 4 to 6 hours as needed. The total dosage of atropine should not exceed 4 mg. The effect of the drug is usually prompt.
      b) Atropine may be given subcutaneously if the intravenous route is not feasible immediately.
      c) Oral administration of atropine has been used, but its effectiveness is less predictable.
  3. Side Effects and Toxicity
      a) Serious toxic effects of atropine are uncommon, but VPCs or ventricular tachyarrhythmias may be induced.
      b) Common side effects or mild toxicity includes a dry mouth, urinary retention, exacerbation of glaucoma, hallucination, hyperpyrexia, and marked sinus tachycardia.

B. ISOPROTERENOL
  Before artificial pacemakers were available for clinical use, the treatment of choice for complete AV block was the administration of isoproterenol. The drug is still useful in the treatment of Adams-Stokes syndrome during an emergency or temporarily until an artificial pacemaker can be inserted. Isoproterenol is, at present, still the drug of choice in the treatment of Adams-Stokes syndrome due to bradyarrhythmias, primarily complete AV block. Isoproterenol is capable of accelerating both the supraventricular and the ventricular pacemakers and of improving AV conduction. It possesses a potent inotropic action leading to an increment in the stroke volume, the amplitude of myocardial contraction, and the coronary blood flow.
  1. Indications
      a) The primary indication of isoproterenol is in the treatment of Adams-Stokes syndrome due to complete AV

block or ventricular standstill until an artificial pacemaker is inserted.

> b) For secondary indication, isoproterenol may be used in place of atropine in the treatment of symptomatic sinus bradycardia, sinus arrest, and SA block.

2. Administration and Dosage

> a) Isoproterenol can be given by direct intracardiac, intravenous, intramuscular, or subcutaneous injection, or it may be given by intravenous infusion.
>
> b) In emergency situations, such as severe Adams-Stokes syndrome or ventricular standstill, isoproterenol can be given by intracardiac or intravenous injection.
>
> c) The usual dosage is between 0.02 and 0.05 mg, but up to 0.1 mg may be administered. Otherwise the drug can be given subcutaneously or intramuscularly in a dosage of 0.1 to 0.4 mg every 2 to 6 hours as needed.
>
> d) Continuous intravenous infusion of isoproterenol is indicated in severe cases in order to maintain the ventricular rate around 50 to 60 bpm until an artificial pacemaker can be inserted. The usual method is to dilute 0.1 mg of isoproterenol in 200 ml of 5% dextrose in water, and the initial infusion rate is 1 to 4 μg per minute. The infusion rate may be increased to 5 to 10 μg per minute, and, occasionally, up to 40 μg per minute may be required to maintain an ideal ventricular rate.
>
> e) The most popular route for this drug is sublingually, and the usual dosage is 10 to 30 mg every 1 to 6 hours. It can occasionally be given as often as every 30 minutes as needed.

3. Side Effects and Toxicity

> a) Side effects or mild toxicity of isoproterenol include tremor, nervousness, sweating, nausea, weakness, headache, dizziness, palpitation, and hypotension.
>
> b) A serious toxic effect is the production of ventricular tachyarrhythmias, which may occur equally with small or large doses.

C. EPINEPHRINE

Epinephrine has been almost as popular as isoproterenol in the treatment of Adams-Stokes syndrome. However, epinephrine is considered inferior to isoproterenol because the former drug produces significant hypertension and is prone to provoke ventricular irritability, particularly VF.

Epinephrine is capable of accelerating the atrial, as well as the ventricular, rate. The degree of acceleration of the atrial rate has no relationship to the initial atrial rate, whereas the degree of the acceleration of the idioventricular rate is closely related to the initial ventricular rate. Specifically, the degree of acceleration of the idioventricular rate is the greatest when the

initial ventricular rate is slow, while the enhancement of the ventricular rate is insignificant when the initial ventricular rate is relatively rapid.
1. Indications
    a) The primary indication for epinephrine is in the treatment of ventricular standstill, particularly that associated with acute MI.
    b) The secondary indication for epinephrine is in the treatment of Adams-Stokes syndrome due to high degree or complete AV block, until an artificial pacemaker is inserted.
2. Administration and Dosage
    a) In urgent situations, as in ventricular standstill, epinephrine 0.3 to 0.6 ml of 1:1000 solution may be given by intravenous, intramuscular, subcutaneous, or intracardiac injection. Slow injection over a period of several minutes is recommended under the ECG monitoring; the rate of injection should be regulated according to the patient's response.
    b) For long-term therapy, 0.5 to 1 mg, 1:1000 solution of epinephrine diluted in 250 ml of 5% dextrose in water can be given by a continuous intravenous infusion. The initial rate of the intravenous drip is usually 1 to 4 µg per minute, and the rate may be increased to 4 to 8 µg per minute according to the patient's response.
3. Side Effects and Toxicity
    a) Side effects or mild toxicity of epinephrine include nervousness, trembling, pallor, and hypertension.
    b) A serious toxic effect is the production of ventricular tachycardia and fibrillation.
X. MANAGEMENT OF TACHYARRHYTHMIAS ASSOCIATED WITH WOLFF-PARKINSON-WHITE SYNDROME

When tachyarrhythmias of transient and short duration occur in the patient with WPW syndrome, treatment is usually not indicated. However, WPW syndrome characteristically produces recurrent supraventricular tachyarrhythmias in many patients. Therefore, every physician should be fully familiar with the diagnostic criteria as well as the management of WPW syndrome.

There are several ways to approach the management of WPW syndrome-related tachyarrhythmias (see Table 12–5).

Detailed descriptions regarding the management of various tachyarrhythmias in WPW syndrome are found elsewhere in this book (see Chapter 9).

SUGGESTED READING

Alboni, P., Shantha, N., Pirani, R., et al.: Effects of amiodarone on supraventricular tachycardia involving bypass tracts. Am. J. Cardiol. 53:93, 1984.

Antonaccio, M.J. and Gomoll, A.: Pharmacology, pharmacodynamics and pharmacokinetics of sotalol. Am. J. Cardiol. 65:12A, 1990.

Belhassen, B. and Horowitz, L.N.: Use of intravenous verapamil for vetricular tachycardia. Am. J. Cardiol. 54:1131, 1984.

Benson, D.W., Jr., Dunnigan, A., Green, T.P., et al.: Periodic procainamide for paroxysmal tachycardia. Circulation 72:147, 1985.

Bissett, J.K., et al.: Electrophysiology of atropine. Cardiovasc. Res. 9:73, 1975.

Brodsky, M.A., Allen, B.J., Abate, D. and Henry, W.L.: Propafenone therapy for ventricular tachycardia in the setting of congestive heart failure. Am. Heart J. 110:794, 1985.

Brown, A.K., Primhak, R.A. and Newton, P.: Use of amiodarone in bradycardia-tachycardia syndrome. Br. Heart J. 40(10):1149, 1978.

Browne, K.F., Prystowsky, E.N., Zipes, D.P., et al.: Clinical efficacy and electrophysiologic effects of cibenzoline therapy in patients with ventricular arrhythmias. J. Am. Coll. Cardiol. 3:857, 1984.

Brugada, P. and Wellens, H.J.J.: Effects of intravenous and oral disopyramide on paroxysmal atrioventricular nodal tachycardia. Am. J. Cardiol. 53:88, 1984.

Chilson, D.A., Heger, J.J., Zipes, D.P., et al.: Electrophysiologic effects and clinical efficacy of oral propafenone therapy in patients with ventricular tachycardia. J. Am. Coll. Cardiol. 5:1407, 1985.

Chow, M.S.S., Kluger, J., DiPersio, D.M., et al.: Antifibrillatory effects of lidocaine and bretylium immediately postcardiopulmonary resuscitation. Am. Heart J. 110:938, 1985.

Connolly, S.J. and Hoffert, D.L.: Usefulness of propafenone for recurrent paroxysmal atrial fibrillation. Am. J. Cardiol. 63:817, 1989.

Danilo, P., Jr.: Mexiletine. Am. Heart J. 97(3):399, 1979.

Danilo, P., Jr.: Tocainide. Am. Heart J. 97(2):259, 1979.

De Bono, G., Kaye, C.M., Roland, E. and Summers, J.H.: Acebutolol: Ten years of experience. Am. Heart J. 109:1211, 1985.

Deedwania, P.C.: Suppressant effects of conventional beta blockers and sotalol on complex and repetitive ventricular premature complexes. Am. J. Cardiol. 65:43A, 1990.

De Soyza, N., Terry, L., Murphy, M.L., et al.: Effects of propafenone in patients with stable ventricular arrhythmias. Am. Heart J. 108:285, 1984.

Dubner, S.J., Elencwajg, B.D., Palma, S., et al.: Efficacy of flecainide in the management of ventricular arrhythmias: Comparative study with amiodarone. Am. Heart J. 109:523, 1985.

Duff, H.J., Roden, D.M., Carey E.L., et al.: Spectrum of antiarrhythmic response to encainide. Am. J. Cardiol. 56:887, 1985.

Duff, H.J., Wyse, D.G., Manyari, D., and Mitchell, L.B.: Intravenous quinidine: Relations among concentration, tachyarrhythmia suppression and electrophysiologic actions with inducible sustained ventricular tachycardia. Am. J. Cardiol. 55:92, 1985.

Dumoulin, P., Jaillon, P., Kher, A., et al.: Long term efficacy and safety of oral encainide in the treatment of chronic ventricular ectopic activity: Relationship to plasma concentrations—a French multicenter trial. Am. Heart J. 110:575, 1985.

Dunn, M. and Glassroth, J.: Pulmonary complication of amiodarone toxicity. Prog. Cardiovas. Dis. 31:447, 1989.

Falk, R.H.: Flecainide-induced ventricular tachycardia and fibrillation in patients treated for atrial fibrillation. Ann. Inter. Med. 111:107, 1989.

Flowers, D., O'Gallagher, D., Torres, V., et al.: Flecainide: Long-term treatment using a reduced dosing schedule. Am. J. Cardiol. 55:79, 1985.

Goy, J.J., Kaufmann, U., Kappenberger, L. and Sigwart, U.: Restoration of sinus rhythm with flecainide in patients with atrial fibrillation. Am. J. Cardiol. 62:38D, 1988.

Hohnloser, S.H., Zabel, M., Zehender, M., et al.: Comparison of twice daily with thrice daily administered encainide for benign or potentially lethal ventricular arrhythmias. Am. J. Cardiol. *63*:73, 1989.

Huang, S.K. and Marcus, F.I.: Antiarrhythmic drug therapy of ventricular arrhythmias. Curr. Probl. Cardiol. *11*:178–240, 1986.

Huikuri, H.V., Cox, M., Interian, A., Jr., et al.: Efficacy of intravenous propranolol for suppression of inducibility of ventricular tachyarrhythmias with different electrophysiologic characteristics in coronary artery disease. Am. J. Cardiol. *64*:1305, 1989.

Huycke, E.C., Sung, R.J., Dias, V.C., et al.: Intravenous diltiazem for termination of reentrant supraventricular tachycardia: A placebo-controlled, randomized, double-blind, multicenter study. J. Am. Coll. Cardiol. *13*:538, 1989.

Hwang, M.H., Danoviz, J., Pacold, I., et al.: Double-blind crossover randomized trial of intravenously administered verapamil. Its use for atrial fibrillation and flutter following open heart surgery. Arch. Intern. Med. *144*:491, 1984.

Josephson, M.E., Kastor, J.A., Kitchen, J.G., III: Lidocaine in Wolff-Parkinson-White syndrome with atrial fibrillation. Ann. Intern. Med. *84*:44, 1976.

Josephson, M.E.: Antiarrhythmic agents and the danger of proarrhythmic events. Ann. Intern. Med. *111*:101, 1989.

Kadish, A.H., Weisman, H.F., Veltri, E.P., et al.: Paradoxical effects of exercise on the QT interval in patients with polymorphic ventricular tachycardia receiving type Ia antiarrhythmic agents. Circulation *81*:14, 1990.

Kappenberger, L.J., Fromer, M.A., Steinbrunn, W. and Shenasa, M.: Efficacy of amiodarone in the Wolff-Parkinson-White syndrome with rapid ventricular response via accessory pathway during atrial fibrillation. Am. J. Cardiol. *54*:330, 1984.

Kim, S.G., Seiden, S.W., Matos, J.A., et al.: Combination of procainamide and quinidine for better tolerance and additive effects for ventricular arrhythmias. Am. J. Cardiol. *56*:84, 1985.

Koch-Weser, J.: Drug therapy: Bretylium. N. Engl. J. Med. *300*:473, 1979.

Koch-Weser, J.: Drug therapy: Disopyramide. N. Engl. J. Med. *300*:957, 1979.

Koch-Weser, J.: Drug therapy: Metoprolol. N. Engl. J. Med. *301*:698, 1979.

Kopelman, H.A. and Horowitz, L.N.: Efficacy and toxicity of amiodarone for the treatment of supraventricular tachyarrhythmias. Prog. Cardiovas. Dis. *31*:355, 1989.

Kuck, K.H., Kunze, K.P., Schluter, M. and Duckeck, W.: Encainide versus flecainide for chronic atrial and junctional ectopic tachycardia. Am. J. Cardiol. *62*:37L, 1988.

Levine, J.H., Michael, J.R. and Guarnieri, T.: Treatment of multifocal atrial tachycardia with verapamil. N. Engl. J. Med. *312*:21, 1985.

Mattioni, T.A., Zheutlin, T.A., Dunnington, C. and Kehoe, R.F.: The proarrhythmic effects of amiodarone. Prog. Cardiovas. Dis. *31*:439, 1989.

Mattioni, T.A., Zheutlin, T.A., Sarmiento, J.J., et al.: Amiodarone in patients with previous drug-mediated torsade de pointes: Long-term safety and efficacy. Ann. Intern. Med. *111*:574, 1989.

Mitchell, L.B., Wyse, D.G., Gillis, A.M. and Duff, H.J.: Electropharmacology of amiodarone therapy initiation: Time courses of onset of electrophysiologic and antiarrhythmic effects. Circulation *80*:34, 1989.

Miura, D.S., Keren, G., Torres, V., et al.: Antiarrhythmic effects of cibenzoline. Am. Heart J. *109*:827, 1985.

Morganroth, J.: Safety and efficacy of a twice-daily dosing regimen for moricizine (ethmozine). Am. Heart J. *110*:1188, 1985.

Morganroth, J., Nestico, P.F. and Horowitz, L.N.: A review of the uses and limitations of tocainide—a class IB antiarrhythmic agent. Am. Heart J. *110*:856, 1985.

Morganroth, J., Oshrain, C., Steele, P.P.: Comparative efficacy and safety of oral tocainide and quinidine for benign and potentially lethal ventricular arrhythmias. Am. J. Cardiol. *56*:581, 1985.

Morganroth, J., Bigger, J.T. and Anderson, J.L.: Treatment of ventricular arrhythmias by

United States cardiologists: A survey before the cardiac arrhythmia suppression trial results were available. Am. J. Cardiol. *65*:40, 1990.

Morganroth, J., Pearlman, A.S., Dunkman, W.B., et al.: Ethmozin: A new antiarrhythmic agent developed in the USSR. Efficacy and tolerance. Am. Heart J. *98*:621, 1979.

Mueller, R.A. and Baur, H.R.: Flecainide: A new antiarrhythmic drug. Clin. Cardiol. *9*:1, 1986.

Myerburg, R.J., Kessler, K.M., Cox, M.M., et al.: Reversal of proarrhythmic effects of flecainide acetate and encainide hydrochloride by propranolol. Circulation *80*:1571, 1989.

Myers, M., Peter, T., Weiss, D. et al.: Benefit and risks of long-term amiodarone therapy for sustained ventricular tachycardia/fibrillation: Minimum of three-year follow-up in 145 patients. Am. Heart J. *119*:8, 1990.

Naccarella, F., Bracchetti, D., Palmieri, M., et al.: Comparison of propafenone and diso-pyramide for treatment of chronic ventricular arrhythmias: Placebo-controlled, double-blind, randomized crossover study. Am. Heart J. *109*:833, 1985.

Nademanee, K. and Singh, B.N.: Effects of sotalol on ventricular tachycardia and fibril-lation produced by programmed electrical stimulation: Comparison with other antiar-rhythmic agents. Am. J. Cardiol. *65*:53A, 1990.

Perry, J.C., McQuinn, R.L., Smith, R.T., et al.: Flecainide acetate for resistant arrhythmias in the young: Efficacy and pharmacokinetics. J. Am. Coll. Cardiol. *14*:185, 1989.

Pollak, P.T., Sharma, A.D. and Carruthers, S.G.: Correlation of amiodarone dosage, heart rate, QT interval and corneal microdeposits with serum amiodarone and desethyl-amiodarone concentrations. Am. J. Cardiol. *64*:1138, 1989.

Ravid, S., Podrid, P.J., Lampert, S. and Lown, B.: Congestive heart failure induced by six of the newer antiarrhythmic drugs. J. Am. Coll. Cardiol. *14*:1326, 1989.

Rutledge, J.C., Harris, F., Amsterdam, E.A. and Skalsky, E.: Clinical evaluation of oral mexiletine therapy in the treatment of ventricular arrhythmias. J. Am. Coll. Cardiol. *6*:780, 1985.

Saksena, S., Klein, G.J., Kowey, P.R., et al.: Electrophysiologic effects, clinical efficacy and safety of intravenous and oral nadolol in refractory supraventricular tachyar-rhythmias. Am. J. Cardiol. *59*:307, 1987.

Schutzenberger, W., Leisch, F., Kerschner, K., et al.: Clinical efficacy of intravenous amiodarone in the short term treatment of recurrent sustained ventricular tachycardia and ventricular fibrillation. Br. Heart J. *62*:367, 1989.

Stamato, N.J., Frame, L.H., Rosenthal, M.E., et al.: Procainamide-induced slowing of ventricular tachycardia with insights from analysis of resetting response patterns. Am. J. Cardiol. *63*:1455, 1989.

Strasburger, J.F., Smith, R.T., Jr., Moak, J.P., et al.: Encainide for resistant supraventricular tachycardia in children: Follow-up report. Am. J. Cardiol. *62*:50L, 1988.

Suttorp, M.J., Kingma, J.H., Lie-A-Hwen, L. and Mast, E.G.: Intravenous flecainide versus verapamil for acute conversion of paroxysmal atrial fibrillation or flutter to sinus rhythm. Am. J. Cardiol. *63*:693, 1989.

The Cardiac Arrhythmia Suppression Trial (CAST): Preliminary report: Effect of encainide and flecainide on mortality in a randomized trial of arrhythmia suppression after myocardial infarction. N. Engl. J. Med. *321*:406, 1989.

Veltri, E.P. and Reid, P.R.: Amiodarone pulmonary toxicity: Early changes in pulmonary function tests during amiodarone rechallenge. J. Am. Coll. Cardiol. *6*:802, 1985.

Wasty, N., Saksena, S. and Barr, M.J.: Comparative efficacy and safety of oral cibenzoline and quinidine in ventricular arrhythmias: A randomized crossover study. Am. Heart J. *110*:1181, 1985.

Zipes, D.: A consideration of antiarrhythmic therapy. Circulation *72*:949, 1985.

DIRECT CURRENT SHOCK

Edward K. Chung

Direct current (DC) shock is widely used to terminate supraventricular as well as ventricular tachyarrhythmias in various clinical circumstances. Direct current shock is often a life-saving measure in the termination of ventricular tachycardia (VT) or fibrillation (VF). Because of the ready availability of DC cardioverters, the use of large dosages of various antiarrhythmic drugs (Chapter 12), especially quinidine and procainamide, is no longer necessary in most clinical situations. About 90% of the cases of AF are successfully converted to sinus rhythm, whereas 95 to 97% of cases of VT can be terminated by the procedure. Also 90 out of 100 patients who have AF refractory to large doses of quinidine could be converted to sinus rhythm by DC shock. Electrical cardioversion is much safer than various antiarrhythmic drugs when the procedure is applied properly.

For successful cardioversion, it is important to apply the procedure properly, and all possible contraindications should be eliminated. It should be emphasized that DC shock may not only be ineffective for digitalis-induced tachyarrhythmias, but it also may be fatal, because ventricular tachyarrhythmias or ventricular standstill may be induced. In general, when digitalis-induced tachyarrhythmias are treated, DC shock may be attempted only as a last resort after all available measures have been exhausted (Chapter 18).

An automatic implantable mini-defibrillator has been tried in human beings in recent years with favorable results (discussed later in this chapter).

The use of the DC cardioverter may be divided into two major categories: (1) the treatment of acute tachyarrhythmias; and (2) elective cardioversion for chronic AF and flutter.

I. TECHNICAL CONSIDERATIONS, PREPARATIONS, AND PRECAUTIONS

A. Maintenance care is necessary to be certain that DC shock equipment is in good working condition.

1. In general, the electrical integrity of the equipment should be checked every month by the biomedical engineering personnel.

2. Paddles must be large enough to stimulate most of the heart muscle fibers simultaneously. Otherwise small paddles may deliver high electric-current density in a localized pathway that may cause myocardial damage.

3. For the external DC shock, anterior and posterior paddles are ideal, but two anterior paddles are an alternative choice. Anterior and posterior paddles are preferable because the patient lies on the flat posterior paddle and only the anterior one needs to be held by the operator (a physician or nurse). This method is an important safety measure, particularly with the equipment in which one paddle is grounded. The anterior-posterior paddle position is said to lower considerably the amount of electrical energy necessary for the electric shock treatment in comparison with using the two anterior paddles.

4. As a rule, food should be withheld from the patient for at least several hours before applying DC shock (except for emergency treatment) to avoid vomiting.

5. Induced transient amnesia is necessary during application of DC shock (except for emergency treatment), and the amnesia can be easily produced by IV injection of diazepam (Valium) in a dosage of 5 to 10 mg. General anesthesia or premedication is unnecessary. The duration of the action of diazepam (Valium) is only 3 to 4 min, and additional doses may be given, if necessary, within several minutes after the first injection.

6. The treatment room in which DC shock is applied should be fully equipped for a continuous cardiac monitoring and full CPR facilities including all cardiac emergency medications and an artificial cardiac pacemaker.

7. Recording of specific ECG leads should be possible as needed, before, during, and after the electric shock treatment. Before DC shock treatment, a short heart-rhythm strip (lead V_1 or II) should be recorded in order to confirm the underlying heart rhythm so that it is obvious when a normal sinus rhythm is restored after DC shock treatment.

8. Paste (ECG paste is commonly used) should be applied liberally to the patient and should be rubbed well into his skin to reduce electrical resistance.

9. It should be certain that no part of the patient's skin is in direct contact with the metal of the trolley or the bed on which he is lying. No one should touch the patient, his bed, or any equipment to which the patient is attached at the moment of application of DC shock.

10. For elective cardioversion, all types of digitalis preparations should be withheld for at least 24 to 48 hours before the electric shock treatment.

11. If the shock treatment cannot be postponed in patients who are taking digitalis, 100 to 250 mg of phenytoin (Dilantin) should be given by IV injection before DC shock. Alternatively, 50 to 75 mg of lidocaine (Xylocaine) or 50 to 100 mg of procainamide (Pronestyl) may be injected IV in place of phenytoin (Dilantin). These medications may reduce the incidence of serious arrhythmias considerably in this circumstance.

12. Because the thromboembolic phenomenon is relatively high in certain high-risk groups, anticoagulants may be beneficial before and after DC shock. Anticoagulant therapy is highly recommended for patients with recent MI, cardiomyopathies, rheumatic heart disease (RHD), artificial heart valves, previous history of thromboembolic phenomenon and for elderly people. Many physicians recommend anticoagulant therapy at least a few day to one week before DC shock and 3 to 4 weeks after the shock treatment in these cases. True efficacy of the routine use of anticoagulant therapy for DC shock treatment is not certain, however.

13. After the termination of the tachyarrhythmia by DC shock, the 12-lead ECG should be recorded. The ECG should be monitored at least for the next 24 hours.

14. In addition, blood pressure (BP) should be measured every half hour until it becomes stable and until it reaches the control value before the shock treatment.

15. A chest X-ray film may be taken within 24 hours to exclude the possibility of pulmonary edema, especially when a high-energy-level shock was applied.

16. Even when normal heart rhythm is restored by DC shock, various medications may be needed thereafter.

II. DC CARDIOVERSION FOR ACUTE TACHYARRHYTHMIAS

1. For the treatment of various supraventricular and ventricular tachyarrhythmias with acute onset, DC cardioversion is often a life-saving measure (Figs. 13–1 to 13–3).

2. When a clinical situation is extremely urgent, such as in the treatment of life-threatening VT or VF (Fig. 13–3), premedication for transient amnesia or anesthesia is not needed. Thus, 100 to 200 watt sec of DC shock can be applied directly. If the arrhythmias persist, DC shock with increased energy (200 to 400 watt sec) should be applied immediately following the first shock.

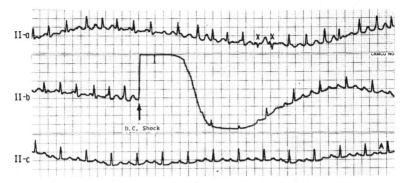

FIG. 13–1. Leads II-a, b, and c are continuous. Atrial fibrillation has been converted to sinus rhythm by direct current shock. Note the occasional aberrant ventricular conduction (marked X) and the one atrial premature beat (marked A).

3. On the other hand, if the clinical situation is not urgent, small amounts of thiopental sodium (Pentothal) or diazepam (Valium) may be administered in order to induce a transient anesthesia or amnesia immediately before the application of DC shock.
4. Premedication may not be indicated when only a small energy discharge is required, particularly in the treatment of atrial flutter.
5. Following termination of ventricular tachyarrhythmias (Figs. 13–2 and 13–3), continuous IV infusion of lidocaine (Xylocaine) and, less commonly, procainamide is usually indicated, followed by oral maintenance therapy with procainamide (Pronestyl), quinidine, or disopyramide (Norpace).

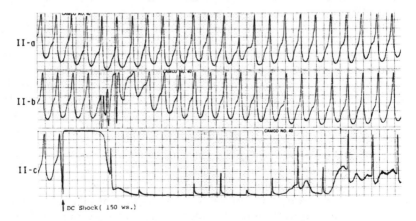

FIG. 13–2. Leads II-a, b, and c are continuous. Ventricular tachycardia (150 beats/min) is terminated by direct current shock (150 Wsec).

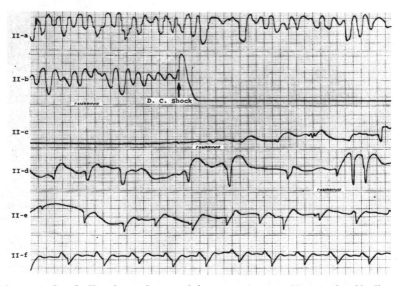

FIG. 13–3. Leads II-a, b, c, d, e, and f are continuous. Ventricular fibrillation is terminated by direct current shock, and sinus rhythm is restored. Note that there are ventricular premature contractions and unstable AV junctional escape rhythm in leads II-d and e before sinus rhythm is established.

6. When AF or flutter is terminated by DC shock (Fig. 13–1), maintenance doses of oral quinidine and digitalis are needed in most instances.
7. Various tachyarrhythmias associated with the WPW syndrome can be terminated successfully by DC shock (Chapter 9).

III. CONTRAINDICATIONS OR NONINDICATIONS OF DIRECT CURRENT SHOCK

One of the most important aspects in considering the indications for DC cardioversion is the probability of restoration of sinus rhythm and of its maintenance for a reasonable period of time. In general, a heart that is difficult to convert to sinus rhythm is also difficult to maintain in sinus rhythm. The success of conversion is *not* directly influenced by the type of heart disease, prior resistance to quinidine therapy, age or sex of the patient, presence or absence of CHF, occurrence of thromboembolism, or degree of ventricular chamber enlargement.

In the following situations, DC shock is either contraindicated or is not indicated:

1. Digitalis toxicity or hypokalemia (Chapter 18).
2. Severe mitral insufficiency or marked left atrial hypertrophy.
3. AF or flutter with advanced or complete AV block (often a manifestation of SSS).
4. Chronic AF with duration of 5 years or longer.

5. Imminent valvular surgery.
6. Lone AF with slow ventricular rate (often a manifestation of SSS).
7. Marked first-degree AV block (the P-R interval more than 0.28 sec) before the onset of AF.
8. Recurrence of AF or flutter during adequate digitalis and quinidine therapy.
9. Sick sinus syndrome (SSS).
10. Terminal stages of cancer patients or similar clinical circumstances.

In general, chronic AF with advanced or complete AV block is a manifestation of advanced SSS (Chapter 11).

IV. COMPLICATIONS OF DIRECT CURRENT SHOCK

Complications can be reduced to a minimum or can even be avoided in most instances when the patient is properly selected and when the procedure is properly applied. In general, complications of DC cardioversion are directly related to technical errors during the procedure, severity of the atrial damage, and improper use or over-dosage of antiarrhythmic drugs. Technical errors in using a DC cardioverter include failure to synchronize the discharge, disregard for ECG artifacts that may trigger electrical discharge during the vulnerable period and that may lead to the development of ventricular fibrillation, and excessive energy settings. In addition, excessive dosage of digitalis or various antiarrhythmic agents produces various and sometimes more serious postcardioversion arrhythmias.

1. DC shock may unmask digitalis-induced arrhythmias (Chapter 18).
2. Ventricular tachyarrhythmias may develop following DC shock, particularly during digitalis therapy (Chapter 12).
3. Pre-existing advanced or complete AV block, or ventricular standstill may occur following DC shock. When a markedly prolonged ventricular standstill is present after termination of any ectopic tachyarrhythmia, the diagnosis of SSS is strongly suspected providing that the arrhythmia is not drug-induced (e.g., DI). When any bradyarrhythmia (marked sinus bradycardia, advanced or complete AV block, ventricular standstill, AV junctional or ventricular escape rhythm) is observed following termination of any tachyarrhythmia, these arrhythmias represent bradytachyarrhythmias in which an artificial pacemaker is indicated in most cases (Chapter 14).
4. When the stable sinus rhythm fails to appear following termination of any ectopic tachyarrhythmia (particularly AF or flutter) by DC shock, the finding indicates a marked sinus-node dysfunction (SSS—Chapter 11) or a marked sinus node depression from digitalis or antiarrhythmic agents (e.g., quinidine).
5. DC cardioversion may induce *new* atrial tachyarrhythmias.

This change is considered to occur when the electric discharge is given during the atrial vulnerable period. Cardioversion-induced atrial tachyarrhythmias can be terminated by an additional DC shock in most cases.

6. Occurrence of thromboembolism, particularly cerebrovascular accidents in elderly individuals, within 24 to 48 hours following DC shock is not uncommon.

7. Intense and repeated DC shocks in dogs produce myocardial damage that is associated with increased serum MB creatine phosphokinase (CPK), but conventional DC shock does not cause such change in human beings.

8. Superficial burn of the skin under the paddle may be induced by repetitive applications of DC shock, especially when sufficient jelly is not applied.

V. CARDIAC ARRHYTHMIAS RELATED TO DC SHOCK

Although DC shock is indispensable in the termination of various supraventricular as well as ventricular tachyarrhythmias in many patients, certain cardiac arrhythmias may develop following the procedure. Some cardiac arrhythmias may be observed immediately following DC shock, even during ideal situations. Serious arrhythmias tend to develop from the procedure when DI or electrolyte imbalance (especially hypokalemia) is present, when the patient is elderly with advanced heart disease or pre-existing conduction defect, and when the procedure is improperly performed.

1. It is very common to observe atrial or AV junctional premature contractions following the termination of supraventricular tachyarrhythmias (AF, flutter or tachycardia, and AV junctional tachycardia), and in some cases, ventricular tachyarrhythmias.

2. Similarly, occasional appearances of AV junctional escape beats or a period of AV junctional escape rhythm with or without AV dissociation are not uncommon during the first 1 to 3 sec (sometimes longer) following cardioversion.

3. In addition, sinus bradycardia and sinus arrhythmia preceded by a short period of sinus arrest are also not infrequently encountered 1 to 2 sec after the termination of a tachyarrhythmia. Irregular and slow sinus activity in this circumstance is simply due to the sinus node's requirement of a warm-up period following a depression by a rapid ectopic-impulse discharge. A failure of the sinus node to take over cardiac activity for a long period of time, such as is seen in AV junctional escape rhythm without discernible P waves, or with extremely slow and irregular sinus activity, indicates that the sinus node is diseased (SSS—Chapter 11) or markedly depressed by digitalis or antiarrhythmic agents.

4. When the heart is severely damaged and the sinus node as well as ectopic escape pacemakers are unable to produce impulses following cardioversion, an atrial as well as a ventricular standstill is produced.

5. Varying degrees of AV block may be observed following DC shock when a pre-existing AV conduction defect occurs. First-degree AV block is extremely common following the termination of chronic AF or flutter. In this case, recurrence of the AF or flutter is common and repeated cardioversion has little value.

6. Cardioversion may change a pre-existing AF to an atrial flutter or a tachycardia or vice versa instead of a sinus rhythm. The reason for the development of new atrial tachyarrhythmias following DC shock is probably the fact that the electrical discharge may fire during the vulnerable period of the atria. This is particularly true when the P-R intervals are long and the AV conduction ratios vary. Cardioversion-induced atrial tachyarrhythmias can be terminated by an additional DC shock in most cases.

7. The appearance of occasional VPCs immediately following DC shock is relatively common and is insignificant clinically.

8. Frequent VPCs and runs of VT or VF, however, are serious problems.

9. The most common cause of VF that develops immediately following DC shock is improper synchronization, that is, the electrical discharge falls during the vulnerable period of the ventricles (the R-on-T phenomenon).

10. In addition, the development of ventricular tachyarrhythmias immediately after DC shock is often attributed to digitalis or quinidine intoxication, even in the presence of proper synchronization.

11. Frequent VPCs or even short runs of VT may be provoked when DC shock is applied to a patient with hypoventilation during deep anesthesia.

12. In general, unnecessarily high-energy discharges are prone to induce various cardiac arrhythmias.

VI. ELECTIVE CARDIOVERSION

A. Elective cardioversion is indicated for the treatment of chronic tachyarrhythmias, primarily AF or flutter, when restoration of sinus rhythm is considered beneficial.

B. Less commonly, elective cardioversion is applied to terminate other tachyarrhythmias such as atrial or AV junctional tachycardia.

C. Purpose of Elective Cardioversion. Elective cardioversion is indicated when a restoration of sinus rhythm is considered beneficial. In general, cardioversion is expected to provide:

1. Increment of cardiac output leading to improvement of CHF and increase in exercise tolerance.

2. Better control of the ventricular rate.

3. Reduction of thromboembolic phenomenon.

D. Preparation for Elective Cardioversion

1. Before DC cardioversion is attempted, all possible contraindications and nonindications must be carefully avoided.

2. Every patient with chronic AF or flutter must be digitalized and quinidinized 24 hours to 1 week prior to DC cardioversion. At least 15% of cases of chronic AF can be converted to sinus rhythm by digitalis alone or by a combination of digitalis and of quinidine (oral maintenance dose).

3. It is important to remember that short-acting digitalis preparations such as digoxin should be withheld for 24 to 48 hours immediately before DC shock is applied.

4. If a long-acting digitalis preparation such as digitoxin is used, the drug should be discontinued for 3 to 5 days prior to cardioversion.

5. The use of an anticoagulant for 1 to 2 weeks before and after DC cardioversion is emphasized by many investigators in order to prevent thomboembolism, but its practical value is uncertain. Anticoagulation, however, is recommended in patients who have prior or recent systemic emboli.

6. Pentothal or diazepam (Valium) may be used prior to cardioversion especially when high energy discharge is required.

7. It should be noted that cardioversion is contraindicated for AF with slow ventricular rate due to advanced or complete AV block (often a manifestation of advanced SSS). When DC shock is applied in this case, the procedure may induce markedly slow and unstable escape rhythm or ventricular standstill, which may be fatal.

VII. AUTOMATIC IMPLANTABLE CARDIOVERTER DEFIBRILLATOR

A remarkable new development has been made by a team of physicians and scientists at Johns Hopkins University Hospital in Baltimore, and favorable therapeutic achievements have been demonstrated after in-depth studies in the past 20 years. At present, automatic implantable cardioverter defibrillator (AICD) has been widely utilized at many other medical centers with a good clinical outcome. The AICD was approved by the FDA for clinical use on October 4, 1985.

1. The new implantable device, called a "mini-defibrillator" or "automatic implantable cardioverter defibrillator," is implanted under the skin of the abdomen and is attached to the heart by two electrodes—one through the veins to the right atrium and the other to the apex of the right ventricle.

2. This mini-defibrillator senses the onset of VF and automatically delivers the electric shocks (700 v) to the heart to terminate the arrhythmia and restore sinus rhythm.

3. The size of the new device is comparable to that of a cigarette pack and it weighs about 180–300 grams.

4. The electric shocks can be delivered in 15 to 20 sec after the initiation of VF, and a conscious patient feels a sharp tingling sensation from the shock.

5. When VF persists and normal heart rhythm is not restored

by the first electric shock, this mini-defibrillator commands up to three more shocks.

6. The device has a capacity of delivering as many as 100 electric shocks during the 3 to 5 year life of its lithium batteries.

7. The way in which the automatic mini-defibrillator works is somewhat comparable to that of an artificial cardiac pacemaker.

8. As expected, there are some untoward effects of the AICD. For example, the arrhythmia recognition by the device has not been perfected. Erroneous discharge of the AICD has been reported in the presence of AF and other forms of supraventricular tachyarrhythmias.

9. Infection following implantation of the AICD occasionally occurs, but malfunction of the device is a rare occurrence.

10. The energy discharge is often painful to the patient, especially when repetitive shocks are necessary.

11. The AICD cannot be used as a single therapy in patients with frequent episodes of VF because rapid drainage of power will be produced.

12. Some patients may require one or more antiarrhythmic agents even after the AICD implantation, because frequent shock will cause rapid battery depletion.

13. This new device, AICD, should be available worldwide so that sudden death due to VF, which often occurs outside the hospital, may be prevented. The AICD will be particularly valuable to high risk patients with a previous history of VF with or without evidence of CAD.

14. The combination of programmable multiple pacing and cardioverter-defibrillator modalities in a single compact unit will be a major advance in the management of refractory ventricular tachycardia as well as ventricular fibrillation.

SUGGESTED READINGS

Aarons, D., Mower, M. and Veltri, E.: Use of the elective replacement indicator in predicting time of automatic implantable cardioverter-defibrillator battery depletion. PACE 12:1724, 1989.

Ali, N., Dias, K., Banks, T. and Sheikh, M.: Titrated electrical cardioversion in patients on digoxin. Clin. Cardiol. 5:417, 1982.

Atkins, J.M.: New option: Automated defibrillation for sudden cardiac death. Contemp. Intern. Med. 11, 1990.

Bardy, G.H., Ivey, T.D., Allen, M.D., et al.: Evaluation of electrode polarity of defibrillation efficacy. Am. J. Cardiol. 63:433, 1989.

Bardy, G.H., Ivey, T.D., Allen, M. and Johnson, G.: A prospective, randomized evaluation of effect of ventricular fibrillation duration of defibrillation thresholds in humans. J. Am. Coll. Cardiol. 13:1362, 1989.

Bardy, G.H., Ivey, T.D., Allen, M.D., et al.: Prospective comparison of sequential pulse and single pulse defibrillation with use of two different clinically available systems. J. Am. Coll. Cardiol. 14:165, 1989.

Carlson, M.D., Freeman, C.S., Garan, H. and Ruskin, J.N.: Sensitivity of an automatic external defibrillator for ventricular tachyarrhythmias. Cardiology Board Review 6:73, 1989.

De Belder, M.A. and Camm, A.J.: Implantable cardioverter-defibrillators, (ICDs) 1989: How close are we to the ideal device? Clin. Cardiol. 12:339, 1989.

De Belder, M.A. and Camm, A.J.: Implantable electrical devices in the management of tachyarrhythmias. Clin. Cardiol. 12:461, 1989.

Eisenberg, M.S., Moore, J., Cummins, R.O., et al.: Use of the automatic external defibrillator in homes of survivors of out-of-hospital ventricular fibrillation. Am. J. Cardiol. 63:443, 1989.

Fogoros, R.N., Elson, J.J. and Bonnet, C.A.: Actuarial incidence and pattern of occurrence of shocks following implantation of the automatic implantable cardioverter defibrillator. PACE 12:1465, 1989.

Fujimura, O., Jones, D.L. and Klein, G.J.: The defibrillation threshold: How many measurements are enough? Am. Heart J. 117:977, 1989.

Geddes, L.A. and Hamlin, R.: The first human heart defibrillation. Am. J. Cardiol. 52:403, 1983.

Hopson, J.R., Hopson, R.C. and Kerber, R.E.: The role of energy and current in successful defibrillation and cardioversion. Cardiology Board Review 6:31, 1989.

Jaffe, G.N.: Automated defibrillation: A problem, a challenge, and an opportunity. Contemporary Intern. Med. 8, 1990.

Kay, G.N., Plumb, V.J., Dailey, S.M. and Epstein, A.E.: Current role of the automatic implantable cardioverter-defibrillator in the treatment of life-threatening ventricular arrhythmias. Am. J. Med. 88:1–25N, 1990.

Kalbfleisch, K.R., Lehmann, M.H., Steinman, R.T., et al.: Reemployment following implantation of the automatic cardioverter defibrillator. Am. J. Cardiol. 64:199, 1989.

Kavanagh, K.M., Tang, A.S.L., Rollins, D.L., et al.: Comparison of the internal defibrillation thresholds for monophasic and double and single capacitor biphasic waveforms. J. Am. Coll. Cardiol. 14:1343, 1989.

Kerber, R.E., Jensen, S.R., Gascho, J.A., et al.: Determinants of defibrillation: prospective analysis of 183 patients. Am. J. Cardiol. 52:739, 1983.

Kerber, R.E., Jensen, S.R., Grayzel, J., et al.: Elective cardioversion: influence of paddle-electrode location and size on success rates and energy requirements. N. Engl. J. Med. 305:658, 1981.

Kerber, R.E., Martins, J.B., Kelly, K.J., et al.: Self-adhesive preapplied electrode pads for defibrillation and cardioversion. J. Am. Coll. Cardiol. 3:815, 1984.

Kral, M.A., Spotnitz, H.M., Hordof, A., et al.: Automatic implantable cardioverter defibrillator implantation for malignant ventricular arrhythmias associated with congential heart disease. Am. J. Cardiol. 63:118, 1989.

Kuppermann, M., Luce, B.R., McGovern, B., et al.: An analysis of the cost effectiveness of the implantable defibrillator. Circulation 81:91, 1990.

Lehmann, M.H., Steinman, R.T., Schuger, C.D. and Jackson, K.: Defibrillation threshold testing and other practices related to AICD implantation: Do all roads lead to Rome? PACE 12:1530, 1989.

Manolis, A.S., Rastegar, H. and Estes, N.A.M., III: Automatic implantation cardioverter defibrillator. JAMA 262:1362, 1989.

Mirowski, M., Reid, P.R., Winkle, R.A., et al.: Mortality in patients with implanted automatic defibrillators. Ann. Int. Med. 98:585, 1983.

Mirowski, M.: Management of malignant ventricular tachyarrhythmias with automatic implanted cardioverter-defibrillators. Mod. Conc. Cardiovasc. Dis. 52:41, 1983.

Murakawa, Y., Gliner, B.E., Shankar, B., and Thakor, N.V.: The effect of an unsuccessful subthreshold shock on the energy requirement for the subsequent defibrillation. Am. Heart J. 117:1065, 1989.

Murakawa, Y., Gliner, B.E. and Thakor, N.V.: Success rate versus defibrillation energy: Temporal profile and the most efficient defibrillation threshold. Am. Heart J. *118*:451, 1989.

Myerburg, R.J., Luceri, R.M., Thurer, R., et al.: Time to first shock and clinical outcome in patients receiving an automatic implantable cardioverter-defibrillator. J. Am. Coll. Cardiol. *14*:508, 1989.

Patton, J.N., Allen, J.D. and Pantridge, J.F.: The effects of shock energy, propranolol, and verapamil on cardiac damage caused by transthoracic countershock. Circulation *69*:357, 1984.

Pozen, R.G., Pastoriza, J., Rozanski, J.J., et al.: Determinants of recurrent atrial flutter after cardioversion. Br. Heart J. *50*:92, 1983.

Reid, P.R., Mirowski, M., Mower, M.M., et al.: Clinical evaluation of the internal automatic cardioverter-defibrillator in survivors of sudden cardiac death. Am. J. Cardiol. *51*:1608, 1983.

Saksena, S., Tullo, N.G., Krol, R.B. and Mauro, A.M.: Initial clinical experience with endocardial defibrillation using an implantable cardioverter/defibrillator with a triple-electrode system. Arch. Intern. Med. *149*:2333, 1989.

Troup, P.J.: Implantable cardioverters and defibrillators. Curr. Probl. Cardiol. 14:675, 1989.

Veltri, E.P., Mower, M.M., Mirowski, M., et al.: Follow-up of patients with ventricular tachyarrhythmia treated with the automatic implantable cardioverter defibrillator: Programmed electrical stimulation results do not predict outcome. J. Electrophysiol. 3:467, 1989.

Walls, J.T., Schuder, J.C., Curtis, J.J., et al.: Adverse effects of permanent cardiac internal defibrillator patches on external defibrillation. Am. J. Cardiol. *64*:1144, 1989.

chapter

ARTIFICIAL CARDIAC PACING

Edward K. Chung

It is well documented that artificial cardiac pacing is one of the most important and reliable ways to manage various cardiac arrhythmias, particularly bradyarrhythmias. Until 15 to 20 years ago, the primary indication of permanent artificial pacing had been for the treatment of complete AV block (Fig. 14–1). The most common indication of permanent artificial pacemakers, at the present time, however, is in the treatment of the sick sinus syndrome (SSS). In addition, artificial pacing with over-driving pacing rate (faster than usual pacing rate) is often a life-saving measure for refractory tachyarrhythmias. The term "brady-tachyarrhythmia syndrome" (BTS) is used when the abnormal heart rhythms consist of a component of rapid rhythm as well as a slow rhythm. In this case, artificial cardiac pacing has an important role because drug therapy alone is usually ineffective. Bradytachyarrhythmia syndrome is often a late manifestation of SSS (Chapter 11).

Artificial pacing for various tachyarrhythmias (antitachycardia pacing) will be discussed in detail later in this chapter. Automatic implantable cardioverter-defibrillator (AICD) is fully described in Chapter 13.

The artificial cardiac pacemaker functions in a manner very similar to the natural pacemaker to initiate the electrical impulses generated by small batteries. The electrical impulses travel through the pacing electrodes to the heart from the pulse generator. The artificial pacemaker is timed to produce the electrical impulses (usually about 70 to 72 beats/min) just like the cardiac impulses initiated by the natural pacemaker (sinus node). In most cases, the heart is capable of pumping adequate amounts of blood under the control of an artificial pacemaker.

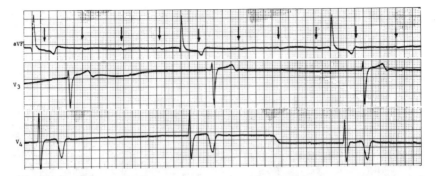

FIG. 14–1. Arrows indicate sinus P waves. The rhythm is sinus (arrows) with ventricular escape (idioventricular) rhythm (rate: 17 beats/min) due to complete AV block (complete infranodal block).

Approximately 250,000 people (500,000 according to some reports) live with artificial cardiac pacemakers in the United States of America alone, and 25,000 to 40,000 (100,000 to 110,000 according to some medical reports) new patients require artificial pacemaker implantations annually. Although it is difficult to know exactly how many people live worldwide with artificial pacemakers, the estimated number is at least 500,000 people (750,000 to 1,000,000 according to some reports). The total number of artificial pacemakers sold within the last 20 years is estimated to be approximately at least 1.5 to 2 million, possibly more. It is clearly evident that artificial cardiac pacing can provide not only the prolongation of human lives, but can also provide a significant improvement in the quality of life. Long-term administration of various drugs (e.g., isoproterenol, atropine, epinephrine) for bradyarrhythmias is no longer necessary because of a ready availability of artificial pacemakers in most civilized countries.

The fundamental principles for the use of an artificial pacemaker were established as early as 1932, and external cardiac pacing was introduced into clinical medicine in 1952. In 1957, temporary direct myocardial stimulation in the treatment of complete AV block was introduced, and a transistorized, self-contained, implantable pacemaker for long-term correction of chronic complete AV block was established in 1960. Mercury-zinc cells were used for the energy source until 15 to 20 years ago, but a lithium battery has now replaced the mercury-zinc battery entirely for all types of artificial pacemakers. In general, a lithium battery lasts 10 to 12 years in most clinical circumstances. The earlier pacemakers lasted only 15 to 18 months, and therefore frequent replacement of the pulse generator was required at that time. The nuclear-powered pacemaker was introduced about 25 years ago in clinical medicine, but it is not commonly used because it has no particular advantage compared with the lithium-powered pacemaker.

Many types of artificial pacemakers are on the market, but the most commonly used model is a demand-ventricular pacemaker (Fig. 14–2).

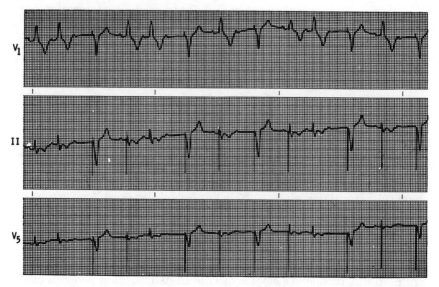

FIG. 14–2. Sinus rhythm (rate: 100 beats/min) with 3:2 Mobitz type II AV block and intermittent ventricular demand pacemaker rhythm associated with RBBB.

The demand pacemaker has a sensing device that cuts the pacemaker off if the natural heart rhythm is faster than the preset pacing rate. When the patient's own rhythm becomes slower than the preset pacing rate, the sensing device turns the artificial pacemaker on again, which is the reason that the term "demand" or "standby" pacemaker is used. In other words, the demand-artificial pacemaker works only when it is needed. When the atrial contribution is considered desirable, coronary (or atrial) sinus pacing or bifocal (AV sequential) pacing should be carried out. Coronary sinus-pacing rhythm exhibits retrograde P waves initiated by the pacemaker spikes, and the P waves are followed by the QRS complexes (Fig. 14–3). Typical bifocal pacemaker rhythm shows two artificial pacemaker spikes. One pacing spike initiates the P wave and another pacing spike initiates the QRS complexes so that the atria and the ventricles are activated sequentially (Fig. 14–4). Needless to say, an AV sequential pacemaker is indicated when significant AV conduction disturbance is present.

In the past few years, multi-programmable pacemakers have been introduced in clinical medicine. In this new type of artificial pacemaker, various functions (e.g., pacing rate, energy output, sensitivity) of the pacemaker can easily be controlled and adjusted noninvasively after implantation in order to provide the best pacing for an individual. The multi-programmable pacemakers are going to eventually replace all non-programmable pacemakers.

A fixed-rate ventricular pacemaker is seldom used today because ven-

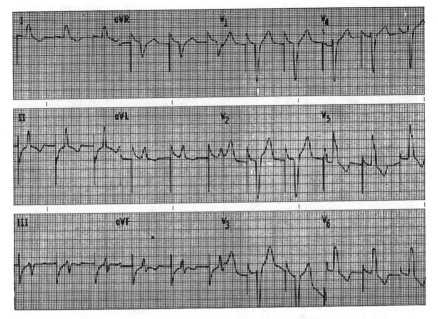

FIG. 14–3. Coronary sinus pacemaker rhythm with LBBB.

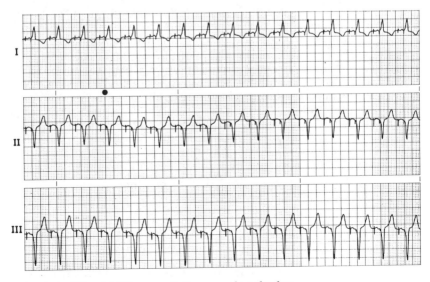

FIG. 14–4. Bifocal (AV sequential) pacemaker rhythm.

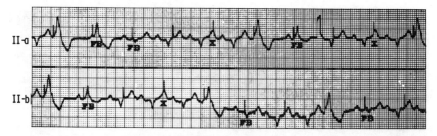

FIG. 14–5. Sinus rhythm with first-degree AV block and intermittent fixed-rate ventricular pacemaker rhythm. Note frequent ventricular fusion beats (marked FB) and the R-on-T phenomena (marked X). Leads II-a and b are *not* continuous.

tricular fibrillation may be provoked by the R-on-T phenomenon (Fig. 14–5).

Following implantation of an artificial pacemaker, every patient should have periodic medical check-ups and should carry out necessary daily care because the artificial pacemaker needs care like any other mechanical device, and complications or malfunctions may occasionally occur.

I. INDICATIONS FOR ARTIFICIAL PACEMAKERS

The precise criteria for the use of a temporary or a permanent pacemaker vary slightly from institution to institution, but the following conditions are generally accepted.

A. Short-Term Pacing (Temporary Pacing)
1. Symptomatic second-degree or third-degree AV block, especially during acute MI, requires temporary pacing. It should be noted that AV block per se does not require artificial pacing.
2. Symptomatic and drug-resistant sinus arrhythmias including sinus bradycardia, sinus arrest, sinoatrial (SA) block, and AV junctional bradyarrhythmias (often manifestations of SSS).
3. Bifascicular and incomplete trifascicular block associated with acute anterior MI (Fig. 14–6) usually requires short-term pacing (prophylactic pacing) because these findings are often followed by a slow ventricular escape rhythm due to complete AV block (infra-nodal AV block or complete bilateral bundle branch block—BBBB—Table 14–1).
4. Emergency treatment for Adams-Stokes syndrome, symptomatic BBBB and SSS.
5. Before or during implantation of a permanent pacemaker when the patient is symptomatic (e.g., syncope or near-syncope).
6. Prophylactic pacing during major surgery when Adams-Stokes syndrome or marked bradyarrhythmias are anticipated.
7. Drug-resistant tachyarrhythmias or bradytachyarrhythmias by overdriving pacing rate (Figs. 14–7 and 14–8).

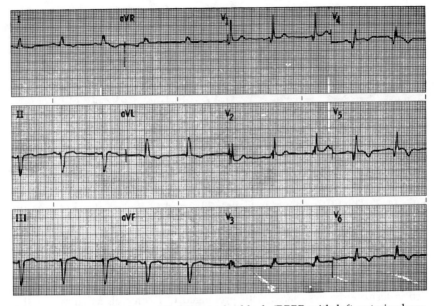

FIG. 14–6. Sinus rhythm with bifascicular block (RBBB with left anterior hemiblock) associated with recent extensive anterior MI.

At present, the most commonly used pacemaker for a short-term pacing is the temporary transvenous type. In almost all situations, a demand unit is preferable to a fixed-rate unit because normal AV conduction may be present during the insertion of a pacemaker (especially when it is used prophylactically) and because it is not uncommon to observe normal AV conduction occurring intermittently following the development of complete AV block. A bipolar or unipolar catheter electrode is inserted, via a jugular or arm vein, into the right ventricle, preferably in the apical region, under direct

Table 14–1. Diagnostic Criteria of Bilateral Bundle Branch Block (Bifascicular and Trifascicular Block)

1. Right bundle branch block with left anterior hemiblock
2. Right bundle branch block with left posterior hemiblock
3. Alternating left and right bundle branch block
4. Left or right bundle branch block with first-degree or second-degree AV block (not every case)
5. Left or right bundle branch block with prolonged H-V interval > 55 msec
6. Left bundle branch block on one occasion and right bundle branch block on another occasion
7. Mobitz type II AV block
8. Any combination of the above findings
9. Complete AV block with ventricular escape rhythm

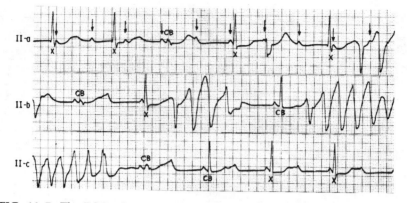

FIG. 14–7. The ECGs shown in Figures 14–7 and 14–8 were obtained from the same patient on different occasions. In Figure 14–7, leads II-a, b, and c are continuous. The tracing shows sinus rhythm with intermittent ventricular escape rhythm (marked X) due to high-degree AV block and frequent ventricular premature contractions with short runs of ventricular tachycardia. Note the occasional ventricular captured beats (marked CB). This type of arrhythmia is called the bradytachyarrhythmia syndrome. In addition, multiformed (atypical) ventricular tachycardia associated with prolonged Q-T interval, as shown in this tracing, has been termed "torsade de pointes."

vision using fluoroscopy with an image intensifier. Otherwise, the blind-float technique may be used in certain cases. In this method, the catheter electrode is advanced gently into position as the location of the tip is monitored by ECG. The usual pacing rate is around 70 to 72 beats/min.

When a physiologic pacing is desired, of course, AV sequential (bifocal) pacing mode is preferable. One of the important beneficial effects of atrial pacing is its ability to suppress a variety of ectopic tachyarrhythmias, particularly those of supraventricular origin. Thus, atrial pacing, coronary-sinus pacing, and AV sequential pacing (Figs. 14–3 and 14–4) are advantageous in the treatment of bradytachyarrhythmia syndrome or drug-resistant tachyarrhyth-

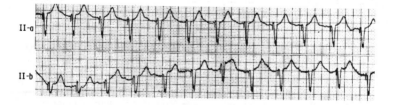

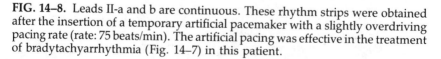

FIG. 14–8. Leads II-a and b are continuous. These rhythm strips were obtained after the insertion of a temporary artificial pacemaker with a slightly overdriving pacing rate (rate: 75 beats/min). The artificial pacing was effective in the treatment of bradytachyarrhythmia (Fig. 14–7) in this patient.

mias. When significant AV conduction disturbance is present in these circumstances, AV sequential pacing (bifocal pacing) must be carried out.

B. Long-Term Pacing (Permanent Pacing)

The decision as to whether long-term pacing is indicated or not is serious, because the patient must live with an artificial pacemaker all his life and must observe various necessary cautions and daily care. In addition, the pulse generator should be changed every 8 to 12 years in most cases (every 3 to 6 years in older models), depending upon the model. One of the most serious problems following permanent pacemaker implantation is the malfunction of the unit, which may be fatal. At times, it is difficult to judge whether a permanent artificial pacemaker is definitely required, because some controversy exists among physicians in certain clinical cases. In general, in the following situations, long-term pacing is considered to be indicated.

1. Symptomatic or advanced SSS (Chapter 11).
2. Symptomatic, chronic second-degree (usually Mobitz type II) or third-degree (infra-nodal) AV block (Figs. 14–1 and 14–2).
3. Complete AV block in acute MI (regardless of the location of MI) lasting more than 2 to 3 weeks.
4. Congenital complete AV block.
5. Symptomatic bilateral bundle branch block (Table 14–1).
6. Recurrent Adams-Stokes syndrome (usually due to Mobitz type II, advanced or complete AV block and SSS).
7. Recurrent drug-resistant tachyarrhythmias benefited by temporary pacing.
8. Carotid sinus syncope (may or may not be due to SSS).

When the indication of a permanent pacemaker has been determined, the type of pacemaker suitable for the specific patient must be chosen in view of the patient's age, his general condition, and the underlying disease. When physiologic pacing is desired, AV sequential (bifocal) pacing is preferable because the artificial pacing can provide almost identical hemodynamic consequences compared to the natural sinus rhythm so that the maximal cardiac output can be maintained (Fig. 14–4). For this reason, bifocal pacing has become the most commonly used method of artificial pacing in most clinical circumstances today. One of the major advantages of atrial pacing is its capability to suppress various ectopic tachyarrhythmias, particularly those of supraventricular origin. Drug-resistant tachyarrhythmias or bradytachyarrhythmias are often best treated with atrial pacing, coronary sinus pacing, or AV sequential pacing. Of course, the AV sequential pacing must be used when significant AV conduction disturbance is evident under these circumstances. A fixed-rate ventricular pacemaker (Fig. 14–5) is seldom used today because various complications occur frequently. Most pacemaker manufacturers continuously produce the fixed-rate ventricular pacemakers primarily for foreign countries.

Ordinary-demand ventricular pacing (Fig. 14–2) is adequate in the treatment of complete AV block when physiologic artificial pacing is considered unessential.

C. Artificial Pacemakers in Acute Myocardial Infarction

A special comment is in order regarding the use and abuse of artificial pacemakers in acute MI, because there is significant controversy among physicians on this topic.

1. Temporary Pacing in Acute MI, Regardless of Location
    a) Symptomatic and drug resistant bradyarrhythmias of any origin or mechanism.
        (1) Sinus bradycardia, sinus arrest, SA block
        (2) AV block (second-degree, high-degree and complete)
        (3) AV junctional and ventricular escape rhythm
        (4) Bilateral bundle branch block (Table 14–1)
    b) SSS and bradytachyarrhythmia syndrome.
    c) Drug-resistant tachyarrhythmias.
    d) DC shock-resistant tachyarrhythmias.
    e) Ventricular standstill.

2. Temporary Pacing in Acute Diaphragmatic MI
    a) Drug-resistant symptomatic, second-degree, high-degree or complete AV block, sinus bradycardia, sinus arrest, SA block, and AV junctional escape rhythm.
    b) Extremely slow ventricular rate (below 40 beats/min) due to any mechanism (even when the exact underlying mechanism is uncertain).
    c) SSS and bradytachyarrhythmia syndrome.
    d) Refractory ectopic tachyarrhythmias.
    e) Ventricular standstill.

3. Indications for Temporary Pacing in Acute Anterior MI
    a) Complete AV block—pacing (often permanent) is indicated in every case regardless of symptoms.
    b) Mobitz type II AV block (usually permanent pacing is indicated).
    c) Drug-resistant symptomatic sinus bradycardia, sinus arrest, SA block, slow-escape rhythm with or without AV block.
    d) SSS and bradytachyarrhythmia syndrome.
    e) Various forms of BBBB (bifascicular and trifascicular block) with acute onset (Table 14–1, Fig. 14–6).
    f) Refractory ectopic tachyarrhythmias.
    g) Ventricular standstill.

4. Indications of Permanent Pacing in Acute Myocardial Infarction
    a) Mobitz type II AV block, regardless of symptoms.
    b) Complete AV block (complete trifascicular block) in acute anterior MI regardless of symptoms.
    c) Symptomatic or advanced SSS and bradytachyarrhythmia syndrome regardless of location of MI.
    d) Symptomatic and drug-resistant bradyarrhythmias with

slow ventricular rate (less than 40 beats/min) in acute diaphragmatic MI lasting more than 2 to 3 weeks.

  e) Recurrent or persisting drug-resistant or DC shock-resistant ectopic tachyarrhythmias benefited by temporary pacing.

  f) Acute bifascicular block with intermittent complete AV block in acute anterior MI regardless of symptoms.

5. No Value of Artificial Pacing in Acute MI

  a) First-degree AV block alone (acute or pre-existing).

  b) Asymptomatic Wenckebach AV block (acute or pre-existing).

  c) Asymptomatic or transient sinus or AV junctional bradyarrhythmias.

  d) Nonparoxysmal AV junctional or ventricular tachycardia, and ventricular parasystolic tachycardia.

  e) Left anterior hemiblock alone (acute or pre-existing).

  f) Pre-existing RBBB or LBBB alone or left posterior hemiblock alone.

6. Equivocal or Questionable Value of Artificial Pacing in MI

  a) Acute RBBB alone.

  b) Acute LBBB alone.

  c) Acute left posterior hemiblock alone.

  d) Transient acute bifascicular block (asymptomatic).

  e) Acute LBBB or RBBB, or left anterior or posterior hemiblock with first-degree AV block or prolonged H-V interval.

  f) Late (more than 1 week after the onset of acute episode) development of acute bifascicular block (asymptomatic).

  g) Pre-existing bifascicular or incomplete trifascicular block (asymptomatic).

D. Antitachycardia Pacing

Although artificial pacemakers have been used primarily in the treatment of various bradyarrhythmias, antitachycardia pacing has become a very important pacing mode in the management of various tachyarrhythmias in recent years. The approval of the first implantable cardioverter-defibrillator in 1985 for general clinical application was a major step in the treatment of life-threatening ventricular tachycardia (VT) and ventricular fibrillation (VF). Automatic implantable cardioverter-defibrillator (AICD) has received increasing popularity ever since 1985 as a long-term therapy for recurrent VT and VF in recent years, but implantable devices for the treatment of supraventricular tachyarrhythmias have *not* achieved comparable popularity. AICD was described in detail in chapter 13.

Antitachycardia pacing can be used in the acute care setting as well as in the chronic long-term clinical setting. Acute antitachycardia pacing should be considered when patients suffer from clinically significant tachyarrhythmias in the emergency room, intensive and cardiac care units, and post-operative recovery room. Since acute antitachycardia pacing is employed routinely during electrophysiologic studies (EPS), the subject has been discussed in detail in chapter 22.

In this chapter, clinically pertinent information regarding antitachycardia pacing will be briefly described.

1. Following open heart surgery, various atrial tachyarrhythmias are relatively common, especially during the first several postoperative days. In this clinical setting, antitachycardia pacing is often useful.

2. In most medical centers, it is now routine to leave temporary epicardial ventricular pacing wires in place following open heart surgery. In addition, leaving an atrial pacing wire in place provides the option of atrial pacing.

3. Atrial pacing is effective in terminating various atrial tachyarrhythmias, and this therapeutic method is often preferable when various complications associated with anti-arrhythmic drug therapy and digitalis toxicity are anticipated (see Chapters 12 and 18).

4. Ventricular tachyarrhythmias are less common than atrial tachyarrhythmias postoperatively, but the former are the major problems in the cardiac care units, emergency room and similar acute clinical settings.

5. Transthoracic pacing can be used to terminate relatively slow, well-tolerated VT, without using general anesthesia.

6. In some patients, VT may be associated with complete AV block which becomes apparent only after termination of VT. Needless to say, a combination of VT and complete AV block is one of the most serious bradytachyarrhythmias. Under the circumstances, the pacing technique is extremely beneficial by providing antibradycardia support as well.

7. Antitachycardia pacing should be strongly considered for recurrent VT, particularly in patients suffering from acute myocardial infarction (MI).

8. Antitachycardia pacing is usually effective in terminating monomorphic VT at moderately rapid rates (less than 200 beats per minute).

9. On the other hand, antitachycardia pacing is not so effective in terminating a very rapid VT (rates faster than 200 beats/min) which often degenerates into ventricular flutter or VF.

10. For **torsade de pointes** (drug-induced or congenital Q-T syndrome), ventricular antitachycardia pacing at rates 90 to 120 beats per minute is usually effective in preventing further episodes of this VT (see Chapters 10 and 12).

11. For ventricular pacing, the most stable location is in the right ventricular apex and the best long-term results are achieved when the pacing threshold is well below 1 mA.

12. By and large, the stimulus amplitude should be higher for antitachycardia pacing than for antibradycardia pacing. At faster rates, the threshold rises.

13. In addition, at any given pacing rate, there is a greater likelihood of terminating the tachycardia with higher stimulus amplitudes. For transvenous pacing with a threshold of 1 mA, amplitudes of 10 to 15 mA should be used for antitachycardia pacing. With esophageal and transthoracic pacing, such excesses of stimulation over threshold amplitudes are generally not possible because of either limitations of the pacing device or discomfort to the patient. Nevertheless, attempts should be made to exceed the threshold by as much as clinically appropriate or tolerated.

14. For a long-term chronic therapy, the risk-benefit ratios and the prediction of the efficacy of antitachycardia pacing should be carefully evaluated in each given patient. By and large, antitachycardia pacing provides an effective long-term therapy, with low-risk surgery and minimal need for the patient's compliance. Various antiarrhythmic agents and their side effects can often be reduced or even eliminated completely.

15. Pacemaker implantation in patients with VT raises serious concerns because the rate of acceleration may lead to life-threatening ventricular arrhythmias and even sudden death. Thus, exhaustive drug trials should be carried out before considering pacemaker implantation.

16. Combination of AICD and antitachycardia pacemaker in the same unit should be an ideal device in the treatment of a very rapid VT associated with syncopal episodes, episodes of acceleration or episodes of VF (see also Chapter 13).

17. In the treatment of supraventicular tachycardia, continuous reprogramming of the pacemaker is necessary until the device functions properly according to the patient's clinical need.

18. Many young patients are reluctant to receive pacemaker implantation because of cosmetic and psychological concerns.

19. Antitachycardia pacing has received less-than-enthusiatic attention among many physicians for various reasons. Many physicians are *not* fully familiar with the device, and some patients may require various antiarrhythmic agents even after pacemaker implantation. Thus, many physicians would prefer to exhaust the antiarrhythmic drug therapy before considering antitachycardia pacing.

20. No doubt, however, antitachycardia pacing and AICD will be the most important therapeutic modality for recurrent and life-threatening ventricular tachyarrhythmias in many patients.

II. TYPES OF ARTIFICIAL PACEMAKERS
   A. Fixed-Rate Ventricular Pacemaker
      1. The fixed-rate pacemaker is designed to function regardless of the patient's own natural rhythm (Fig. 14–5).

2. A fixed-rate ventricular pacemaker can be used with relative safety in patients who have established chronic complete AV block when normal AV conduction is unlikely to occur, even temporarily.

3. In addition, older patients who have relatively good cardiac function using a fixed-rate pacemaker are able to carry out their ordinary activities quite adequately, because a maximum cardiac output is not important to sustain their limited physical requirements.

4. In approximately 25% of patients who require permanent pacing for Adams-Stokes syndrome, normal AV conduction (either normal sinus rhythm or second-degree AV block) may return either temporarily or even for long periods of time. In this case, the patient's own rhythm competes with the pacemaker rhythm so that the patient may develop ventricular fibrillation (VF) as a result of the R-on-T phenomenon. Primarily because of this, a demand pacemaker is preferable for many patients in whom normal AV conduction may return even momentarily.

5. A fixed-rate pacemaker is often used when overdriving pacing is indicated for treatment of drug-resistant ectopic tachyarrhythmias.

6. It is seldom used today because other newer pacemakers possess various superior aspects.

B. Demand (Standby) Ventricular Pacemaker

1. In the past 15 to 20 years, demand pacemakers have gradually replaced fixed-rate pacemakers because of a definitive superiority in the former so that competition between the natural rhythm and the artificial pacemaker rhythm can be avoided.

2. The demand ventricular pacemaker functions only when the R-R intervals of the natural rhythm exceed a preset limit (Fig. 14–2). A demand pacemaker, therefore, is particularly ideal for temporary pacing when bradyarrhythmias are transient or intermittent.

3. It is important to recognize "hysteresis" (the interval from the natural beat to the immediately following paced beat is longer than the consecutively-occurring pacing interval) in some models of demand units. Otherwise, the finding may be misdiagnosed as a malfunction.

4. Some disadvantages in the use of transvenous catheter electrodes include perforation of the ventricles, failure of pacing due to migration or exit block, infection, and fracture.

C. Atrial-Synchronized Pacemaker

1. A more physiologic type of artificial pacemaker is the atrial-synchronized pacemaker.

2. In this type of pacemaker, the pulse generator is triggered by the natural P wave of atrial depolarization and ventricular stimulation follows after an optimal delay corresponding to

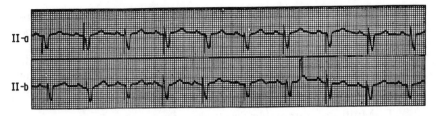

II-a

II-b

FIG. 14–9. Atrial-synchronized pacemaker rhythm. Leads II-a and b are *not* continuous.

the P-R interval (Fig. 14–9). In other words, an atrial-synchronized pacemaker functions as an electronic bundle of His.

3. The major advantage of this type of pacemaker is its ability to provide maximum augmentation of the cardiac output at changing atrial rates in order to meet varying physiologic requirements.

4. Another benefit is its utilization of the atrial contribution to ventricular filling to further augment cardiac output.

5. Thus, an atrial-synchronized pacemaker becomes extremely valuable in younger or more active patients.

6. When atrial tachycardia or flutter occurs, the pacemaker induces AV block of varying degree so that an optimum ventricular rate is maintained.

7. Although the advantages of an atrial-synchronized pacemaker are definitely known, electronic failure is frequent, and thoracotomy takes longer because of the complexity of the device.

8. An atrial-synchronized pacemaker is contraindicated in AF, marked sinus bradycardia, unstable atrial activity such as SA block, sinus arrest, and atrial standstill.

D. Bifocal (AV Sequential) Demand Pacemaker

1. Bifocal (AV sequential) demand pacemaker consists of two demand units, a conventional QRS-inhibited ventricular pacemaker and a QRS inhibited atrial pacemaker (Fig. 14–4).

2. In this model, the escape interval of the atrial pacemaker is designed to be shorter than that of the ventricular pacemaker. Thus, the difference between these two escape intervals is a determining factor for the AV sequential delay.

3. The bifocal demand pacemaker can stimulate both atria and ventricles in sequence, or it may stimulate the atria alone, or it may remain totally dormant. Thus, the pacemaker functions automatically according to the individual patient's needs.

4. In general, the bifocal demand pacemaker is considered to be indicated in the following situations:

   a) Sick sinus syndrome.

    b) Significant atrial bradyarrhythmias associated with intermittent high-degree or complete AV block (symptomatic).

    c) High-degree or complete AV block (symptomatic), in that atrial contribution to the ventricular output is essential.

  5. The bifocal demand pacemaker does not compete with spontaneous ventricular contractions.

E. Multi-Programmable Pacemaker

  1. The purpose of multi-programmability of artificial pacing is to provide the optimal cardiac function to an individual with a specific clinical circumstance by modifying and controlling various pacemaker parameters (functions) noninvasively after pacemaker implantation.

  2. The primitive idea of the programmability of artificial pacing was introduced as early as 1960, but modern programmable pacemakers were introduced in early 1973 for the first time. Initially, only two pacemaker functions (pacing rate and energy output) were programmed.

  3. Newer multi-programmable pacemakers have the capability to modify many parameters including:

    a) Pacing rate.

    b) Energy output (pulse amplitude or duration).

    c) Sensitivity (sensing threshold).

    d) Refractory period.

    e) Hysteresis.

    f) Pacing mode.

    g) AV delay.

  4. Almost all pacemaker manufacturers that produce artificial pacemakers in the United States of America provide models that possess multi-programmability.

  5. The pacing rate can be adjusted from 30 to 120 beats/min (up to 400 beats/min in some temporary pacing models).

  6. The programmable pacemaker is useful in patients with SSS and with bradytachyarrhythmia syndrome (Figs. 14–7 and 14–8) by selecting the optimal pacing rate for the patient's exact need.

  7. In elderly individuals and patients with angina pectoris, relatively slow pacing rate is desirable. Depending upon the patient's cardiac status, the pacing rate may be increased or reduced.

  8. For refractory tachyarrhythmias, overdrive pacing is indicated. In this case, the best effective pacing rate may be selected exactly for the patient's need, noninvasively.

  9. The energy source for the multi-programmable pacemaker is lithium, which usually lasts 10 to 12 years.

  10. Disadvantages of the programmable pacemaker may include the following:

    a) Higher probability of malfunction because of complexity.

    b) Higher cost.

c) Greater educational burdens for physicians, technicians, and all involved personnel because of complex design.

d) Increased reluctance of all cardiac patients with programmable pacemakers to take a trip overseas or to small towns where sophisticated medical facilities and highly trained cardiologists or cardiac surgeons are not readily available.

F. Miscellaneous Remarks

Pacing site may be in the atria or coronary sinus region in order to utilize the atrial contribution and normal activation of the entire heart. In *coronary sinus pacemaker rhythm*, the retrograde P wave is initiated by the pacing spike and followed by the optimal P-R interval and normal QRS complex (Fig. 14–3).

Nuclear-powered artificial pacemakers were introduced more than a decade ago into clinical medicine, particularly in many European countries, but they are not frequently used today because the nuclear-powered pacemaker has no clear advantage when compared with various other pacemakers with lithium-energy source. In addition, the usual problems associated with the nuclear-powered pacemaker prevent its usage in clinical medicine.

III. COMPLICATIONS OF ARTIFICIAL PACING

During the insertion or implantation of an artificial pacemaker, the danger of inducing ventricular fibrillation is always possible and, therefore, a cardioverter must be available immediately. In addition, various commonly used anti-arrhythmic agents (Chapter 12) also should be available immediately. Common complications are as follows:

A. Malfunctioning Artificial Pacemakers

Because of complicated designs of newer pacemakers, malfunctioning pacemakers are difficult to diagnose with a certainty unless the exact characteristics of a given pacemaker are carefully studied.

A malfunctioning unit may be manifested in the following ways:

1. Acceleration of Pacing Rate (Runaway Pacemaker)
    a) Runaway pacemaker is common when a fixed-rate pacemaker is used (Fig. 14–10).
    b) When the runaway pacemaker runs extremely fast, the pre-existing bradyarrhythmia reappears (Fig. 14–11).
    c) In advanced cases of runaway pacemaker, VF may occur, on the other hand VF can occur even in a pacemaker that is functioning normally (Fig. 14–12).
    d) Runaway pacemaker is a medical emergency. In this case, the malfunctioning unit should be disconnected from the heart promptly. The electrode wires can be cut near their attachments to the pacer. A replacement unit with a temporary pacemaker connected to the bare electrode ends results usually in a prompt recovery.

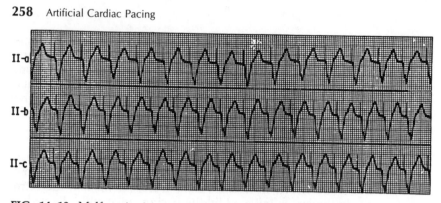

FIG. 14–10. Malfunctioning pacemaker is manifested by runaway pacemaker (rate: 107–125 beats/min). Leads II-a to c are *not* continuous.

        e) Antitachyarrhythmic agents are ineffective for a runaway
           pacemaker.
    2. Slowing of Pacing Rate
       a) Slowing of pacing rate is a common form of malfunction
          when a demand unit is used (Fig. 14–13).
       b) Slowing of pacing may be associated with irregular pac-
          ing (Fig. 14–14).

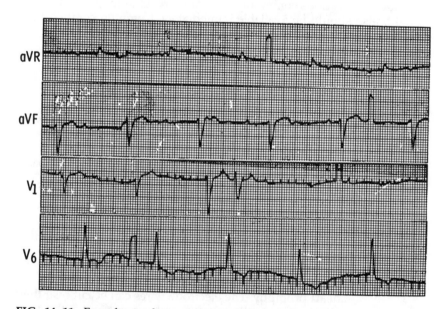

FIG. 14–11. Far advanced runaway pacemaker shows the pacing rate of 480 beats/min. Because none of the pacing stimuli capture the ventricles, the preexisting complete AV block is the underlying cardiac rhythm and one VPC.

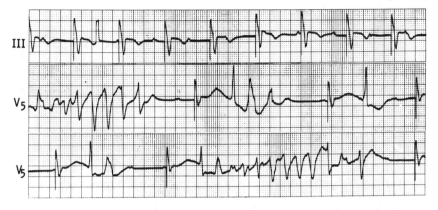

FIG. 14–12. Ventricular fibrillation is initiated by frequent VPCs with the R-on-T phenomenon. Note that an artificial pacemaker function is normal. There is the pacemaker hysteresis (the R-R interval from the last natural beat to the immediately following pacing beat is longer than the consecutively occurring pacing intervals).

3. Irregular Pacing
   a) Irregular pacing is usually observed in advanced or late state of malfunction (Fig. 14–14).
   b) Irregular pacing may be associated with slowing or acceleration of the pacing rate.
4. Failure of Cardiac Capture
   a) Failure of cardiac capture is a very common problem (Fig. 14–15).
   b) Failure of cardiac capture may be associated with a runaway pacemaker or slowing of pacing rate.
   c) Failure of capture may occur in a normally functioning pacemaker because of various causes (e.g., quinidine or

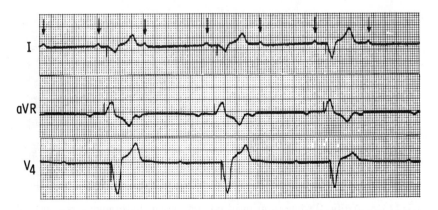

FIG. 14–13. Arrows indicate sinus P waves. Malfunctioning pacemaker is manifested by markedly slow pacing rate (rate: 32 beats/min).

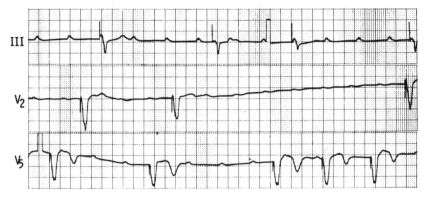

FIG. 14–14. Malfunctioning pacemaker is manifested by markedly slow and irregular ventricular pacemaker rhythm.

procainamide toxicity, hyperkalemia, advanced underlying heart disease).

5. Failure of Sensing
   a) Failure of sensing may occur alone, but it often coexists with failure of cardiac capture.
   b) Failure of sensing may be associated with other manifestations of malfunction.
   c) Failure of sensing may, of course, occur in normally functioning pacemakers for various reasons (e.g., low amplitude of QRS complex of the natural beats).

6. Perforation of the Ventricles
   a) Perforation of the ventricles can occur when a transverse catheter electrode is used.
   b) Perforation of the ventricles may be suspected when the following findings occur unexpectedly:

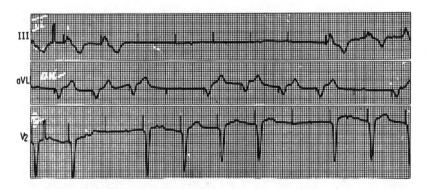

FIG. 14–15. Artificial pacemaker-induced ventricular rhythm with frequent failure of ventricular capture causing intermittent ventricular standstill.

          (1) RBBB.

          (2) Recurrent diaphragmatic contraction.

          (3) Pericarditis or pericardial effusions.

          (4) A pansystolic murmur (due to rupture of the ventricular septum).

    7. Other Findings

        a) Electrode fracture.

        b) Infection.

        c) Thrombosis or embolism.

        d) Knotting of the wire.

        e) Various cardiac arrhythmias, which may be due to malfunction of the unit or which may simply coexist with the normally functioning pacemaker rhythm.

IV. POSSIBLE INTERFERENCE WITH ARTIFICIAL PACEMAKER FUNCTION

    The following items may interfere with artificial pacemaker function:

  A. Electric shavers.

  B. Automobile motors.

  C. Motorcycles.

  D. Malfunctioning television sets.

  E. Direct contact with an ungrounded electrical appliance.

  F. Indirectly by proximity to equipment producing strong, rapidly fluctuating magnetic fields.

  G. Muscle stimulator for home use.

  H. Electric motors fitted with brushes and with commutators.

   I. Motor-operated hospital beds.

  J. Electrosurgical and physical therapy equipment.

  K. Direct current shock.

V. FACTORS MODIFYING PACEMAKER FUNCTION

    Various factors may modify the artificial pacemaker function:

  A. Sympathomimetic amines may increase myocardial irritability.

  B. Hyperkalemia may cause failure of cardiac capture.

  C. Fibrosis around the pacemaker electrode may cause failure of cardiac capture.

  D. Advancement of underlying heart disease may cause failure of cardiac capture.

  E. Quinidine or procainamide toxicity may cause failure of cardiac capture.

VI. AFTERCARE OF PATIENTS WITH ARTIFICIAL PACEMAKERS

  A. What the Patient Has To Do

    1. Every patient who has a permanent pacemaker should check the pulse 1 or 2 times/day to be certain that the pacemaker's preset rate remains constant.

    2. In case of alteration of the pulse rate (either slowing or increasing) a physician should be notified immediately because this pulse rate change may be indicative of malfunction of the pacemaker.

    3. When any new symptoms or signs, such as chest pain, syn-

copal episode, dizziness, or wound infection occur, a physician should be notified immediately.

B. What the Physician Has To Do
1. The patient should be fully instructed regarding the usual **daily care,** including common signs of a malfunctioning pacemaker, following the pacemaker implantation and before discharge.
2. The patient should be given an **identification card** indicating: the name of the patient, the date of the pacemaker implantation, the name of the surgeon who performed the pacemaker implantation or the physician who follows the pacemaker care after discharge, the name of the institution in which the pacemaker was implanted, the type and the model number of the pacemaker and the manufacturer's name, and a medical summary, including medications (optional).
3. Pacemaker Follow-up Care
   a) First visit (1 month after discharge):
      (1) Check surgical wound.
      (2) Detect gross evidence of malfunction.
      (3) Ask about usual pulse rate and about any complaint, such as chest pain or syncopal episode.
   b) Routine visit (every 3 to 6 months). Perform such procedures as ECG analysis.
   c) Elective hospitalization: for battery change.
   d) Emergency hospitalization: for replacing malfunctioning unit.
4. Pacemaker Follow-up Procedure for Each Visit
   a) Complete check-up of patient's cardiac status and status of pacemaker implantation site and the pacemaker function.
   b) Long rhythm strips (leads II and V_1) to check the pacing rate and to compare with preset rate.
   c) A 12-lead ECG (at least once or twice per year) to detect any unexpected or new ECG abnormality.
   d) When the patent's own sinus rhythm returns following implantation of a demand pacemaker, certain maneuvers, such as reducing the patient's own heart rate by carotid sinus stimulation or by edrophonium chloride (Tensilon) injection, or by accelerating the artificial pacemaker rate by using a magnet, should enable one to check the function of the pacemaker.
   e) Ask about any unusual or new complaint, such as chest pain or fainting episodes.
   f) Arrange elective or emergency surgery as needed.
5. ECG Analysis of Pacemaker Function
   a) Long rhythm strip (lead II) and preferably 6-lead ECG at each visit.
   b) A 12-lead ECG every 12 months (routine check-up), when

Table 14–2. Pacemaker Codes

First letter: chamber paced
   A—Atrium
   V—Ventricle
   D—Double chambers

Second letter: chamber sensed
   A—Atrium
   V—Ventricle
   D—Double chambers
   O—None

Third letter: mode of response
   T—Triggered
   I—Inhibited
   D—Dual (triggered and inhibited)
   O—Not applicable

malfunction is suspected, and when the patient has unusual or new symptoms.
  c) Measure pacing rate to compare with preset rate.
  d) Measure pacemaker artifact amplitude to compare with preset amplitude (often special equipment is needed).
  e) Detect cardiac arrhythmias.
6. Radiographic Analysis of Pacemaker Function
  a) Chest radiographs (sometimes of abdomen) are taken before discharge, 6 to 9 months after discharge, and yearly films thereafter. In addition, films should be taken immediately when malfunction is suspected.
  b) Check the position of the pacemaker and of the lead system. Malposition, twisting, angulation, and rotation of electrode or pulse generator should be checked.
7. Pacemaker Clinic
  a) When the pacemaker clinic with a specially designed pacemaker follow-up device is available, various pacemaker functions can be tested.
  b) These tests can be done on each patient's visit to the clinic, but the follow-up care can be provided through a long-distance telephone (a specially designed transtelephonic monitoring system).
  c) Various pacemaker functions (e.g., pacing rate, energy output) can be adjusted as needed when the pacemaker has a multiprogrammable capability.
8. Pacemaker Codes
  In recent years, artificial pacemaker codes (see Table 14–2) have been introduced into clinical medicine. The pacemaker codes provide useful information (e.g., chamber paced, chamber sensed, and mode of pacing response).

SUGGESTED READINGS

Austin, J.L., Preis, L.K., Crampton, R.S., et al.: Analysis of pacemaker malfunction and complications of temporary pacing in the coronary care unit. Am. J. Cardiol. 49:301, 1982.

Besley, D.C., McWilliams, G.J., Moodie, D.S. and Castle, L.W.: Long-term follow-up of young adults following permanent pacemaker placement for complete heart block. Am. Heart J. 103:332, 1982.

Breivik, K., Ohm, O. and Engedal, H.: Long-term comparison of unipolar and bipolar pacing and sensing, using a new multiprogrammable pacemaker system. PACE 6:592, 1983.

Broadbent, J.C., Nishimura, R.A. and Harrison, C.E.: Reentrant tachycardia associated with atrial synchronous pacing; report of a case with intact ventriculo-atrial conduction. Mayo Clinic Proc. 58:620, 1983.

Combs, W.J., Reynolds, D.W., Sharma, A.D. and Bennett, T.D.: Cross talk in bipolar pacemakers. PACE 12:1613, 1989.

Den Dulk, K., Bertholet, M., Brugada, P., et al.: A versatile pacemaker system for termination of tachycardias. Am. J. Cardiol. 52:731, 1983.

Den Dulk, K., Lindemans, F.W., Bar, F.W. and Wellens, H.J.J.: Pacemaker related tachycardias. PACE 5:476, 1982.

Dreifus, L.S.: Pacemaker Therapy. Cardiovasc. Clin. Philadelphia, F.A. Davis Co., 1983.

Elmqvist, H.: Prevention of pacemaker mediated arrhythmias. PACE 6:382, 1983.

Falk, R.H., Knowlton, A.A. and Battinelli, N.J.: The effect of propranolol and verapamil on external pacing threshold: A placebo-controlled study. PACE 11:1429, 1988.

Famularo, M.A. and Kennedy, H.L.: Ambulatory electrocardiography in the assessment of pacemaker function. Am. Heart J. 104:1086, 1982.

Feuer, J.M., Shadling, A.H. and Messenger, J.C.: Influence of cardiac pacing mode on the long-term development of atrial fibrillation. Am. J. Cardiol. 64:1376, 1989.

Fisher, J.D., Kim, S.G., Furman, S. and Matos, J.A.: Role of implantable pacemakers in control of recurrent ventricular tachycardia. Am. J. Cardiol. 49:194, 1982.

Freedman, R.A., Rothman, M.T. and Mason, J.W.: Recurrent ventricular tachycardia induced by an atrial synchronous ventricular-inhibited pacemaker. PACE 5:490, 1982.

Furman, S. and Gross, J.: Dual-chamber pacing and pacemakers. Curr. Probl. Cardiol. 15:119, 1990.

Gardner, M.J., Waxman, H.L., Buxton, A.E. et al.: Termination of ventricular tachycardia: evaluation of a new pacing method. Am. J. Cardiol. 50:1338, 1982.

Geddes, J.S.: Editorial: "Physiological" pacing. Brit. Heart J. 50:109, 1983.

Goldschlager, N.F.: Cardiac Pacemakers. Cardiol. Clin. 3:499, 1985.

Guarnerio, M., Furlanello, F., Del Greco, M., et al.: Transesophageal atrial pacing: A first-choice technique in atrial flutter therapy. Am. Heart J. 117:1241, 1989.

Hanley, P.C., Vlietstra, R.E., Merideth, J., et al.: Two decades of cardiac pacing at the Mayo Clinic (1961 through 1981). Mayo Clin. Proc. 59:268, 1984.

Harthorne, J.W.: Indications for pacemaker insertion: types and modes of pacing. Prog. Cardiovasc. Dis. 23:393, 1981.

Harthorne, J.W.: Cardiac Pacemakers. Curr. Probl. Cardiol. 12:651, 1987.

Hayes, D.L. and Furman, S.: Stability of AV conduction in the sick sinus node syndrome patients with implanted atrial pacemakers. Am. Heart J. 107:644, 1984.

Kastor, J.A.: Preventive pacing. N. Engl. J. Med 307:180, 1982.

Kappenberger, L., Valin, H. and Sowton, E.: Multicenter long-term results of antitachycardia pacing for supraventricular tachycardias. Am. J. Cardiol. 64:191, 1989.

Karbenn, U., Borggrefe, M. and Breithardt, G.: Pacemaker-induced ventricular tachycardia in normally functioning ventricular demand pacemakers. Am. J. Cardiol. 63:120, 1989.

Katzenberg, C.A., Marcus, F.I., Heusinkveld, R.S. and Mammana, R.B.: Pacemaker failure due to radiation therapy. PACE 5:156, 1982.

Keren, G., Miura, D.S. and Somberg, J.C.: Pacing termination of ventricular tachycardia: Pacing termination of ventricular tachycardia: influence of antiarrhythmic-slowed ectopic rate. Am. Heart J. 107:638, 1984.

Kerr, C.R., Tyers, G.F.O. and Vorderbrugge, S.: Atrial pacing: efficacy and safety. PACE 12:1049, 1989.

Lerman, B.B., Waxman, H.L., Buxton, A.E., et al.: Tachyarrhythmias associated with programmable automatic atrial antitachycardia pacemakers. Am. Heart J. 106:1029, 1983.

Levine, P.A., Brodsky, S.J. and Seltzer, J.P.: Assessment of atrial capture in committed atrioventricular sequential (DVI) pacing systems. PACE 6:616, 1983.

Levine, P.A., Seltzer, J.P., and Pirzada, F.A.: The "pacemaker syndrome" in a properly functioning physiologic pacing system. PACE 6:279, 1983.

Littleford, P.O., Curry, R.C., Jr., Schwartz, K.M. and Pepine, C.J.: Pacemaker-medicated tachycardias: a rapid bedside technique for induction and observation. Am. J. Cardiol. 52:287, 1983.

Littleford, P.O., Schwartz, K.M. and Pepine, C.J.: A temporary external DDD pacing unit. Am. J. Cardiol. 53:1041, 1984.

Madigan, N.P., Flaker, C.C., Curtis, J.J., et al.: Cartoid sinus hypersensitivity: beneficial effects of dual-chamber pacing. Am. J. Cardiol, 53:1034, 1984.

Newman, D.M., Lee, M.A., Herre, J.M., et al.: Permanent antitachycardia pacemaker therapy for ventricular tachycardia. PACE 12:1387, 1989.

Parsonnet, V.: The proliferation of cardiac pacing: medical, technical, and socioeconomic dilemmas. Circulation 65:841, 1982.

Parsonnet, V. and Bernstein, A.D.: Pseudomalfunctions of dual-chamber pacemakers. PACE 6:376, 1983.

Parsonnet, V., Crawford, C.C. and Bernstein, A.D.: The 1981 United States Survey of cardiac pacing practices. J. Am. Coll. Cardiol. 3:1321, 1984.

Parsonnet, V., Bernstein, A.D. and Lindsay, B.: Pacemaker-implantation complication rates: An analysis of some contributing factors. J. Am. Coll. Cardiol. 13:917, 1989.

Rozanski, J.J., Blankstein, R.L. and Lister, J.W.: Pacer arrhythmias: myopotential triggering of pacemaker mediated tachycardia. PACE 6:795, 1983.

Rubin, J.W., Frank, M.J., Boineau, J.P. and Ellison, R.G.: Current physiologic pacemakers: a serious problem with a new device. Am. J. Cardiol. 52:88, 1983.

Sakasena, S. and Goldschalager, N.F.: Electrical Therapy for Cardiac Arrhythmias: Pacing, Antitachycardia Devices, Catheter Ablation. Philadelphia, W.B. Saunders Co., 1990.

Sapire, D.W., Casta, A., Safley, W., et al.: Vasovagal syncope in children requiring pacemaker implantation. Am. Heart J. 106:1406, 1983.

Singer, I., Olash, J., Brennan, A.F. and Kupersmith, J.: Initial clinical experience with a rate responsive pacemaker. PACE 12:1458, 1989.

Van Gelder, L.M. and El Gamal, M.I.H.: Undersensing in VVI-pacemakers detected by Holter monitoring. PACE 11:1507, 1988.

Volosin, K.J., O'Connor, W.H., Fabiszewski, R. and Waxman, H.L.: Pacemaker-mediated tachycardia from a single chamber temperature sensitive pacemaker. PACE 12:1596, 1989.

c h a p t e r

15

CARDIOPULMONARY RESUSCITATION

Edward K. Chung

I. GENERAL CONSIDERATIONS

A sudden and unexpected cessation of effective cardiopulmonary performance is a cardiac emergency that requires immediate recognition and proper management. A rapid and effective institution of measures to maintain the delivery of oxygen to vital organs and to reverse the initiating pathophysiologic derangements is essential. Although the techniques for sustaining critical tissues and returning cardiac performance to a level adequate to sustain life are now universally practiced, they have been generally accepted and practiced only within the past 24 years. Before that time, cardiac resuscitation was performed, if at all, primarily by thoracotomy with open-chest cardiac massage. The demonstration by Kouwenhoven and his co-workers in 1960 of the effectiveness of closed-chest cardiac massage made it possible for all appropriately trained physicians and paramedical personnel to successfully perform cardiac resuscitation. Even before the demonstration of the efficacy of closed-chest cardiac massage, the development of an external alternating-current cardiac defibrillator capable of reverting ventricular fibrillation to a normal sinus rhythm was reported by Zoll and his co-workers. Since then, the direct current defibrillator is the preferred mode of cardiac defibrillation.

Appropriate use of those modalities has saved countless lives.

Table 15–1.   Etiology of Cardiovascular Collapse*

Causative Factor	Number of Patients
Coronary artery disease	239
Respiratory failure	55
Pulmonary embolism	18
Stokes-Adams syndrome	11
Cardiomyopathy	7
Uremia	32
Reaction to angiography	6
Miscellaneous	184
Total	552

* Johnson, A.L., Tanser, P.H., Ulan, R.A., and Wood, T.E.: Results of cardiac resuscitation in 552 patients. Am. J. Cardiol. 20:831, 1967.

Perhaps the most important factors (aside from those related to the underlying cause) in determining the outcome of a sudden cardiac catastrophe is the presence of personnel skilled in cardiac resuscitation. Every physician, regardless of his subspecialty or interest, should make the acquisition and maintenance of cardiac resuscitation skills an essential part of his training and practice. Education of the general public in CPR has also been demonstrated to enhance survival when CPR is required.

It is important to note any special attending physician's order requesting no CPR on certain patients who are terminally ill because of advanced cancer, irreversible stroke, etc. Under this special circumstance, CPR should *not* be performed.

II. ETIOLOGY OF THE CESSATION OF CARDIAC PERFORMANCE

The primary causes of sudden and unexpected cessation of effective cardiac performance and cessation of spontaneous respiratory activity may be neurologic, pulmonary, or cardiovascular disorders. Table 15–1 lists the findings of Johnson and his co-workers, who evaluated the causes of cardiovascular collapse in a review of 552 patients for whom cardiopulmonary resuscitation (CPR) was attempted. Similar distributions of causes have been reported by others.

The likelihood of recovery is determined by the underlying primary pathophysiologic derangements and by how rapidly effective CPR is instituted. Although cardiovascular stability may be achieved following anatomic damage, the phenomena most likely to be reversible are those associated with abnormal cardiac electrical events (cardiac arrhythmias). When it can be determined, the nature of the cardiac arrhythmia causing cardiopulmonary collapse is either a tachyarrhythmia (usually ectopic) or a bradyarrhythmia, ventricular fibrillation being the most common tachyarrhythmia and ventricular standstill being the most common bradyarrhythmia. It is possible, but less common, for a rapid supraventricular tachyarrhythmia to cause cardiovascular collapse; likewise, a severe degree of bradyarrhythmia of various potential mechanisms may result in cardiovascular collapse.

The inciting cardiac arrhythmia may have disparate causes. Experience in cardiac care units has demonstrated a high incidence of such an arrhythmia related to acute myocardial infarction or ischemia. Catastrophic arrhythmia, however, may develop de novo or in the presence of chronic but self-limited arrhythmia. Thus chronic ventricular ectopic beats may be observed before the development of ventricular tachycardia or fibrillation and may be related to myocardial fibrosis, cardiomyopathy, mitral valve prolapse syndrome, electrolyte disturbance, or drug intoxication, particularly digitalis intoxication.

III. INDICATIONS

Cardiopulmonary resuscitation should be instituted immediately on recognition of the sudden cessation of effective cardiopulmonary performance. The following findings are manifested on loss of cardiopulmonary performance:
1. Loss of consciousness.
2. Loss of carotid and femoral pulses.
3. Loss of respiration.
4. Loss of heart tones.
5. Loss of blood pressure.

Unless cardiac monitoring is continuous, recognition of the arrest of cardiopulmonary function may be delayed. Thus in a cardiac or intensive care unit in which continuous monitoring is available, the need for CPR should be immediately recognized. In a general hospital ward, the recognition of cardiovascular collapse depends on the presence of medical personnel who may be alerted by hospital personnel or visitors. In that setting, the recognition of cardiovascular catastrophe may be delayed because no observer was present. Outside the hospital even more critical delays are likely to be encountered before adequate resuscitative measures are initiated.

IV. ORGANIZATION

Cardiopulmonary resuscitation can be performed by one person, but it is best performed by a team. In the hospital, where a team is likely to be present, a plan must be made so that the people needed for CPR can be immediately summoned to the scene. The members of the team should be assigned clearly defined duties. A suggested plan of organization follows:
1. Senior physician. Assumes overall responsibility for the resuscitative efforts and directs all necessary procedures and drug therapy.
2. Junior physician or nurse. Performs closed-chest cardiac resuscitation and artificial ventilation.
3. Junior physician. Starts IV line.
4. Nurse. Has access to and prepares the required drugs, administers IV medications, and monitors cardiac rhythm and blood pressure.

5. Laboratory technician. Is available for performing required laboratory procedures.

V. CANDIDATES

For whom should CPR be performed? The question can be a difficult one. There are four considerations which must be assessed when deciding whether to perform CPR. These considerations are: (1) the choice of the patient if he is mentally competent, or the family if he is not. Little would seem to be gained by prolonging an individual's suffering against his will; (2) the likelihood of success. The following deals with this issue; (3) the quality of life to be anticipated if CPR is successful. For patients who have an incurable or terminal disease such as terminal cancer, and for patients who have severe neurologic disturbances, particularly those involving loss of higher cortical function, CPR would seem inappropriate. Cardiopulmonary resuscitation should be aimed primarily at the patient in whom restoration of cardiopulmonary stability results in a potential for a continued productive life and not in a perpetuation of preterminal agony or a vegetative existence; (4) the legal status and rights of physicians and families to withhold CPR in certain circumstances. This issue raises a very complicated question that has been reviewed by courts with varying opinions. While a compassionate approach to the patient and family must guide the physician, unfortunately the legal consideration may not be ignored. In the hospital setting, if the decision not to resuscitate a patient is made jointly with either patient or family that fact should be clearly indicated as part of the orders in the patient's chart. If there is a definite order from the attending physician indicating that CPR should *not* be performed in certain terminally ill patients as a result of advanced cancer, irreversible stroke, etc., CPR may not be performed. The foregoing discussion relates to situations in which adequate time is given for the decision-making process. If the medical status of a patient is not known before cardiopulmonary collapse, it is mandatory to proceed with CPR without hesitation.

VI. INITIAL MEASURES AND TECHNIQUES

The goals of initial emergency measures for CPR are to maintain ventilation of the lungs and to deliver adequate amounts of oxygenated blood to tissues. The initial measures have been described as the ABCs of therapy: A = Clearing the airway, B = Instituting breathing, C = Restoring circulation. It has been reported that a direct blow to the sternum can revert ventricular fibrillation, ventricular tachycardia, and asystole to normal sinus rhythm. It is thus appropriate to attempt that maneuver first; it should take only 1 to 2 sec. A forceful blow should be delivered to the sternum with the heel of the hand. It may be repeated once or twice if no response occurs. If the maneuver is not successful, one should immediately proceed to measures required to support life, as follows:

A. A = Clear the Airway

Place the patient in a supine position (Fig. 15–1). Place one

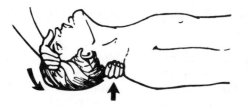

FIG. 15–1. Head tilt method of opening the airway. (Reprinted with permission from the Journal of the American Medical Association.)

hand behind the neck and the other on the forehead. Tilt the head back; that maneuver lifts the tongue from the back of the throat and results in an intrinsically unobstructed airway. At the same time, remove any obvious foreign body or obstructions in the mouth or nasal passages. Those maneuvers alone may lead to a restoration of breathing and to recovery. In some individuals, chin lift and forehead tilt may be more effective than head tilt and neck lift (Fig. 15–2). The tips of the fingers of one hand are placed under the lower jaw on the bony part near the chin, bringing the chin forward, supporting the jaw, and helping to tilt the head back. The other hand continues to press on the forehead to tilt the head back.

B. B = Institute Ventilation
   1. Mouth-to-Mouth Technique. Maintain the backward tilt of the head with one hand (Fig. 15–3). Pinch the nostrils closed

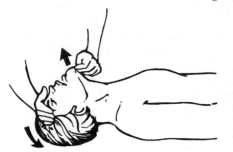

FIG. 15–2. Chin lift and head tilt method of opening the airway. (Reprinted with permission from the Journal of the American Medical Association.)

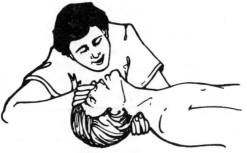

FIG. 15–3. Mouth to mouth resuscitation. (Reprinted with permission from the Journal of the American Medical Association.)

with the other hand. Place the mouth over the patient's mouth, completely sealing the patient's mouth, so that air does not leak. At the end of inspiration, exhale a larger than normal breath into the patient's mouth. If the procedure is performed correctly, a rise should be noted in the patient's chest as the intrathoracic volume is increased. No air should be lost through the nose or mouth while the lungs are inflated. After inflation of the lungs, remove your mouth from the patient's mouth, allowing his lungs to deflate. Air should be heard escaping from the lungs during that period.

2. Mouth-to-Nose Technique. Maintain the backward head tilt with one hand. Close the patient's jaw and seal his mouth with your hand. Place your mouth over the patient's nose, and after inhaling deeply, again exhale through the patient's nose. The indications for a successful maneuver are the same as those described for mouth-to-mouth techniques. Two quick full breaths without allowing time for full lung deflation between breaths, are delivered after each cycle of 15 compressions in single rescuer CPR. One breath every 5 sec is performed either for nonbreathing victims with a pulse (rescue breathing alone), or during 2-rescuer CPR. During 2-rescuer CPR the breath is interposed during the upstroke of the fifth chest compression.

3. Problems with Ventilation. If inflation of the lungs is resisted, suspect a foreign body in the airway. Roll the patient onto his side and deliver a firm blow between the shoulder blades in an attempt to dislodge the foreign body. The patient's mouth and oropharynx should then be explored for a foreign body. Another maneuver for the removal of a foreign body is the Heimlich maneuver. The patient can be either upright or supine. If the patient is upright, grasp him from behind, below the rib cage with your fist against his abdomen (Figs. 15–4 and 15–5). If the patient is supine, place your hands one on top of the other on the patient's abdomen, between the rib cage and the navel (Fig. 15–6). In both cases the hand is thrust quickly into the patient's abdomen. The thrust increases the pressure within the large airway and thus "pops" out the foreign body.

Gastric distension may be limited by maintaining ventilation volumes that just cause a rise in the chest, thereby avoiding exceeding esophageal opening pressures. Gastric distension is most likely to occur if there is excessive inflation pressure or if the airway is partially or completely obstructed. If despite these precautions gastric distension results in inadequate ventilation, the patient should be placed on his side and pressure over the epigastrium should be applied. This maneuver should be performed with caution because of the risk of inducing regurgitation. If regur-

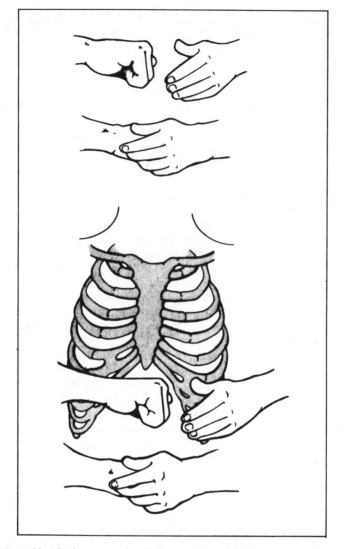

FIG. 15–4. Hand placement for abdominal thrust. (Reprinted with permission from the Journal of the American Medical Association.)

gitation does occur, then turn the patient to the side and wipe out the mouth before resuming CPR. If functioning suction equipment is available, an indwelling nasogastric tube may be inserted to avoid gastric distension and decrease the likelihood of vomiting.

The first two steps of CPR aim to institute ventilation. The procedures may be performed in any setting even by one person. In the hospital setting, in which more help and more facilities may be available, there may be some modifications,

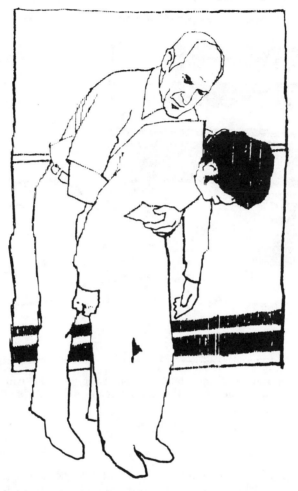

FIG. 15–5. Application of the Heimlich maneuver with the patient upright. (Reprinted with permission from the Journal of the American Medical Association.)

but the basic approach is the same. In the hospital, a bag-and-mask technique may be used instead of either of the expired-air techniques. The prime advantages of that technique are that oxygen may be added to the intake and that some physicians find it is esthetically less distressing.

C. C = Restore Circulation

The final step of the initial resuscitative measures is the institution of cardiac massage. Except when the patient is already in the operating room or when chest wounds preclude open-chest massage, there is virtually no situation in which one would not perform closed-chest massage rather than open-chest massage.

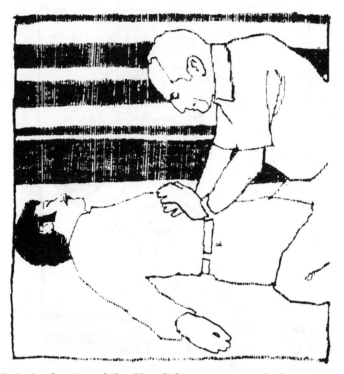

FIG. 15–6. Application of the Heimlich maneuver with the patient supine. (Reprinted with permission from the Journal of the American Medical Association.)

Although the traditional concept of CPR is that the heart is squeezed between the sternum and the spine to force blood from the heart, studies have questioned this viewpoint. Closed-chest massage may rather be effective because chest compression causes a generalized increase in intrathoracic pressure. This generalized increase in intrathoracic pressure causes collapse of thin-walled venous structures beyond a critical-closure pressure thus preventing retrograde flow of venous blood into the superior vena cava. At the same time, a pressure gradient between the intrathoracic arterial vessels and the lower pressure in the extrathoracic great vessels is created. This pressure results in antegrade flow through the aorta as long as the intrathoracic pressure is not so high as to cause collapse of the thick-walled aorta. During the relaxation phase, the reduction in intrathoracic pressure results in opening of the intrathoracic venous structures and antegrade flow occurs into the right atrium, right ventricle, pulmonary arteries, and pulmonary veins. The left ventricle according to this theory acts as a con-

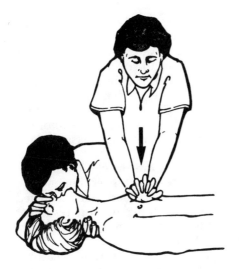

FIG. 15–7. Position for closed chest cardiac massage. (Reprinted with permission from the Journal of the American Medical Association.)

duit for blood rather than as a bellows that is passively closed and opened.

On a practical standpoint these studies suggest that maintaining a high-intrathoracic pressure during cardiac compression results in an augmentation of cardiac output during CPR. Further studies have demonstrated that cardiac output may be further increased if compression of the chest takes up 60% of the cardiac cycle instead of the traditional recommendation of 50% of the cardiac cycle.

A consensus of the best technique for CPR has not yet integrated these newer concepts into practical recommendations. The current recommendations of the American Heart Association follow:

1. Closed-Chest Massage
   a) Position. The patient's back must be on a firm surface. Place a hard board under the patient's back if he is on a soft surface such as a bed. Position yourself alongside the patient. Place the heel of one hand over the lower third of the patient's sternum (but not on the xyphoid process). Your hand should not be in touch with the patient's chest except for the heel of the hand. The other hand may rest on the first hand or may grasp the wrist of the hand on the lower sternum. The elbows are straightened by locking them and the body is positioned so that the shoulders are directly over the hands so that the thrust is straight down (Fig. 15–7).
   b) Compression. Depress the patient's chest 1.5 to 2 in. (approximately one-fifth of the AP thickness). The pressure should be smooth and uninterrupted. Following compression, release the sternum and make ready the

hand for the next compression. As aforementioned the duration of compression and relaxation is a controversial issue. Although the current American Heart Association standards for CPR recommend equal durations of chest compression and relaxation as already described, if compression occupies 60% of the cardiac cycle the cardiac output may further be increased. Additionally, if positive airway pressure is maintained during chest compression, the resultant increase in intrathoracic pressure may further augment cardiac output.

  c) Rate. Compress the chest approximately 60 times/min. If only one resuscitator is present, it is recommended that 15 chest compressions should be performed followed by two quick lung ventilations. If two or more resuscitators are present, every fifth chest compression should be followed by a lung inflation.

  d) Pulse. Although it is not an ideal way to measure the efficiency of closed-chest cardiac massage, palpation of peripheral pulses during chest compression may provide a rough guideline. If an indwelling arterial line is present, the contour of the pressure pulse obtained may be of value in assessing the efficiency of cardiac compression.

2. Complications of Cardiac Massage. Although cardiac massage is a safe procedure, one must not be overly vigorous in sternal compression, particularly in children. Reported complications, primarily those caused by inappropriate application of cardiac massage techniques, include fractures of the ribs and sternum, hemothorax, hemopericardium, pneumothorax, bone-marrow emboli, gastric rupture, lacerations of the spleen and liver, and rupture of the aorta.

3. Mechanical Devices. Several mechanical devices, some manual and some automatic, are available for closed-chest massage. In the hands of trained persons, they may make cardiac massage easier and facilitate resuscitative efforts. They should never be used, however, by inexperienced personnel. Misapplication of those devices may result not only in ineffective resuscitation but also in further injury to the patient.

VII. EVALUATION OF SUCCESS

During the emergency measures, one must check for the presence or absence of several signs that indicate the success or failure of your efforts. Those signs are essentially those that were initially affected in cardiovascular collapse.

1. Pulses in the femoral or carotid arteries
2. Heart tones
3. Spontaneous respiratory efforts
4. Palpable or recordable blood pressure

One should also be alert to any change in neurologic status. If the resuscitative efforts have been successful, one may stop and observe the patient for several seconds. If a reversal of cardiovascular collapse has been achieved, the patient should continue to be observed closely, and the cause of the collapse should be determined. If, however, the patient's status does not change, artificial ventilation and cardiac massage must be continued while further, more sophisticated diagnostic and therapeutic approaches are sought. During that period, cardiac massage and ventilation must be continuous, and they should not be halted for longer than 5 seconds.

VIII. SECONDARY MEASURES

If initial resuscitative measures are given no response, perform the following measures while artificial support is continued:

1. Quickly review the chart (if you are not familiar with the patient's condition) to extract any relevant information.
2. Obtain an ECG to assess cardiac rhythm and to evaluate the possibility of abnormalities, including acute myocardial infarction, pulmonary embolism, electrolyte imbalance, and digitalis intoxication.
3. Obtain an arterial blood gas analysis to assess the acid balance and the adequacy of ventilation.
4. Obtain a venous or arterial blood sample for the determination of serum electrolytes.
5. If an IV infusion site is not already available, one should be established. A subclavian or internal jugular sheath allows for infusion of drugs and the potential for pacemaker or Swan-Ganz catheter insertion as well.

When those steps have been taken, further therapeutic intervention may be instituted. Determination of cardiac rhythm is based on either a conventional 12-lead ECG or an oscilloscopic-monitored ECG tracing. The treatment of the various cardiac arrhythmias is described in the following paragraphs (Table 15–2).

A. Treatment of Ventricular Fibrillation

Ventricular fibrillation should be treated as follows:

1. Attempt electrical cardioversion with a direct current defibrillator at 200 to 300 J of delivered energy. If successful in restoring sinus rhythm institute IV lidocaine. If a cardiac rhythm other than sinus rhythm ensues, institute appropriate therapy.
2. If direct current cardioversion is unsuccessful initially, repeat the procedure. Although the use of high or low energy levels is controversial, several studies suggest that energy levels of 175 to 200 J are as effective as energy levels of 320 J or greater. Higher levels of delivered energy may have deleterious effects of refibrillation, heart block, and asystole. Nonetheless, in cases refractory to defibrillation at lower energy levels, levels of 300 to 400 J should be attempted.

If coarse ventricular-fibrillatory waves are present, administer lidocaine 1 mg/kg in an IV bolus, and start an infusion of 4 mg/min. Lidocaine boluses may be repeated every 10 min to

Table 15–2. Drugs Commonly Used in Cardiopulmonary Resuscitation

Indication	Drug	Dosage
Asystole	Isoproterenol	200 μg–1000 μg IV or IC bolus; infusion of 2–12 μg/min
	Epinephrine	200 μg–1000 μg IV or IC bolus; infusion of 2–12 μg/min
	Calcium chloride	10 ml (10% solution) IV to a total of 30 ml
Bradycardia	Atropine	0.3–1.2 mg IV bolus
	Isoproterenol	IV infusion of 2–6 μg/min
Ventricular tachycardia/ fibrillation	Lidocaine	50–100 mg bolus to a total of less than or equal to 300 mg
		IV infusion of 2–4 mg/min
	Procainamide (Pronestyl)	100 mg bolus to a total of less than 1000 mg
		IV infusion of 2–4 mg/min
	Bretylium tosylate	5 mg/kg IV bolus repeated at 10 mg/kg every 15–30 min to a maximum total dose of 30 mg/kg IV infusion of 1–2 mg/min
	Phenytoin (Dilantin)	100 mg over 5 min
		Repeated to a total of less than 500 mg
	Propranolol	1 mg IV q 5–10 min to a total of 5–10 mg

a total of 300 mg if needed. Repeat direct current cardioversion at 400 J. If fine ventricular fibrillatory waves are present, attempt to induce coarser high-amplitude waves by administering epinephrine (0.2 to 1 ml/1:1000 dilution i.e., 200 to 1000 μg) IV or by intracardiac injection. Calcium chloride, 10 ml administered IV or by intracardiac injection, may have a similar effect on the fibrillatory waves. Following the development of high-amplitude fibrillatory waves, electrical cardioversion should be repeated.

In refractory ventricular fibrillation procainamide or bretylium tosylate may be effective.

If ventricular fibrillation cannot be terminated, assess metabolic factors such as acidosis or hypoxia. Sodium bicarbonate may be required to reverse acidosis. These factors may make cardioversion difficult.

The use of automatic implantable cardioverter-defibrillator (AICD) should be strongly considered in patients with recurrent ventricular fibrillation (see Chapter 13).

  B. Treatment of Ventricular Tachycardia
    1. Quickly assess the patient's stability. If ventricular tachycardia results in significant hypotension or congestive heart failure, immediate direct current cardioversion should be performed as just described. Following the restoration of sinus rhythm, IV lidocaine should be administered as just described.
    2. If the patient is hemodynamically stable, initiate pharmacologic cardioversion.

a) The preferred drug is lidocaine. It should be given as just described for ventricular fibrillation. If ventricular tachycardia persists or recurs, give repeated boluses up to a total of 300 mg and start a continuous IV infusion.

b) If ventricular tachycardia is refractory to lidocaine, administer procainamide (Pronestyl) in IV boluses of 100 mg given slowly. Boluses of 100 mg may be administered every 5 min, up to a total of 1000 mg or until hypotension or successful cardioversion occurs. A procainamide drip of 2 to 4 mg/min may likewise be instituted if ventricular irritability persists.

c) Bretylium tosylate administered as an IV bolus followed by a continuous infusion has proven to be effective in some cases refractory to lidocaine or procainamide.

d) Other drugs that may be effective for persistent ventricular tachycardia include quinidine and propranolol (Inderal). Phenytoin (Dilantin) is the drug of choice for digitalis-induced ventricular tachycardia.

e) If ventricular tachycardia persists even after injection of lidocaine and bretylium, other new antiarrhythmic agents (e.g., amiodarone) should be tried (see Chapter 13).

3. If pharmacologic conversion is unsuccessful or if recurrent bouts of ventricular tachycardia occur, artificial pacing with an overdriving rate should be considered. Antitachycardia pacing in the treatment of refractory ventricular tachycardia has been described in detail elsewhere (see Chapter 15).

C. Treatment of Supraventricular Tachyarrhythmias

In elderly patients who have an underlying impairment of cardiovascular performance, rapid supraventricular tachyarrhythmias may cause profound hypotension and cardiovascular collapse. If a profound degree of cardiovascular decompensation is caused by a supraventricular tachyarrhythmia, direct current cardioversion is appropriate. But if in the presence of such an arrhythmia the patient has no evidence of a lack of organ perfusion, no significant neurologic change, and an adequate blood pressure, one may use appropriate drugs including verapamil, digoxin, and propranolol that may require varying periods of time to take effect.

D. Treatment of Bradyarrhythmias

1. Mild-to-Moderate Sinus Bradycardia (More than 40 beats/min). As an isolated phenomenon, mild-to-moderate sinus bradycardia unaccompanied by other cardiovascular abnormalities may not require treatment. On the other hand if associated hypotension is present, atropine, 0.5 to 1 mg, may be administered IV. Administration of a volume load may be of value if hypotension persists.

2. Severe Sinus Bradycardia (Less than 40 beats/min) or second-degree or advanced AV block. The clinical setting dictates

the therapeutic approach. If increased vagal tone seems to play a role in the genesis of the bradyarrhythmias, as it does in patients who have acute diaphragmatic (inferior wall) myocardial infarction, the administration of atropine would be valuable in increasing the heart rate. Administer atropine as a bolus of 0.5 mg IV. If the heart rate does not increase within 3 min, administer an additional bolus of 0.5 mg. If no response occurs to atropine, proceed as with complete AV block.

When marked and persisting sinus bradycardia is refractory to atropine or isoproterenol (Isuprel), the presence of the sick sinus syndrome should be strongly considered.

The use of an artificial pacemaker is generally recommended in all patients with Mobitz type II AV block regardless of the presence or absence of significant symptoms.

3. Intraventricular Block. Prophylactic artificial pacing is recommended for all patients who develop acute left bundle branch block, left posterior hemiblock, or bifascicular block (a combination of right bundle branch block and left anterior or posterior hemiblock) with or without coexisting AV block as a result of acute anterior wall myocardial infarction.

4. Complete AV Block. Start an IV infusion of isoproterenol of 2 to 4 μg/min. If the ventricular rate is slow, a 100 μg bolus of isoproterenol may be given IV while the infusion is continued.

If no response occurs to isoproterenol, an epinephrine 100 μg bolus, and an infusion of 2 to 4 μg/min may be effective.

If despite the measures just described the bradycardia is not reversed, insertion of a transvenous pacemaker is indicated.

When complete AV block is chronic, especially when the block is considered in the infranodal region (complete trifascicular block), permanent implantation of an artificial pacemaker is indicated.

5. Asystole. Administer epinephrine (Adrenalin) or isoproterenol as a 500 μg bolus IV or by intracardiac injection. Calcium chloride may have a synergistic-chronotropic effect. Calcium chloride should likewise be administered IV or by intracardiac injection. If the patient has been treated with propranolol and is likely to have continuing beta-blockade, IV injection of 10 mg of glucagon may also be effective. If it is technically and logistically feasible to insert an artificial pacemaker, that also should be done. A balloon-flotation electrode is the most expeditious means of such emergency pacemaker insertion. A pacemaker with transcutaneous external pacing electrodes has been described. Although it is too early to know what role this device may play, it could facilitate pacing in emergent circumstances.

If an underlying rhythm is restored, an epinephrine or isoproterenol drip may be required to maintain such rhythm.
E. Hemodynamic Status

When a stable cardiac rhythm is restored, attention must be directed toward the adequacy of perfusion. Significant depression of cardiac performance may occur during the period of resuscitation as well as from the underlying cause of the cardiovascular collapse. A long-term approach to ensure adequacy of cardiac performance must be formulated, based on the underlying primary problems. The short-term approach to maintaining cardiac performance may include the use of a variety of inotropic drugs, including isoproterenol, epinephrine, dopamine, dobutamine, calcium chloride, and glucagon.

IX. OTHER MEASURES
A. Ventilation

If continued resuscitative efforts are required following the institution of artificial ventilation, consideration should be given to the insertion of an endotracheal or nasotracheal tube. Such a tube permits more effective pulmonary expansion, the administration of oxygen in high concentration, and the removal of secretions or vomitus from the bronchi by suction. Although such an airway is desirable, it should be inserted only by someone who can do so quickly and adequately. It should not be inserted by a novice whose fumbling efforts may stop resuscitation for a prolonged period. Following the insertion of a tracheal airway, the cuff should be inflated to prevent any further aspiration of vomitus. Manual ventilation co-ordinated with cardiac massage should continue. Self-triggering ventilators should not be used unless they are fully co-ordinated with cardiac massage. The adequacy of ventilation should be determined by serial assessments of the arterial blood gases.

B. Treatment of Acidosis

Metabolic acidosis is a result of inadequate tissue perfusion and oxygenation. Respiratory acidosis occurs if there is significant underlying pulmonary disease, airway obstruction, or inadequate artificial ventilation. If resuscitative efforts are initiated without delay, only minimal metabolic acidosis may occur. The best way to assess the need for bicarbonate replacement is to sample arterial blood to determine the pH, HCO_3, PCO_2, and PO_2. Acidosis with an elevated PCO_2 and a normal or slightly decreased HCO_3 indicates respiratory acidosis. In such a case, bicarbonate replacement is not of major value, and more effective ventilation is required. But if acidosis is accompanied by a normal PCO_2 and a decrease in bicarbonate, metabolic acidosis is present. Bicarbonate should be administered with serial assessment of the arterial blood gases to evaluate the efficacy of the treatment and continuing needs. If arterial blood gas values cannot be determined, it is difficult to assess the need for bicarbonate. Several regimens are prescribed in the literature as guides to bicarbonate therapy. Sodium bicarbonate should be given if the arrest is longer than 1 minute. The initial amount is 1 mEq/kg sodium bicarbonate followed by 0.5 mEq/kg sodium bicarbonate every 10 min. It is important to correct acidosis because it decreases cardiac and peripheral responses to catecholamines, lowers the threshold of ventricular fibrillation, and may induce cardiac asystole.

C. Treatment of Electrolyte Imbalance

Significant derangements of serum electrolytes may lead to various cardiac arrhythmias. Either hyperkalemia or hypokalemia may cause various cardiac arrhythmias, including ventricular irritability. In particular, hypokalemia frequently predisposes to digitalis-induced cardiac arrhythmias. Serum electrolyte values should be determined, and appropriate corrective therapy is essential. Hyperkalemia may be recognized on the electrocardiogram by tall, peaked T waves.

X. TERMINATION OF CARDIOPULMONARY RESUSCITATION

Cardiopulmonary resuscitation should be terminated for two major reasons: the first reason is failure to restore an appropriate cardiac rhythm and adequate pump performance; the second reason is evidence of severe and irreversible cerebral damage. Cardiopulmonary resuscitation should be continued until all the methods of restoring cardiopulmonary stability have been tried. If at that point the heart appears to be unable to maintain an adequate cardiac rhythm and mechanical performance, CPR should be terminated.

Determination of the severity of the neurologic damage is often difficult (and it can have medicolegal ramifications). Severe neurologic damage is suggested by unconsciousness, absence of spontaneous movement, absence of spontaneous respiration, absence of spontaneous eye movements, pupillary dilatation without response to light, and "boxcarring" of the retinal vessels. Although those are not absolute signs of permanent neurologic impairment they suggest severe, potentially irreversible damage and they point toward termination of CPR.

XI. CARE AFTER CARDIOPULMONARY RESUSCITATION

Following successful CPR, assessment of the initial cause and recognition of any persistent risk factors are essential. If any premonitory abnormalities of cardiac rhythm are present they should be treated prophylactically. If an acute myocardial infarction is evident, assessment of the patient's hemodynamic status and cardiac rhythm should be continued in a cardiac care unit. If pulmonary insufficiency is evident, careful attention should be directed to assuring adequacy of ventilation by monitoring the blood gases. If a pulmonary embolism is suspected, the patient must be given anticoagulation therapy with heparin.

A complete assessment of the degree of recovery should be part of post-CPR care. Particular attention should be directed to the patient's neurologic status. If cerebral edema is suspected the following measures may be of value: maintenance of arterial perfusion pressure from 70 to 110 mm Hg, hyperventilation to increase P_{O_2} and to decrease P_{CO_2} to 25 to 35 mm Hg, osmotic or loop diuretics, and corticosteroid administration.

All patients who have been revived with CPR should be observed for several weeks to ensure their stability. During that time, emergency resuscitative facilities should be immediately available. An evaluation of the underlying mechanism should be performed to try to avoid recurrent episodes. A study of the underlying coronary anatomy and left ventricular pump function is helpful in selected patients. Evaluation of primary arrhythmic disturbances should be performed and has been facilitated by electrophysiologic evaluation. If electrophysiologic studies are not available, suppression of any obvious arrhythmias is mandatory.

XII. RESULTS OF CARDIOPULMONARY RESUSCITATION

Many factors determine the success of CPR. The speed with which CPR is instituted and the underlying cause of the cardiopulmonary collapse are important in determining ultimate recovery. Survival has been enhanced in out-of-hospital cardiac arrest in which there is bystander initiated CPR. This of course requires a vast community education effort. Survival has also been enhanced by the immediate availability of defibrillation if emergency rescue personnel are trained to defibrillate in addition to initiating basic life support. The best survival rates seem to occur in coronary artery disease in which a nonrecurring arrhythmia initiated the cardiac arrest. Such would be the case with acute myocardial infarction. The likelihood of success is greatest if ventricular tachycardia is the underlying rhythm and least if asystole or bradycardia is the observed rhythm. Ventricular fibrillation has an intermediate likelihood of success. Higher rates of survival are also noted with drug overdose or in patients undergoing anesthesia. Variable success has been reported with cardiomyopathy, pulmonary embolism, and respiratory insufficiency. Although one would expect that the best results are noted in an intensive or coronary care unit because of the constant attention given the patients, this has actually not been the case. Because only the sickest patients are in the intensive care unit, survival has been as good (if not better) in a well staffed medical ward in which patients are generally less acutely ill. Age and sex are not major determinants of success in CPR.

Survival figures vary from series to series, and they are difficult to compare because of different patient subgroups and different criteria of success. Discharge rates of from 4 to 23% have been reported. Of those patients who survive to be discharged from the hospital, 49% have subsequently been reported on one study to subsequently survive for 4 additional years. An evaluation of the quality of life following successful CPR demonstrated that 93% of the survivors were mentally intact at the time of discharge. Although depression was generally present at the time of discharge, it tended to resolve subsequently. All patients, however, reported some decrease in functional capacity. Both physical limitation and fear caused these limitations. The 38 mentally competent survivors in this study were questioned as to whether they would choose to be resuscitated in the future if necessary. Twenty-one (55%) said yes, sixteen (42%) said no, and one was ambivalent.

XIII. SUMMARY

1. Unexpected cardiopulmonary collapse is a medical emergency that requires immediate institution of artificial measures to support life and to reverse the initiating pathophysiologic event. To approach the problem efficiently, one must have a plan that can be implemented at a moment's notice.

2. The initial goals of CPR are to establish an airway, to institute artificial breathing, and to restore circulation. If those measures do not result in immediate recovery, assessment of cardiac rhythm, cardiac pump performance, ventilatory adequacy, acid-base balance, and serum electrolytes is required.

3. The primary therapeutic modalities are direct current defibrillation, intervention to restore sinus rhythm and normal blood pressure, and procedures to restore normal oxygenation and acid-base balance.

4. If CPR is successful, continued surveillance of the patient is required for complete assessment and for immediate intervention if cardiopulmonary collapse recurs.

5. Successful resuscitation, as defined by hospital discharge, has been reported in various series to occur in 4 to 23% of the patients who undergo CPR.

6. Every physician, nurse, and paramedical person should be capable of delivering CPR, regardless of his specialty. Ideally, this capability should be extended to the lay public.

7. For recurrent ventricular fibrillation, the use of AICD should be strongly considered. Likewise, anti-tachycardia pacing is indicated for refractory ventricular tachycardia.

8. Even after successful CPR, it is essential to investigate and treat any underlying heart disease and cardiac arrhythmias which caused cardiopulmonary arrest.

SUGGESTED READINGS

Bedell, S.E., Delbanco, T.L., and Cook, E.F.: Survival after cardiopulmonary resuscitation in the hospital. N. Engl. J. Med. *309*:569, 1983.

Brunetti, L.L., Weiss, M.J., Studenski, S.A. and Clipp, E.C.: Cardiopulmonary resuscitation policies and practices. Arch. Intern. Med. *150*:121, 1990.

Chandra, N., Rudikoff, M. and Weisfeldt, M.L.: Simultaneous chest compression and ventilation at high airway pressure during cardiopulmonary resuscitation. Lancet *1*:175, 1980.

Curran, W.J., Hyg, S.M.: Law-Medicine notes, the Saikewicz decision. N. Engl. J. Med. *298*:499, 1978.

Eisenberg, M.S., Hallstrom, A., and Bergner, L.: Long-term survival after out-of-hospital cardiac arrest. N. Engl. J. Med. *306*:1340, 1982.

Falk, R.H., Zoll, P.M and Zoll, R.H.: Medical Intelligence. Safety and efficacy of noninvasive cardiac pacing. A preliminary report. N. Engl. J. Med. *309*:1166, 1983.

Fox, M., and Lipton, H.L.: The decision to perform cardiopulmonary resuscitation. N. Engl. J. Med. *309*:607, 1983.

Gascho, J.A., Crampton, R.S., Sipes, J.N., et al.: Energy levels and patient weight in ventricular defibrillation. JAMA *242*:1380, 1979.

Gilston, A., and Leeds, M.B.: Clinical and biochemical aspects of cardiac resuscitation. Lancet *II*:1039, 1965.

Goldberg, A.H.: Cardiopulmonary arrest. N. Engl. J. Med. *290*:381, 1974.

Harwood-Nash, D.C.F.: Thumping of precordium in ventricular fibrillation. S. Afr. Med. J. *36*:280, 1962.

Heimlich, H.J.: A life-saving maneuver to prevent food-choking. JAMA *234*:398, 1975.

Herre, J.M.: Management of patients resuscitated from cardiac arrest. Cardiovas. Rev. & Rep. *11*:33, 1989.

Hollingsworth, J.H.: The results of cardiopulmonary resuscitation. A 3-year university hospital experience. Ann. Intern. Med. *71*:459, 1969.

Johnson, A.L., Tanser, P.H., Ulan, R.A., and Wood, T.E.: Results of cardiac resuscitation in 552 patients. Am. J. Cardiol. *20*:831, 1967.

Kamer, R.S., Dieck, E.M., McClung, J.A., et al.: Effect of New York State's do-not-resuscitate legislation on in-hospital cardiopulmonary resuscitation practice. Am. J. Med. *88*:108, 1990.

Kellermann, A.L., Hackman, B.B., Somes, G.: Dispatcher-assisted cardiopulmonary resuscitation. Circulation *80*:1231, 1989.

Kouwenhoven, W.B., Ing, J.J.R., and Knickerbocker, G.G.: Closed-chest cardiac massage. JAMA *173*:94, 1960.

Linko, E., Koskinen, P.J., Siitonen, L., et al.: Resuscitation in cardiac arrest. An analysis of 100 successful medical cases. Acta Med. Scand. *182*:611, 1967.

Lown, B., Neuman, J., Amarasingham, R., and Berkovits, B.V.: Comparison of alternating current with direct current electroshock across the closed chest. Am. J. Cardiol. *10*:223, 1962.

Luce, J.M., Cary, J.M., Ross, B.K., et al.: New developments in cardiopulmonary resuscitation. JAMA *244*:1366, 1980.

McCrea, W.A., Hunter, E., and Wilson, C.: Integration of ambulance staff trained in cardiopulmonary resuscitation with a medical team providing prehospital coronary care. Br. Heart J. *62*:417, 1989.

Murphy, D.J., Murray, A.M., Robinson, B.E. and Campion, E.W.: Outcomes of cardiopulmonary resuscitation in the elderly. Ann. Intern. Med. *111*:199, 1989.

Myerburg, R.J., Kessler, K.M., Zaman, L., et al.: Survivors of prehospital cardiac arrest. JAMA *247*:1485, 1982.

Nelson, D., and Ashley, P.F.: Rupture of the aorta during closed-chest cardiac massage. JAMA *193*:115, 1965.

Pantridge, J.F., and Geddes, J.S.: A mobile intensive-care unit in the management of myocardial infarction. Lancet *II*:271, 1967.

Pennington, J.E., Taylor, J., and Lown, B.: Chest thump for reverting ventricular tachycardia. N. Engl. J. Med. *283*:1192, 1970.

Relman, A.S.: The Saikewicz Decision: Judges as physicians. N. Engl. J. Med. *298*:508, 1978.

Safar, P.: Pathophysiology and resuscitation after global brain ischemia. Int. Anesthesiol. Clin. *17*:239, 1979.

Saphir, R.: External cardiac massage. Prospective analysis of 123 cases and review of the literature. Medicine *47*:73, 1968.

Scharf, D., and Bonnemann, C.: Thumping of the precordium in ventricular standstill. Am. J. Cardiol. 5:30, 1960.

Standards and Guidelines for Cardiopulmonary Resuscitation (CPR) and Emergency Cardiac Care (ECC). JAMA 244:453, 1980.

Taylor, G.J., Rubin, R., Tucker, M., et al.: External cardiac compression. A randomized comparison of mechanical and manual techniques. JAMA 240:644, 1978.

Taylor, G.J., Tucker, W.M., Greene, H.L., et al.: Importance of prolonged compression during cardiopulmonary resuscitation in man. Medical Intelligence 296:1515, 1977.

Thompson, R.G., Hallstron, A.P., and Cobb, L.A.: Bystander-initiated cardiopulmonary resuscitation in the management of ventricular fibrillation. Ann. Intern. Med. 90:737, 1979.

Tresch, D.D., and Thakur, R.K.: Issues in resuscitation of the elderly after cardiac arrest. Cardiology Board Review 7:20, 1990.

Weaver, W.D., Cobb, L.A., Copass, M.K., et al.: Ventricular defibrillation—A comparative trial using 175-J and 320-J shocks. N. Engl. J. Med., 307:1101, 1982.

Wildsmith, J.A.W., Dennyson, W.G., and Myers, K.W.: Results of resuscitation following cardiac arrest. Br. J. Anaesthesiol. 44:716, 1972.

Zoll, P.M., Paul, M.H., Linenthal, A.J., et al.: The effects of external electrical currents on the heart. Circulation 14:745, 1956.

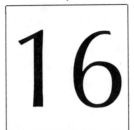

ENDOCARDITIS, MYOCARDITIS AND PERICARDITIS

Jae Ki Ko and Edward K. Chung

The heart is composed of three layers: the endocardium, the myocardium, and the pericardium. Infectious diseases and inflammatory processes can involve either one of these layers or a combination of them. Infectious diseases of the heart are rarely an emergency with the exception of acute infective endocarditis, and cardiac tamponade. However, some of these cardiac disorders should be included in the differential diagnosis of true cardiac emergencies because of their clinical significance.

I. ENDOCARDITIS
    A. General Considerations
        Endocarditis is a microbial infection of the endocardium. It can occur on the valve leaflets (native or prosthetic), endocardial surface, or extracardiac endothelial surfaces (e.g., arteriovenous fistula). Traditionally, endocarditis has been classified as "acute" and "subacute" according to the infecting organism, disease course, and its prognosis. Acute bacterial endocarditis is caused primarily by virulent staphylococci with a short course (days to weeks rather than months), and is fatal if left untreated. On the other hand, subacute bacterial endocarditis (SBE), caused primarily by *streptococcus viridans*, shows a longer (for months) and milder course. By and large, the prognosis is favorable with appropriate therapy.

Over the years, early recognition and antimicrobial therapy have altered the courses of these 2 forms of endocarditis so that an overlap exists between the acute and subacute forms in terms of etiologic agents, clinical course, and prognosis. Thus, the use of the term, "infective endocarditis" has been suggested. At times, however, it is clinically more convenient to classify endocarditis according to causative agents (e.g., Staphylococcal endocarditis, or *Streptococcus viridans* endocarditis).

Significant changes have occurred in the pattern of infective endocarditis in the past 3 decades.

1. The incidence of infective endocarditis has increased among the old age group.
2. The frequency of underlying rheumatic heart disease (RHD) has decreased, whereas degenerative heart diseases and prosthetic valves have taken on a more important role as underlying conditions.
3. There is an increasing incidence of infective endocarditis found among intravenous drug abusers.
4. The incidence of nosocomial infective endocarditis is increasing. Aforementioned changes have also altered the spectrum of infecting organisms. The frequency of streptococcal endocarditis has decreased, whereas that of staphylococcal endocarditis has increased.

B. Etiology

Infective endocarditis may be caused by a variety of microorganisms (e.g., bacteria, fungi, rickettsiae, and possible viruses).

1. Streptococci
   a) Streptococci are still the most common causative agent of infective endocarditis (40 to 50%) even through there has been a decline in their incidence.
   b) *Streptococcus viridans* is responsible for most streptococcal endocarditis.
   c) Other streptococci (microaerophilic and anaerobic) produce infective endocarditis with increasing frequency.
   d) Streptococci (*S. viridans, S. pneumoniae*) are the most common causative agents of late prosthetic valve endocarditis.
2. Staphylococci
   a) *S. aureus* is the most common causative agent of acute endocarditis.
   b) It is highly invasive, and invades previously normal cardiac valves.
   c) *S. aureus* is the most common agent of infective endocarditis among intravenous (IV) drug abusers.
   d) Coagulase-negative *S. epidermidis* is the most common organism in "early" prosthetic endocarditis.

3. Other Bacteria
   Other bacteria may include pneumococci, Neisseria gonorrhea, hemophilus influenza, salmonella species.
4. Fungi
   a) Candida and aspergillus are most commonly responsible for fungal endocarditis.
   b) Fungal endocarditis is characterized by a longer duration with a large arterial embolic occlusion.
   c) It is more likely to occur in patients with indwelling intravascular catheters who have frequently undergone prolonged treatment with corticosteroids and broad spectrum antibiotics or have undergone open heart surgery.
   d) IV drug abusers have an increased risk of fungal endocarditis.

C. Predisposing Factors
   Predisposing factors may include:
   1. Dental procedures
   2. Oropharyngeal operation
   3. Gastrointestinal diagnostic and therapeutic procedures
   4. Genitourinary diagnostic and therapeutic procedures
   5. Hyperalimentation
   6. Burns

D. Underlying Diseases
   1. Rheumatic heart disease (RHD): The importance of RHD for infective endocarditis has decreased over the past 30 years primarily because the incidence of RHD has been reduced significantly. At present, only 40 to 50% of infective endocarditis are encountered in patients with pre-existing RHD.
   2. Congenital heart diseases: Ventricular septal defect (VSD), tetralogy of Fallot, patent ductus arteriosus (PDA), and coarctation of aorta are most commonly associated with infective endocarditis. Atrial septal defect (ASD) with secundum defect carries a negligible risk.
   3. Mitral valve prolapse syndrome (MVPS) with mitral regurgitation
   4. Idiopathic hypertrophic subaortic stenosis (IHSS)
   5. Degenerative calcific aortic valvular stenosis
   6. Prosthetic valve replacement
   7. Myocardial infarction (MI)

E. Pathophysiology
   1. The primary event in the development of infective endocarditis is the transient invasion of microorganisms in the blood circulation.
   2. Infecting organisms usually originate from the oropharynx, gastrointestinal tract, genitourinary tract, lungs, or skin.
   3. Microorganisms can deposit on either damaged or normal endothelial surfaces and serve as a nidus for the aggregation of fibrin and platelets. Vegetations are formed and may consist of bacteria fibrin, platelets, leucocytes, and red blood cell debris.

    4. Vegetations usually develop on the low pressure side (e.g., the ventricular surface of the aortic valve in aortic regurgitation and the atrial side in mitral regurgitation).

    5. Infective endocarditis involves primarily the left side of the heart. Among IV drug abusers, however, the tricuspid valve is more commonly involved.

    6. Vegetations may extend to adjacent intracardiac structures leading to various complications (e.g., rupture of papillary muscle, ring abscess of the aortic valve, conduction defects, and cardiac tamponade).

    7. Embolization of vegetations may result in a variety of systemic complications (see below).

F. Clinical Manifestations

    Clinical symptoms and signs result from the following pathophysiologic mechanisms.

    1. Bacteremia produces nonspecific constitutional symptoms (e.g., fever, malaise, loss of appetite, anorexia, vomiting) and signs (e.g., anemia and splenomegaly).

    2. Infection on the valve and local invasion may cause valvular regurgitation, congestive heart failure (CHF), rupture of the chordae tendineae or papillary muscles, fistular formation, pericarditis with cardiac tamponade, ring abscess, or conduction defect.

    3. Embolization may involve brain, kidneys, spleen, myocardium, and other sites of the body resulting in stroke, renal infarction, splenic infarction, and MI.

    4. Metastatic infection produces abscesses and mycotic aneurysms. Most commonly, these metastatic emboli travel to brain, spleen, kidneys, superior mesenteric artery, and coronary arteries.

    5. As immunologic phenomena, circulating immune complexes may cause glomerulonephritis, Roth's spot, Janeway lesions, Osler's node, arthritis, and pericarditis.

G. Physical Findings

    1. Fever is the most frequent sign, but may be absent in elderly patients and individuals with CHF, uremia, or intracerebral hemorrhage (10 to 15%).

    2. Pallor and anemia (75 to 80%).

    3. Heart murmurs (80 to 90%).

    4. Skin manifestations:

      a) Petechiae (20 to 40%) are the most common frequent lesions.

      b) Splinter hemorrhage (vertical streaks under the nail).

      c) Osler's nodes (15%) are subcutaneous, tender and erythematous papules in the pulp of the distal fingers.

      d) Janeways lesions (10%) are small, erythematous and nontente macules on the hypothenar eminences of the hands and soles.

      e) Clubbing of fingers (10 to 20%).

5. Ocular manifestations:
Roth's spot (less than 5%) is a flame-shaped hemorrhage with a pale center in the retina.
6. Splenic manifestations:
   a) Splenomegaly (25 to 30%)
   b) Splenic infarction (50%)
   c) Rupture of spleen (rare)
H. Complications
  1. Cardiac complications
    a) CHF is the most common and serious complication, and is the most common cause of death.
    b) Myocardial abscess
    c) Pericarditis with cardiac tamponade
    d) Myocardial infarction (MI)
  2. Extracardiac complications
    a) Renal
      (1) Renal infarction
      (2) Glomerulonephritis (focal or diffuse)
      (3) Renal abscess
      (4) Cortical necrosis
      (5) Renal failure
    b) Neurologic
      (1) Cerebrovascular disease is the most frequent neurologic complication.
      (2) Toxic syndromes; headache, insomnia and vertigo.
      (3) Psychiatric; confusion, psychosis, neurosis and disorientation.
      (4) Spinal cord or peripheral nerves involvement; girdle pain paresis and mononeuritis.
    c) Splenic; infarction, abscess, rupture.
    d) Mycotic aneurysms
    e) Pulmonary; embolism, pneumonia, abscess.
 I. Laboratory Findings
  1. Hematologic findings
    a) Normocytic normochromic anemia (75 to 80%)
    b) Elevated erythrocyte sedimentation rate (90%)
    c) Leucocytosis
    d) Thrombocytopenia
    e) Elevated serum gamma globulin
  2. Urinalysis: Urinalysis is usually normal but patients with renal complication may show microscopic or macroscopic hematuria, proteinuria, or red blood cell casts.
  3. Blood culture: Blood culture is the most important laboratory test to identify the infecting microorganism and determine the most appropriate therapeutic agents. Blood culture should be done 3 separate times (10 to 15 min intervals) 24 hours prior to initiation of antimicrobial therapy. At least 2 weeks of incubation is required both aerobically and anaer-

obically. Culture-negative endocarditis may occur in 10 to 15% of the patients.

4. Electrocardiography: Serial ECGs may be helpful in acute infective endocarditis (i.e., staphylococcal infection) since a septal abscess may form and may produce significant conduction defects.

5. Chest roentgenography: Chest X-ray may show signs of underlying heart diseases. Various complications including CHF, pulmonary embolism, pulmonary infarction, pneumonia, and lung abscess may be detected.

6. Echocardiography: Echocardiography can detect vegetations as well as intracardiac complications in up to 80% of the patients with infective endocarditis. Doppler echocardiography is valuable in detecting early valvular regurgitation and assessing the severity of it.

J. Management
1. General principles
   a) Early recognition and prompt treatment are extremely important. As soon as endocarditis is considered clinically, blood cultures should be obtained 3 to 5 times with 10 to 15 minute intervals. Thereafter empiric antimicrobial therapy should be instituted promptly and continued until the results of the blood cultures become available.
   b) The antimicrobial agent(s) of choice should be:
      (1) Bactericidal
      (2) In sufficient dosage and duration of administration
      (3) Administered parenterally (intravenously)
      (4) Free of toxic side effects during prolonged administration
      (5) Individually curtailed.
   c) No anticoagulant should be used. There is no advantage in preventing embolization. Anticoagulants are hazardous since they may cause severe hemorrhage.
   d) Surgery is another therapeutic modality. It has reduced the mortality of infective endocarditis.
2. Specific treatments
   a) Streptococcal endocarditis
      (1) Penicillin G 10 to 20 million units/day IV in divided dosage every 4 hours for 4 weeks.
      (2) Penicillin G 10 to 20 million units/day in divided doses every 4 hours plus gentamicin 1 mg/kg IV every 8 hours or streptomycin 0.5 g intramuscularly (IM) every 12 hours for 2 weeks.
      (3) In case of penicillin hypersensitivity, vancomycin 500 to 700 mg/kg every 6 hours IV for 4 weeks.
   b) Enterococcal endocarditis
      (1) Penicillin G 20 to 40 million units/day IV in divided doses every 4 hours for 4 to 6 weeks.
      (2) Ampicillin 12 gm/day IV in divided doses every 4

hours plus streptomycin 0.5 gm IM every 12 hours, or gentamicin 1 mg/kg IV for 4–6 weeks.
   (3) In case of penicillin hypersensitivity, vancomycin 500 to 700 mg/kg every 6 hours IV plus gentamicin 1 mg/kg IV every 8 hours or streptomycin 0.5 gm IM every 12 hours for 4 to 6 weeks.
   c) Staphylococcal endocarditis
      (1) Penicillin-sensitive endocarditis: penicillin G 20 to 30 million units/day IV in divided doses every 4 hours for 4 to 6 weeks.
      (2) Penicillinase-producing endocarditis: nafcillin, methicillin, or oxacillin 12 gm/day in divided doses every 4 hours for 6 weeks.
      (3) In case of penicillin hypersensitivity, vancomycin 500 mg IV every 6 hours for 4 to 6 weeks.
   d) Fungal endocarditis
      (1) Amphotericin B 1 to 1.5 mg/kg/day IV.
   e) Culture-negative infective endocarditis
      (1) Penicillin G 20 to 30 million units/day in divided doses every 4 hours plus gentamicin 1 mg/kg IV.
   f) Prosthetic valve endocarditis
      (1) Prosthetic valve endocarditis should be treated according to the etiologic agents with two drugs of synergy for 6 to 8 weeks or in combination with early surgical intervention.
   g) Surgical therapy should be considered in the following conditions.
      (1) CHF refractory to medical therapy
      (2) Recurrent septic embolization
      (3) Persistent presence of the causative organism despite adequate treatment
      (4) Fungal endocarditis
K. Prognosis
   Prognosis depends on the type of the infecting organisms, involved valve, presence of complications, patient's age, and duration of the disease before the initiation of treatment. The following factors are poor prognostic indicators:
   1. Advanced age (over 60 years of age)
   2. Involvement of aortic or prosthetic valves
   3. Infective endocarditis caused by staphylococcal, gram-negative bacteria, or fungi
   4. Presence of significant complications
   5. Presence of debilitating diseases (e.g., diabetes mellitus or cirrhosis of the liver)
   6. Delayed diagnosis and treatment.
II. MYOCARDITIS
   A. General considerations
      Myocarditis is an inflammatory process of the myocardium with necrosis and/or degeneration of adjacent myocytes. It may

be focal or diffuse. Myocarditis may be classified as acute, sub-acute, or chronic depending upon the progress of the disease. Classification may also follow the etiologic factors. The clinical picture ranges from little or no symptom to life-threatening CHF and even sudden death.

B. Etiology

A variety of infectious and noninfectious agents are known to cause myocarditis. In the United States, various viruses are considered to be the most common etiologic agents.

1. Infectious
   a) Viruses: Coxsackie (A and B), echo, polio, adeno, influenza, hepatitis, vaccinia, and human immunodeficiency virus.
   b) Bacteria: Staphylococci, streptococci, pneumococci, meningococci, gonococci, diphtheria, and mycobacteria tuberculosis.
   c) Mycoplasma
   d) Protozoa: Toxoplasma cruzi (Chagas' disease), toxoplasma gondii, and plasmodium falciparum.
   e) Parasites: Trichinella spirallis, and echinococcosis granulosis.
   f) Rickettsiae: R. rickettsii, R. brunettii, and scrub typhus.
   g) Fungi: Aspergillus, candida, and histoplasma.
   h) Spirochetes: Leptospira, Lyme's disease, and relapsing fever.

2. Noninfectious
   a) Drugs: phenothiazine derivatives, penicillin derivatives, cocaine, lithium, and methyldopa, etc.
   b) Connective tissue diseases: systemic lupus erythematosus, and rheumatoid arthritis.
   c) Physical agents: radiation, heat stroke, and hypothermia.
   d) Insect stings.

C. Clinical Manifestations

Symptoms and signs of myocarditis depend on the location and the extent of the lesion and the clinical course of the disease process. Patients with focal myocarditis are totally asymptomatic and may go unrecognized. However, diffuse involvement can cause fulminating CHF and even sudden death.

1. There may be nonspecific, infection-related symptoms (fever, cough, nausea, vomiting, diarrhea, myalgia and pleurodynia, etc.).
2. Chest pain is the most common cardiovascular symptom.
3. Fatigue, exertional dyspnea, and CHF may result from multifocal or diffuse involvement.
4. Even sudden death can ensue.

D. Physical Findings

1. Tachycardia (disproportional to body temperature) is a common finding.
2. The first heart sound is usually soft.

    3. The third or fourth heart sound may be heard.

    4. Pericardial friction rub may be audible if myocarditis extends to the pericardium (myopericarditis).

E. Laboratory Findings

    1. Hematologic findings

        a) Slight to moderate leukocytosis with neutrophilia.

        b) Elevated erythrocyte sedimentation rate.

        c) Elevation of CPK-MB isoenzyme (reflection of the extent of the myocardial enzyme).

    2. Virus isolation and viral antibody titers

        If viral myocarditis is suspected, the diagnosis is confirmed by isolation of the virus and a four-fold increase of viral antibody titers.

    3. Electrocardiography

        The most common characteristic finding is nonspecific ST-T changes. Atrial and ventricular arrhythmias and conduction defects may be observed if conduction system is involved focally or diffusely.

    4. Chest roentgenography

        Patients with CHF may reveal cardiomegaly or pulmonary congestion. It is a useful tool for follow-up study.

    5. Echocardiography

        Two-dimensional echocardiography is valuable in the diagnosis and evaluation of the myocarditis. Echocardiography can detect abnormalities of wall motion and pericardial effusion.

    6. Nuclear imaging

        a) Technetium-99m pyrophosphate scan is useful in identifying focal or diffuse myocardial necrosis.

        b) Gated blood pool scan can be useful in assessing the size, function, and wall motion abnormality of the ventricles.

        c) Indium-111 monoclonal antimycin antibody imaging is a reliable screening method for evaluation of myocarditis.

    7. Endomyocardial biopsy

        a) The procedure is safe and can be repeated.

        b) Endomyocardial biopsy occasionally establishes the specific diagnosis but not its cause.

        c) Serial biopsies may help to evaluate the efficacy of the immunosuppressive therapy.

F. Diagnosis

    Myocarditis should be suspected when there are various symptoms and signs such as unexplained hypotension, tachycardia, fatigue in the setting of new onset of cardiac abnormalities (e.g., CHF and cardiac arrhythmias) without previous heart diseases. Myocarditis can be diagnosed by endomyocardial biopsies.

G. Differential Diagnosis

    1. Pericarditis

    2. Infective endocarditis

3. Coronary atheroslerostic heart diseases
4. Valvular heart diseases.

H. Management

1. In general, the treatment of myocarditis is supportive. Non-viral infectious myocarditis should be treated according to the etiologic agents.
2. As soon as myocarditis is suspected, all patients should be admitted to the hospital for evaluation and proper treatment.
3. Bed rest is recommended until general symptoms as well as signs are improved and all laboratory findings are returned to normal.
4. Continuous ECG monitoring should be performed in early stages in order to detect clinically significant arrhythmias promptly.
5. Symptomatic advanced or complete AV block may require a temporary or even permanent artificial pacemaker.
6. Anticoagulants are indicated for persistent CHF complicated with thromboembolism, but contraindicated when pericarditis is present.
7. The use of corticosteroid and immunosuppressive drugs is still controversial. They should be considered as a last therapeutic measure.
8. For patients with cardiogenic shock, intra-aortic balloon pump may be indicated.
9. Biventricular external cardiac assist devices and cardiac transplantation may be considered if the cardiogenic shock is refractory to aggressive medical therapy and intra-aortic balloon pump.

I. Prognosis

In most cases, myocarditis is benign and self-limited. Some patients, however, may be complicated with conduction defects, malignant arrhythmia, CHF, cardiogenic shock, or even death. Chronic dilated cardiomyopathy may develop in some cases.

III. PERICARDITIS

The pericardium is a closed, flask-shaped sac that consists of an inner serous membrane (visceral pericardium) and an outer fibrous membrane (parietal pericardium). The normal pericardium contains 15 to 50 ml of clear fluid with a composition of plasma ultrafiltrate. Pericarditis is an inflammatory process of the pericardium. It is clinically classified as acute (less than 6 weeks in duration), subacute (6 weeks to 6 months) and chronic (more than 6 months in duration). Acute pericarditis is the most frequent and most important pericardial disease.

A. Acute Pericarditis

Acute pericarditis is characterized by chest pain, pericardial friction rub, and typical ECG changes. It may present as a dry form (pericarditis without effusion) and wet form (pericarditis with pericardial effusion).

1. Etiology
    Acute pericarditis has a variety of etiologies.
    a) Idiopathic.
    b) Infectious.
        (1) Viral: Coxsackie B, echo, influenza, hepatitis B, and mumps
        (2) Bacterial: tuberculosis and other bacteria
        (3) Fungal
        (4) Parasitic
        (5) Rickettsial
        (6) Spirochetal
        (7) Mycoplasma
    c) Connective tissue disease: rheumatoid arthritis, systemic lupus erythematosus, and ankylosing spondylitis.
    d) Hypersensitivity reactions
        (1) Drugs: procainamide, hydralazine, isoniazid, penicillins and methysergide.
        (2) Acute myocardial infarction (MI).
        (3) Dressler's syndrome.
        (4) Postpericardiotomy syndrome.
    e) Metabolic
        (1) Renal failure
        (2) Myxedema
        (3) Cholesterol pericarditis
    f) Trauma
        (1) Penetrating injury
        (2) Nonpenetrating injury
        (3) Cardiac operation
        (4) Cardiac perforation during cardiac catheterization and pacemaker implantation
    g) Neoplasms
        (1) Primary
        (2) Secondary
    h) Radiation
    At present, the most common etiology is idiopathic, and other common causes of acute pericarditis are viruses, uremia, neoplasm, trauma, and acute MI. Coxsackie B virus is the most common etiologic agent of acute viral pericarditis. Antibiotic therapy has made bacterial pericarditis a rare entity. Tuberculous pericarditis was most commonly encountered of all pericarditis in the past, and it is still the most common bacterial pericarditis in the underdeveloped countries.
2. Clinical manifestations
    a) Chest pain is the cardinal symptom of acute pericarditis. The characteristic features are as follows:
        (1) Location: retrosternum or left precordial
        (2) Quality: sharp, stabbing (usually pleuritic and persistent or dull)

   (3) Radiation: trapezius ridge, neck and sometimes left
       arm
   (4) Duration: hours or days
   (5) Aggravating factors: lying supine, coughing, deep
       inspiration, and swallowing
   (6) Alleviating factors: sitting and leaning forward
   b) Dyspnea is noted in the presence of pericardial effusion
      which compresses adjacent bronchi and lungs. Dyspnea
      may be caused by shallow rapid breathing to avoid chest
      pain.
   c) Underlying diseases may cause other specific and non-
      specific complaints.
3. Physical findings
   a) Usually a mild fever is present (37 to 38°C).
   b) The cardinal sign of acute pericarditis is friction rub. It
      is described as "scratching," "grating," or "creaking,"
      and has three components (presystolic, systolic and dia-
      stolic). Friction rub can be best heard by listening with
      the diaphragm of a stethoscope at the left lower sternal
      border with the patient sitting up and leaning forward.
      It may be evanescent or persistent.
   c) If mild pericardial effusion is present, friction rub cannot
      be heard, and heart sounds may be muffled. Ewart's sign
      (dullness to percussion beneath the angle of the left scap-
      ula) may appear due to compression of the lungs by
      effusion. However, it is a rare finding.
4. Laboratory findings
   a) Moderate leukocytosis and increased erythrocyte sedi-
      mentation rate usually are present.
   b) Other laboratory abnormalities may be found depending
      on the underlying etiologies.
   c) Electrocardiography
      ECG abnormalities (Fig. 16–1) occur in 80 to 90% of
      patients with acute pericarditis. Serial ECGs are very
      important in confirming the diagnosis and differentiating
      it from acute myocardial infarction. There are four
      sequential findings.
      (1) S-T segment elevation: In an acute stage, the S-T seg-
          ment shows concave upward elevation in all leads
          except leads aVR and V_1, which are depressed.
      (2) S-T segment returns to baseline and T wave becomes
          flattened when acute phase is over.
      (3) T wave is inverted during subacute stage.
      (4) T wave returns to normal.
   d) Chest roentgenography
      Chest X-ray is, in general, of little value but cardiac
      silhouette may be enlarged if a large pericardial effusion
      is present.

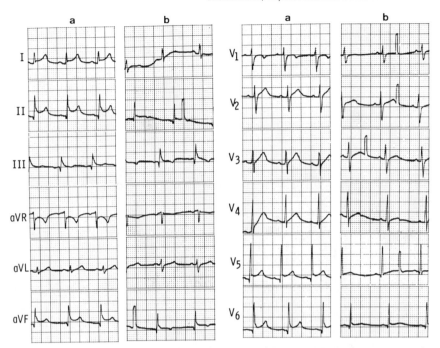

FIG. 16–1. Two ECG tracings (a and b) obtained from the same patient with acute pericarditis. Tracing a shows marked S-T segment elevation in practically all leads (except leads aVR and V_1). Tracing b, taken several days later, reveals much less S-T segment elevation and flattening of T waves in many leads.

 e) Echocardiography
  Echocardiography is the most sensitive and accurate diagnostic method in detection and follow-up of acute pericarditis with pericardial effusion.
5. Diagnosis
  Acute pericarditis can be diagnosed by a characteristic chest pain, friction rub, and typical serial ECG abnormalities. Acute MI is the most important disorder to be differentiated from acute pericarditis. In general, history (characteristics of chest pain), physical examination, cardiac enzymes, ECG findings and other laboratory tests can be useful in the differential diagnosis between them. Other considerations are angina pectoris, pleurisy with or without pleural effusion, pulmonary embolism, aortic dissection, mediastinal emphysema, and chest wall syndromes.
6. Management
  As soon as acute pericarditis is suspected, all patients should be admitted to the cardiac service because a differential diagnosis ought to be made between acute pericarditis and acute MI. Underlying etiologies and their treatment should be pursued.

    a) Nonspecific therapy

      (1) Bed Rest

        Bed rest is essential until pain and fever disappear because physical activity may aggravate the symptoms.

      (2) Pain control

        Pain is well controlled by such nonsteroidal anti-inflammatory agents as aspirin, ibuprofen, or indomethacin. If these drugs fail to alleviate pain and fever, corticosteroids may be considered.

    b) Specific therapy

      Specific treatment regimens should be curtailed according to the underlying etiologies. Acute purulent pericarditis should be treated with specific antibiotics. Surgical treatment is rarely indicated. Tuberculous pericarditis should be treated with antituberculous drugs for 18 to 24 months.

  7. Prognosis

    It depends on the underlying disease. Pericarditis due to idiopathic, viral, postpericardiotomy syndrome, or Dressler's syndrome are usually self-limited and benign. Some patients (20%) may show recurrence.

B. Cardiac Tamponade

  Accumulation of fluid, gas, or both in the pericardium with an increase of intrapericardial pressure may result in cardiac tamponade producing hemodynamic abnormalities (e.g., elevation of intracardiac pressure, limitation of ventricular diastolic filling, and a reduced stroke volume). It is a rare occurrence, but is a true cardiac emergency. It needs prompt diagnosis and treatment.

  1. Etiology

    Cardiac tamponade may result from any cause of pericarditis described previously. Most tamponade arises from, in order of frequency, malignancies, idiopathic pericarditis, uremia, acute MI, and cardiac perforation from diagnostic procedures.

  2. Clinical signs and symptoms

    Clinical features depend on the speed of fluid accumulation and the distensibility of the parietal pericardium. Even a small amount of fluid may cause tamponade if it accumulates very rapidly.

    Claude S. Beck described the classic "triad" of cardiac tamponade: falling arterial pressure, rising venous pressure, and a small quiet heart (acute tamponade). Patients with severe cardiac tamponade may develop stupor and coma leading to death. However, in most patients, cardiac tamponade develops gradually, and a small quiet heart or severe hypotension is rare. The major complaint is dyspnea. Chest

pain, weight loss, anorexia, weakness, and ascites may also be present.
3. Physical findings
   a) Hypotension is common.
   b) Distended neck vein: Jugular venous distension is the most common physical finding with prominent X descent and absent Y descent.
   c) Tachypnea and tachycardia.
   d) Pulsus paradoxus (exaggerated response of normal inspiratory decline of arterial pressure more than 10 mm Hg). It is useful in establishing the diagnosis of cardiac tamponade, but is also found in patients with chronic obstructive pulmonary disease (COPD), hemorrhagic shock, constrictive pericarditis, restrictive cardiomyopathy, and massive pulmonary embolism.
   e) Chest Roentgenogram
      The heart may be normal in "acute" cardiac tamponade, but cardiac silhouette may be enlarged in "chronic" cardiac tamponade.
   f) Echocardiography
      It is the most useful laboratory tool in the diagnosis and follow-up. Echocardiographic findings include:
      (1) Gross swinging motion of the heart.
      (2) An inspiratory increase in right ventricular dimensions with a reciprocal decrease in left ventricular size.
      (3) Right atrial and ventricular diastolic collapse.
      (4) A marked reduction in the E-F slope and excursion of anterior mitral valve leaflet.
      (5) Early systolic notching of anterior right ventricular wall.
   g) Cardiac Catheterization
      It is useful in establishing the hemodynamic significance of pericardial effusion, in confirming clinical diagnosis, and in guiding pericardiocentesis.
4. Management
   There are two general measures in the management of cardiac tamponade.
   a) Removal of Pericardial Fluid
      Cardiac tamponade should be relieved as soon as possible. Pericardial fluid can be drained by following methods:
      (1) Percutaneous pericardiocentesis with a needle or catheter.
      (2) Closed or open pericardiostomy.
      (3) Pericardiectomy.
   b) General Hemodynamic Support
      (1) Intravenous administration of fluid (e.g., saline) can be effective in maintaining cardiac filling.

(2) Inotropic agents (e.g., norepinephrine, dopamine) may be used to improve stroke volume.

After managing an emergent situation, the next step is to search for the underlying cause of cardiac tamponade and its treatment. The recurrence of cardiac tamponade should be prevented.

ACKNOWLEDGMENT

We would like to express our sincere appreciation to Jaeho Lee, M.D., for his valuable assistance in the preparation of this chapter.

SUGGESTED READINGS

GENERAL

Braunwald, E.: *Heart Disease: A Textbook of Cardiovascular Medicine*, 3rd ed. Philadelphia, Saunders, 1988.
Chung, E.K.: *Quick Reference to Cardiovascular Disease*, 3rd ed. Baltimore, Williams & Wilkins Co., 1987.

ENDOCARDITIS

Brandenburg, R.O, Giuliani, E.R., Wilson, W.R., and Geraci, J.E.: Infective endocarditis: A 25 year overview of diagnosis and therapy. J. Am. Coll. Cardiol. *1*:280, 1983.
Cowgill, L.D., Addonizio, V.P., Hopeman, A.R., and Harken, A.H.: Prosthetic valve endocarditis. Curr. Probl. Cardiol., November, 1986.
Kaye, D.: Changing pattern of infective endocarditis. Am. J. Med. *78* (suppl. 6B):157–161, 1985.
Martin, R.P., Meltzer, R.S., Chia, B.L., et al.: Clinical utility of two-dimensional echocardiography in infective endocarditis. Am. J. Cardiol. *46*:379, 1980.
Terpenning, M.S., Buggy, B.P., and Kauffman, C.A.: Hospital-acquired infective endocarditis. Arch. Intern. Med. *148*:1601, 1988.
Weinstein, L., Rubin, R.H.: Infective endocarditis—1973. Prog. Cardiovas. Dis. *16*:239, 1973.

MYOCARDITIS

Kereiakes, D.J., Parmley, W.W.: Myocarditis and cardiomyopathy. Am. Heart J. *108*:1318, 1984.
Kopecky, S.L., Gersh, B.J.: Dilated cardiomyopathy and myocarditis: Natural history, etiology, clinical manifestations, and management. Curr. Probl. Cardiol. October, 1987.
Starling, R.C., Galbraith, T.A., Myero, P.D. et al.: Successful management of acute myocarditis with biventricular assist devices and cardiac transplantation. Am. J. Cardiol. *62*:341, 1988.
Weinstein, C., Fenoglio, J.J.: Myocarditis. Hum. Pathol. *18*:613, 1987.

PERICARDITIS

Guberman, B.A., Fowler, N.O., Engel, P.J., et al.: Cardiac tamponade in medical patients. Circulation *64*:633, 1981.

Permanyer-Miralda, G., Sagrrista-Sauleda, J., Soler-Soler, J.: Primary acute pericardial disease: A prospective series of 231 consecutive patients. Am. J. Cardiol. *56*:623, 1985.

Shabetai, R.: *The Pericardium*. New York, Grune & Stratton, 1981.

Spodick, D.H.: *Pericardial Diseases*. Philadelphia, F.A. Davis, 1976.

Spodick, D.H.: Differential diagnosis of acute pericarditis. Prog. Cardiovas. Dis. *14*:192, 1971.

Reddy, P.S., Curtis, E.I., O'Tool, T.D., Shaner, J.A.: Cardiac tamponade: Hemodynamic observations in man. Circulation *58*:265, 1978.

c h a p t e r

17

HYPERTENSIVE EMERGENCIES

Edward D. Frohlich

I. GENERAL CONSIDERATIONS
   A. Control of arterial pressure is essential in all patients with hypertension; persistent reduction in elevated pressure is associated with a significant decrease in cardiovascular morbidity and mortality.
   B. Selecting appropriate antihypertensive treatment is a complex decision, particularly when the patient has a hypertensive emergency. In this circumstance, pressure reduction is mandatory, although a variety of problems may underlie the crisis. Therefore, the clinical circumstances and the pathophysiologic mechanisms involved with the overall problem must be considered carefully before deciding on the treatment program.
   C. It follows, then, that in order to manage a hypertensive emergency swiftly and effectively the physician must understand the specific conditions that underlie the emergency, the pathophysiologic mechanisms involved that provoked it, and the mechanisms of drug action before therapy is selected. Through this approach the most appropriate means of treatment will be selected.
II. DEFINITIONS
   A. A *hypertensive emergency* is defined as an elevated arterial pressure that is severe enough to require its rapid reduction. Depending on the associated clinical problem, it may be necessary to reduce the elevated pressure *immediately* (i.e., instantly) or *promptly* (less precipitously).

B. *Immediate* reduction of arterial pressure must be achieved within minutes if a patient has severe hypertension associated with acute left ventricular failure or hypertensive encephalopathy.

C. *Prompt* reduction of pressure is required with accelerated or malignant hypertension. Under these circumstances, however, pressure may be reduced over several hours or even a full day.

D. A hypertensive emergency should not be defined in terms of any specific level of arterial pressure above which there is an emergency (i.e., in excess of 120 or 130 mm Hg). Many patients with blood pressure elevations of that magnitude do not present an emergent or life-threatening situation. But, clearly, if these levels persist, the elevated pressure should be reduced.

E. Some authorities have utilized the term *hypertensive urgency* to denote a specific urgency to reduce and control a markedly elevated pressure, per se. However, under the circumstances of this discussion, this neither constitutes a crisis nor an emergency.

F. Some patients may present with associated medical conditions such as cerebral thrombosis, myocardial infarction, or renal failure, that may be life-threatening. These clinical situations are not hypertensive emergencies in and of themselves; the primary medical problem is the stroke, heart attack, or renal failure. This treatment should include control of the elevated arterial pressure as well as other medical concerns—even though the elevated pressure may not be very high. The elevated arterial pressure, therefore, need not be the emergent medical condition.

G. Also excluded from consideration of hypertensive crisis are those patients with hypertension with specific physical findings, such as left ventricular enlargement or an atrial diastolic gallop rhythm. These findings by themselves may very well suggest prolonged hypertensive disease, but they do not denote acute hypertensive left ventricular failure.

III. INITIAL EVALUATION

A. An integral part of the treatment of any patient with hypertension, whether or not the medical problem is a hypertensive emergency, is a complete medical history and physical examination supported by appropriate laboratory evaluation.

B. History. Certain critical questions should be resolved if possible:

1. What was the patient's blood pressure prior to the present situation that now constitutes the hypertensive crisis?

2. Is there a family history of hypertension or a history of premature death?

3. Did the patient complain of any symptoms prior to the illness?

4. Is there evidence of target organ (i.e., brain, heart, kidneys) involvement?

5. What medications (or other drugs) has the patient been receiving? This includes over-the-counter medications.

Table 17–1. Examining the Patient with Hypertensive Crisis for Clues of Target Organ Involvement

System	Symptoms and Signs	
Ocular	Blurred vision Diplopia Extraocular movement abnormalities Retinal arteriolar (and venular) constriction Exudates Hemorrhages Papilledema	
Brain	Headaches Nausea Vomiting Convulsions Localizing sensory or motor deficits	Somnolence Confusion Coma
Cardiovascular	Cardiac awareness Dyspnea Wheezing Edema Rhythm Murmurs Palpitations Paroxysmal nocturnal dyspnea Reduced exercise tolerance Cardiac enlargement Ventricular gallop(s) Abnormal peripheral pulsations (including delay or bilateral comparison) Quality of heart sounds	Chest pain Cough Increasing fatigability Orthopnea Fluid Arrhythmias Ectopic cardiac beats
Renal	Nocturia Peripheral edema Hematuria Renal enlargement Weakness Elevated serum creatinine levels Electrolyte imbalance Urinary sediment Sodium and potassium excretion	Frequent urination Flank pain Oliguria Tenderness, fatigue Appearance of urine Urinary protein

C. Signs and Symptoms. Symptoms and clinical signs that suggest target organ involvement should be thoroughly explored and evaluated (Table 17–1).
   1. Brain involvement may be present if the patient is or has been comatose or if there is a history of convulsions, headaches, nausea, vomiting, or symptoms of sensory or motor deficit.
   2. Reduced exercise tolerance, chest pain, or other symptoms of cardiac awareness, increased fatigability and exertional dyspnea suggest cardiac involvement.

3. Renal involvement is suggested by nocturia, frequent urination, bilateral peripheral edema, fatigue, and weakness. Other symptoms and signs suggesting renal functional impairment include fatigue, weakness, proteinuria, increasing serum creatinine levels, and evidence of anemia.

D. Physical Examination
   1. Carefully evaluate the optic fundi for vascular changes, hemorrhages and exudates, and papilledema.
   2. Listen for cardiovascular abnormalities such as extra heart sounds and murmurs.
      a) Bilateral equality of peripheral arterial pulsations is important.
      b) Note any abnormal pulmonary or other peripheral vascular findings.
      c) Vascular bruits, particularly in the upper abdominal quadrants, having diastolic timing should suggest occlusive renal arterial disease.
      d) Widened abdominal pulsations should suggest an aortic aneurysm.
   3. Neurologic examination
      a) Assess the history of somnolence, confusion, level of consciousness, and sensory or motor deficits.
      b) Quantify any neurologic findings to allow later assessment of how they evolve during the course of the illness.

E. Laboratory Studies. Central to this evaluation are baseline electrolyte and renal function studies, the chest X-ray, and the electrocardiogram.
   1. Hypokalemic alkalosis (in the absence of diuretic therapy) suggests secondary hyperaldosteronism. This may result from renal arterial disease, accelerated or malignant hypertension, or congestive heart failure.
   2. If the patient is unable to assume an upright position for the chest X-ray, it is still possible to estimate cardiac and aortic root sizes by echocardiography. The aortic outflow contour, size of the main pulmonary artery segment, and clarity of the lung fluids may be assessed on a film taken with portable X-ray equipment.
   3. Although it may be difficult to defer treatment for any protracted time period to await more prolonged urinary collection, a quick assessment of renal function may be obtained by the serum creatinine concentration, immediate urinalysis including a study of the urinary sediment, and semiquantitative determination of urinary protein excretion.
      a) If it is possible to defer treatment for 1 to 2 hours, measurements of quantitative urinary protein excretion, endogenous creatinine clearance, and sodium and potassium excretion rates will permit estimation of electrolyte balance and renal function.
      b) Patients with more than 200 to 400 mg protein excreted

per day in the urine suggests parenchymal disease of the kidney.

IV. HEMODYNAMICS OF COMMONLY USED ANTIHYPERTENSIVE AGENTS

A number of different drugs are available for managing hypertensive emergencies (Table 17–2). They differ greatly in their respective modes of action.

A. Vasodilators (direct-acting smooth muscle relaxants).

   1. Diazoxide reduces arterial pressure immediately, primarily through a decrease in arteriolar smooth muscle tone, with little or no change in venous tone. As a result, an intravenous (IV) bolus injection of diazoxide produces a decrease in total peripheral resistance that is associated with a reflexive increase in heart rate, cardiac output, left ventricular contractility, and the shear rate of blood flow.

   2. Nitroprusside (IV infusion) also acts immediately, but it decreases both arteriolar and venular smooth muscle tone. Consequently, vascular resistance and venous return are reduced, thereby lowering arterial pressure through diminished cardiac output and vascular resistance. The reduction in arterial pressure is associated with less reflexive cardiac stimulation, possibly as a result of the associated reduction in venous return.

B. Ganglionic Blocking Agents

   1. Trimethaphan (IV infusion), a ganglionic blocking agent, produces similar hemodynamic effects to nitroprusside. Arterial pressure is reduced immediately; and on cessation of the infusion, like nitroprusside, arterial pressure returns to preinfusion levels.

   2. The reduction in pressure produced by trimethaphan results from a decreased total peripheral resistance.

   3. Because of the greatly diminished venous tone and consequent lowered venous return to the heart associated with both nitroprusside and trimethaphan, a fall in cardiac output and in the left ventricular ejection rate may occur.

C. Angiotensin converting enzyme (ACE) inhibitors are also effective in rapidly reducing arterial pressure, particularly with these agents administered by vein (e.g., lisinopril).

   1. Pressure is reduced through a fall in total peripheral resistance achieved through arteriolar dilation.

   2. This is not associated with reflex cardiac stimulation.

   3. In patients with congestive heart failure, venous return to the heart is also diminished, thereby reducing ventricular preload and improving cardiac output.

   4. Organ blood flows are maintained and renal blood flow may even increase without increasing glomerular filtration rate.

   5. Since generation of angiotensin II is inhibited, aldosterone release from the adrenal cortex is also reduced, thereby

Table 17–2. Antihypertensive Agents Useful for Patients with Hypertensive Crises

A. *Diuretics (intravenous)*
1. Furosemide
2. Bumetanide
B. *Vasodilators direct-acting*
1. Diazoxide (IV)
2. Sodium nitroprusside (IV)
3. Hydralazine (IV, oral)
4. Minoxidil (oral)
5. Magnesium sulfate (IV)
C. *Calcium entry blockers*
1. Diltiazem
2. Isradipine
3. Nifedipine
4. Nimodipine
5. Verapamil
D. *Angiotensin Converting Enzyme Inhibitors*
1. Captopril
2. Enalapril
3. Lisinopril
E. *Adrenergic inhibitors*
1. Ganglion blocker
   Trimethaphan (IV)
2. Central inhibitor
   Cryptenamin (IV)
3. Centrally acting alpha-receptor agonists
   a. Methyldopa (IV, oral)
   b. Clonidine
4. Postganglionic inhibitors
   a. Guanethidine
   b. Bethanidine
   c. Reserpine (subcutaneous, IM)
5. Receptor Antagonists
   a. α-Receptor blockers
      1. Alpha$_1$ and alpha$_2$ receptor blockers:
         a. Phentolamine (IV)
         b. Phenoxybenzamine (oral)
      2. α-Receptor blockers
         a. Prazosin (a)
         b. Terazosin
   b. β-Blocker (for antiarrhythmic or cardiac slowing effect)
      1. Esmolol
      2. Propranolol
      3. Metoprolol
   c. α and β Receptor Blocker (Labetalol)

diminishing the effects of secondary hyperaldosteronism associated with such conditions as congestive heart failure.
D. Calcium Antagonists
   1. Most calcium antagonists reduce arterial pressure very rapidly, usually within 10 to 20 minutes.

    a) Perforated nifedipine capsules have been said to reduce pressure very rapidly. Oral absorption from the gastrointestinal tract is just as fast. This rapid pressure reduction is frequently associated with reflexive cardiovascular stimulation, possibly with unanticipated angina pectoris.

    b) Verapamil can be administered by vein and is useful in slowing cardiac rate, particularly in patients with supraventricular tachycardia.

    c) Nimodipine also reduces pressure rapidly and has been approved for the particular indications of central nervous system hemorrhagic events.

  2. These agents reduce arterial pressure through arteriolar dilation, thereby decreasing total peripheral resistance.

    a) Organ blood flows are preserved; diltiazem and nitrendipine may even increase renal blood flow without increasing glomerular filtration rate.

    b) Reflexive cardiac stimulation, in general, is not found without calcium antagonists (except nifedipine).

E. Physiological Considerations

  1. Reflex considerations. In general, drugs that inhibit adrenergic function do not produce reflex cardiac stimulation. More recent experience with certain other vasodilators (i.e., calcium antagonists and ACE inhibitors) also do not produce reflexive cardiac stimulation. These characteristics should be considered when selecting a potent agent for patients with any type of hypertensive crisis.

    a) For example, patients with congestive heart failure (CHF), severe angina pectoris, or a dissecting aortic aneurysm should not be given a vasodilating drug, such as diazoxide, that will reflexively increase heart rate, cardiac output, left ventricular contractility, and the shear rate of blood flow. These reactions might aggravate the CHF, precipitate or exacerbate angina pectoris, and cause progression of the aortic dissection.

    b) In these patients, selection of nitroprusside, trimethaphan, a calcium antagonist, or an ACE inhibitor may be wiser depending upon the clinical circumstances. On the other hand, diazoxide may be very useful for the patient with acute hypertensive encephalopathy.

  2. Pseudotolerance. In general, when arterial pressure is reduced, capillary hydrostatic pressure also falls, and intravascular volume may expand as fluid moves from the extravascular to the intravascular space. This tends to attenuate the antihypertensive action of the selected drugs and underscores the value of adding a diuretic to the selected agent.

    a) Pseudotolerance is most pronounced with direct-acting smooth muscle relaxant compounds and the adrenergic inhibitors.

    b) Caution is again emphasized for hypokalemia in patients

Table 17–3. Hypertensive Emergencies

1. Hypertensive encephalopathy

2. Malignant and accelerated hypertension

3. Hypertension and intracranial hemorrhage

4. Hypertension and dissecting aortic aneurysm

5. Hypertensive heart failure (with acute pulmonary edema)

6. Myocardial infarction associated with severe hypertension

7. Hypertension following vascular surgery including
   a. "Post-pump" hypertension
   b. Post-coarctation repair

8. Pheochromocytoma crisis

9. Other pressor crisis:
   a. Hypertensive crisis during cardiovascular catheterization procedure
   b. Clonidine-withdrawal hypertension
   c. Guanethidine plus tricyclic antidepressants
   d. Foodstuff-related hypertension associated with MAO-inhibiting drugs
   e. Epinephrine plus β-blockade

10. Acute glomerulonephritis (oliguria or anuria) with hypertension

11. Eclampsia

with hypertensive emergencies that are associated with secondary hyperaldosteronism or cardiac disease.

V. CLINICAL CONDITIONS.

A large number of clinical situations may be associated with severe hypertension that constitutes a hypertensive emergency (Table 17–3). Each hypertensive emergency is characterized by pathophysiologic alterations that demand specific approaches to treatment. Fortunately, there is a broad spectrum of pharmacologic agents available for tailoring therapy to those specific alterations produced by that emergency (Table 17–2).

A. Hypertensive Encephalopathy. This hypertensive emergency may be defined as markedly elevated arterial pressure associated with coma, severe headaches, neurologic symptoms, nausea, and vomiting.

1. Funduscopy reveals severe arteriolar spasm; in fact, the arterioles may not even be seen. The pathophysiology of the patient who has hypertensive encephalopathy should not be considered interchangeable with the patient who has cerebral thrombosis and hypertension.

2. Treatment requires immediate reduction of arterial pressure by a drug that will dilate arterioles.
   a) Injection of diazoxide (IV) or infusion (IV) of nitroprusside will produce immediate disappearance of the headache, nausea, vomiting, and restlessness; emergence from coma; and remission of the neurological symptom.
   b) These symptoms will recur, however, if arterial pressure returns to pretreatment levels.
   c) Other antihypertensive drugs with longer durations of action should be administered concomitantly so that, once pressure is controlled with initial treatment, it can be maintained with a long-term treatment program, preferably with the same antihypertensive agents.
3. Most drugs that reduce arterial pressure through vasodilation or adrenergic inhibition also produce sodium and water retention.
   a) It is most important, at least early in the treatment program with any of these agents, to include a diuretic to prevent this "pseudotolerance."
   b) Fluid retention (or pseudotolerance) is less likely when the ACE inhibitors or the calcium antagonists are used.
   c) Severe hypertensive states may be associated with secondary aldosteronism and hypokalemia. It follows, therefore, that careful monitoring of serum potassium level and its correction, if abnormal, are necessary to prevent the occurrence of cardiac arrhythmias.
B. Accelerated and Malignant Hypertension. If not adequately managed, malignant, or accelerated, hypertension will result in death. Indeed, before the advent of antihypertensive therapy, almost 30% of patients with malignant or accelerated hypertension died within 1 year of diagnosis of their condition.
   1. For the purpose of this discussion, malignant hypertension is the foremost fulminant disease that is manifested by a severely elevated arterial pressure that is associated pathologically with necrotizing arteriolitis and clinically with exudative retinopathy with papilledema, intense renal vasoconstriction with secondary hyperaldosteronism, and immunological changes that may be associated with alterations in circulating globulins, complement and development of microangiopathic hemolytic anemia. Accelerated hypertension is an earlier stage of the disease in which papilledema is not yet manifested.
   2. Associated with the markedly elevated arterial pressures are funduscopic findings of exudative retinopathy (hemorrhages, exudates, and papilledema) and pathognomonic pathologic findings of necrotizing arteriolitis involving all the organs of the body.
   3. When necrotizing arteriolitis involves the kidney, severe renal arteriolar constriction and diminished renal blood flow

promote a release of renin from the kidney and result in increased formation of angiotensin II (i.e., a state of severe secondary aldosteronism). This latter state is manifested by hypokalemic alkalosis.

4. Arterial pressure should be reduced promptly; but, keep in mind 2 therapeutic goals:
    a) The increased total peripheral resistance and renal vasoconstriction should be reduced with minimal cardiac stimulation.
    b) If used, diuretic agents must not further aggravate the secondary aldosteronism.
5. Until recently, the treatment of choice was a potent adrenergic-inhibiting drug (methyldopa or guanethidine) to reduce arterial pressure. The ACE inhibitors have now been shown to be highly effective antihypertensive agents; they are able to decrease total peripheral resistance while improving intrarenal hemodynamics.
    a) As indicated, the ACE inhibitors may be used with or without the addition of a diuretic.
        (1) Be especially cautious with these agents when used with a potassium-retaining agent since dangerous hyperkalemia and its attendant cardiac complications may develop.
        (2) Because malignant hypertension may be exacerbated or develop from unilateral or bilateral occlusive renal arterial disease (or renal arterial disease in a patient with only one kidney), aggravation of the disease with an ACE inhibitor is always a possibility.
6. If an ACE inhibitor is not used, bear in mind that other vasodilators (except calcium antagonists) and adrenergic-inhibiting drugs cause fluid retention.
    a) Thus, diuretics should be prescribed in appropriate dosages to prevent secondary fluid retention.
    b) If the patient is treated with an adrenergic-inhibiting drug, it may be wise to also prescribe spironolactone (a diuretic that antagonizes the renal tubular effects of aldosterone), triamterene or amiloride (agents that also prevent renal potassium wastage), and possibly a thiazide diuretic.
    c) If renal failure further complicates the patient's condition, furosemide (or another potent loop diuretic) could be given in appropriate doses.
    d) In this, or any other, situation, the patient's serum potassium level should be monitored carefully.
7. Calcium entry blocking drugs have also been used to treat patients with accelerated or malignant hypertension.
    a) Some physicians have suggested the additional use of a β-adrenergic blocking drug to prevent the reflex cardiac stimulation, particularly with agents such as nifedipine.

      b) These agents may also inhibit the release of renin from the kidney and thereby attenuate the degree of secondary aldosteronism.

  C. Intracranial Hemorrhage. This hypertensive emergency is associated with headaches, neurologic symptoms, and, frequently, blood in the spinal fluid. It may result from an intracerebral or subarachnoid hemorrhage caused by the rupture of either a Charcot-Bouchard aneurysm, a congenital berry aneurysm of the circle of Willis, or another cerebral vessel.

    1. A computed axial tomography (CAT) scan of the head will help with the diagnosis. However, if this isn't immediately available, lumbar puncture is not contraindicated. If lumbar puncture is performed, it should be done with extreme caution and rapid expediency. Examine the spinal fluid to determine whether blood is present, or whether the fluid is xanthochromic after it is spun down.

    2. If a subarachnoid hemorrhage is considered, cerebral angiography should be performed to locate the arterial aneurysm. This should not be undertaken unless an experienced neurosurgeon is available.

    3. As soon as the suspicion of intracranial hemorrhage is entertained (that is, even before the CAT scan or lumbar puncture), any of the intravenously administered vasodilators or autonomic-inhibiting drugs should be administered to reduce arterial pressure.

      a) If cardiac failure is associated with the intracranial hemorrhage, do not prescribe a direct acting vasodilator (e.g., diazoxide) unless a β-adrenergic blocking drug is given concomitantly and perhaps digitalis is used to protect the myocardium. Under these conditions, an intravenously administered ACE inhibitor is a wise choice.

      b) Because the patient may have coexistent hypokalemia, consider potassium chloride supplementation (in the IV fluid) if a diuretic such as furosemide is used.

    4. Finally, although patients with intracranial hemorrhage are critically ill, immediate treatment should include appropriate physical medicine consultations.

  D. Dissecting Aortic Aneurysm. Most authorities agree that the patient with a dissecting aortic aneurysm should be treated immediately with controlled-rate (IV) hypotensive therapy, regardless of whether the patient has elevated arterial pressure.

    1. In this situation, a vasodilator that produces reflexive cardiac stimulation (e.g., diazoxide) should *not* be used unless the vasodilator's cardiovascular effects are inhibited. This can be accomplished by using an intravenously administered adrenergic-inhibiting drug (usually a β-blocking agent). Otherwise, the increased cardiac output, ventricular ejection rate, and aortic shearing will increase the dissection.

    2. Drugs recommended for the treatment of patients with dis-

secting aortic aneurysms include trimethaphan, nitroprusside, labetalol (IV), and possibly an intravenously-administered ACE inhibitor.

   a) Immediate pressure reduction will instantly relieve the
   pain associated with the dissection.

   b) Again, if a diuretic is administered concomitantly to prevent fluid retention, serum potassium levels should be
   monitored closely.

   3. In addition to immediate pharmacologic therapy, initial
   management of a dissecting aortic aneurysm should include
   diagnostic aortography (and surgical consultation) to identify more precisely the dissection process and to plan for
   surgical correction of the problem should this be feasible.

E. Congestive Heart Failure. Acute pulmonary edema and CHF
associated with hypertension constitute a major hypertensive
emergency.

   1. In this situation, there are 3 precipitating or confounding
   factors for the cardiac failure:

      a) The increased total peripheral resistance (afterload)
      caused by the severely elevated pressure.

      b) The inability of the myocardium to eject the necessary
      stroke volume, which results in a back pressure of blood,
      thereby increasing the ventricular preload.

      c) The secondary aldosteronism (with hypokalemic alka-
      losis) associated with cardiac failure.

   2. Treatment should include an arteriolar and venular vasodilating agent (e.g., nitroprusside or an ACE inhibitor), or
   the sympatholytic agent trimethaphan. In addition, digitalis
   and a diuretic may be considered. These agents will decrease
   both the afterload and the venous return to the heart (which
   reduces preload) and the secondary hyperaldosteronism.

   3. If, however, the pulmonary edema or cardiac failure is not
   that severe, oral administration of an ACE inhibitor is effective and, perhaps, even more physiologic.

      a) This method of pressure reduction by ACE inhibition not
      only reduces left ventricular afterload without reflex car-
      diac stimulation, but it will also interfere with the sec-
      ondary hyperaldosteronism.

      b) In patients without acute pulmonary edema, use of an
      orally administered ACE inhibitor may also be of value
      in avoiding admission to an intensive care unit.

F. Hypertension with Myocardial Infarction (MI) or after Bypass
Surgery. Severely elevated pressures frequently complicate the
treatment of patients who have undergone coronary bypass
surgery, repair of aortic coarctation, or patients with acute MI.
Common to each of these conditions is an adrenergically mediated pressure elevation.

   1. Controlled hypotension, through the use of either trimeth-

aphan or nitroprusside, is the preferred immediate treatment.

2. Diazoxide may aggravate the situation by producing further cardiac stimulation.

3. Longer-acting intravenously-administered agents (e.g., labetalol, ACE inhibitors, calcium antagonists) may complicate the problem if arterial pressure is reduced to inordinately low levels.

4. In most of these patients, the hypertension is self-limited.

  a) But if the hypertension persists, early initiation of long-term antihypertensive therapy is indicated.

  b) Inordinately high pressures may rend open the areas of vessel proximation by sutures.

  c) In patients who have undergone coronary bypass surgery, a possible initiating factor is the sudden discontinuance of β-adrenergic blocking therapy. Appropriate preventive measures may prevent this.

G. Pressor Crisis Associated with Pheochromocytoma. This condition results from release of catecholamines from an adrenal medullary tumor.

1. The catecholamines not only increase vascular resistance through stimulation of alpha-adrenergic receptors, they also may produce cardiac dysrhythmias (due to stimulation of myocardial β-adrenergic receptor sites).

2. In this circumstance, immediate intravenous administration of the alpha-adrenergic blocking drug phentolamine (5 to 10 mg by injection and then by infusion) reduces arterial pressure.

3. Some investigators have used prazosin in these patients if the pressure elevation is less severe.

4. The β-adrenergic blocking drug (propranolol, 1 to 2 mg IV) should also be administered to prevent or manage the catecholamine induced dysrhythmias.

H. Other Pressor Crisis

1. Not infrequently, an alarming rise in arterial pressures occurs during intravascular and intracardiac catheterization studies.

  a) A number of reports have documented the release of catecholamines into the blood stream from a pheochromocytoma once the hypertonic radiopaque contrast material is injected into the blood supply of the tumor. For this reason, monitor arterial pressure in each patient undergoing such studies and have several ampules of an α-adrenergic blocking drug (e.g., phentolamine, 5 to 10 mg IV) available in case a pressor crisis develops.

  b) If phentolamine reduces arterial pressure immediately, a presumptive diagnosis of pheochromocytoma can be made. Withdraw blood samples to measure catecholamine levels and then begin treatment with either phentolamine or phenoxybenzamine, both of which are α-blockers.

   c) It is important that these patients should not receive a rapidly acting IV vasodilator (e.g., diazoxide) or nifedipine sublingually. These patients are usually being studied for coexistent coronary arterial disease.

2. Another type of pressor crisis may develop in patients receiving monoamine oxidase (MAO) inhibitors (e.g., pargyline, iproniazid, or tranylcypromine).

   a) These patients have therapeutically-impaired degradation of endogenously released norepinephrine.

   b) When such patients ingest foods containing tyramine (e.g., certain cheeses, Chianti wine, marinated foods), the tyramine releases normally stored catecholamines from postganglionic sympathetic nerve endings. Arterial pressure rises to extremely critical levels since the norepinephrine is not inactivated.

   c) Treatment consists of administration of the α-adrenergic blocking drug phentolamine, first by IV bolus injection (5 to 10 mg), and then by infusion.

   d) Most authorities also recommend discontinuing the MAO inhibitor and switching to another antihypertensive or antidepressant agent.

3. In contrast, other antidepressant agents (the imipramine and desimipramine derivatives like tricyclic antidepressants) prevent the re-uptake of catecholamines into the postganglionic sympathetic nerve endings.

   a) Since guanethidine and guanadrel act by gaining entrance to the nerve endings, uptake into the nerve ending will be reduced. The drugs may not reduce pressure when administered to a patient who is receiving an imipramine derivative. A pressor emergency may result.

   b) However, if the antidepressant drug is discontinued while the patient continues to take guanethidine or guanadrel, arterial pressure will fall dramatically.

4. Another pressor crisis may be provoked by the sudden cessation of clonidine therapy.

   a) The mechanism that produces this crisis is still incompletely understood, but patients may experience a precipitous rise in arterial pressure associated with symptoms not unlike those encountered in an acute pheochromocytoma crisis.

   b) Appropriate treatment includes the administration of α-adrenergic and β-adrenergic blocking agents to decrease vascular resistance and myocardial irritability. Simultaneously, either reinstitution of the clonidine or introduction of another antihypertensive drug is mandatory.

I. Acute Glomerulonephritis. Another type of hypertensive crisis occurs in pediatric patients with acute glomerulonephritis complicated by either oliguria or anuria.

1. In these circumstances, the high arterial pressure is associated with expanded intravascular volume and increased cardiac output. Patients with severely elevated pressure will generally have severe headaches as well as neurologic symptoms (including convulsions).

2. Intravascular and extracellular fluid volumes must be reduced. In a patient who is oliguric or anuric, this can be done through hemodialysis and its attendant high ultrafiltration.

J. Eclampsia. This hypertensive crisis, which is manifested by a severe elevation of arterial pressure in association with convulsions during the initial and later stages of labor, has been seen less frequently in recent years. A variety of drugs can be used to treat patients with this condition.

1. If diazoxide is used to reduce pressure, the resultant smooth muscle relaxation will also arrest labor by diminishing uterine contractions. Thus, labor will have to be reinstituted pharmacologically with an oxytocic drug.

2. The "cure" for eclampsia, of course, is delivery of the full-term fetus. Hence, not only is immediate reduction of arterial pressure necessary, but prompt delivery of the fetus is also mandatory.

3. Magnesium sulfate or cryptenamine, administered intravenously, may also be used to control the mother's arterial pressure. Alternatively, injection of hydralazine will reduce pressure without arresting labor.

SUGGESTED READINGS

Frohlich, E.D., Messerli, F.H., Re, R.N., Dunn, F.G.: Mechanisms controlling arterial pressure. *In: Pathophysiology: Altered Regulatory Mechanisms in Disease*, E.D. Frohlich (ed): 3rd Ed. Philadelphia, J.B. Lippincott, 1984, pp. 45–81.

Frohlich, E.D.: Haemodynamics of hypertension. *In: Hypertension: Physiopathology and Treatment*, J. Genest, O. Kuchel, P. Hamet, and M. Cantin (eds): 2nd ed. New York, McGraw-Hill, 1983, pp. 791–810.

Frohlich, E.D.: Left ventricular hypertrophy as a risk factor. *In: Cardiology Clinics*, F.H. Messerli, C. Amodeo, (eds), Philadelphia, W.B. Saunders, 1986, pp. 137–144.

Frohlich, E.D.: Evaluation and management of the patient with essential hypertension. *In: Cardiology*, W.W. Parmley and K. Chatterjee (eds). *Cardiovascular Disease*, Philadelphia, J.B. Lippincott Company, 1987, pp. 1–15.

Frohlich, E.D.: Newer antihypertensive drugs, *In: Progress in Cardiology*, P.N. Yu, and J.F. Goodwin (eds). Philadelphia, Lea & Febiger, 1984, pp. 265–290.

Joint National Committee on the Detection, Evaluation and Treatment of High Blood Pressure: The 1988 report of the joint national committee on the detection, evaluation, and treatment of high blood pressure. Arch. Intern. Med. *148*:1023–1038, 1988.

Frohlich, E.D.: *Hypertension, In: Conn's Current Therapy 1989*, R.E. Rakel (ed). Philadelphia, W.B. Saunders, 1989, pp. 225–241.

Frohlich, E.D.: Update on treatment for hypertensive crises. J. Crit. Illness. 1:10–21, 1986.

Oren, S., Grossman, E., Messerli, F.H., Frohlich, E.D.: High blood pressure: Side effects of drugs, poisons, and food. *In: Cardiology Clinics of North America*, C.V.S. Ram (ed). Philadelphia, W.B. Saunders, 1988, pp. 467–474.

c h a p t e r

18

DIGITALIS INTOXICATION

Edward K. Chung

I. GENERAL CONSIDERATIONS

Cardiac glycosides have probably been the most valuable drugs available for treatment of heart disease since 1785, when the British physician William Withering introduced digitalis.[1] It is well documented that cardiac glycosides are essential to the management of congestive heart failure (CHF), regardless of the underlying heart disease and of various supraventricular tachyarrhythmias, particularly atrial fibrillation with rapid ventricular response.[2]

Although digitalis is less commonly used in recent years because of a ready availability of many new drugs for CHF and various cardiac arrhythmias, digitalis toxicity still occurs not uncommonly because of the frequent use of potent purified cardiac glycosides in conjunction with potent diuretics, which predisposes the patient to the development of hypokalemia. The incidence of digitalis intoxication in general hospitals has been estimated to be approximately 20%.[2] Digitalis intoxication is often unavoidable, because the margin between therapeutic and toxic doses is relatively narrow. The margin is further reduced in elderly and seriously ill patients and those with various modifying conditions, such as hypokalemia, myxedema, electrolyte imbalance, hypoxia, renal failure, and pulmonary disease. The therapeutic dose is approximately 60% of the toxic dose.

It has been well documented that the incidence of digoxin toxicity increases when digoxin and quinidine are administered together

320

because the serum digoxin level often rises in this case. No clear synergistic effect exists, however, between digitoxin and quinidine.

Although cardiac glycosides are often indispensable to the treatment of heart failure and various supraventricular tachyarrhythmias, they are no longer beneficial to a patient who has developed manifestations of digitalis intoxication. Frequently, digitalis intoxication may develop in a patient after a relatively small dose that is either therapeutic or inadequate for other patients. That is especially true in the case of various modifying conditions, such as those just listed. Consequently, the digitalis requirement varies from patient to patient and from time to time in the same patient. The use of the standard dosage for digitalization without adjusting to the individual response is a common cause of digitalis intoxication. It is not uncommon for digitalis to reach intoxicating levels without having the desired therapeutic effect, especially in patients who have intractable congestive heart failure. In retrospect, apparently inexplicable death in patients who have refractory congestive heart failure can often be attributed to digitalis intoxication. In addition, digitalis intoxication occasionally occurs as a result of accidental ingestion of large amounts of digitalis or as a result of a suicide attempt.

Although digitalis is one of the oldest and most commonly used drugs, it is not possible for physicians to determine precisely the optimal therapeutic dosage. The determination of serum digoxin or digitoxin levels is widely used at many institutions to assess the therapeutic and toxic doses of digitalis.[3,4] Markedly increased serum digitalis levels usually indicate digitalis intoxication, whereas very low serum digitalis levels often indicate underdigitalization. The determination of serum digitalis levels is extremely valuable in patients suffering from intractable congestive heart failure or complex cardiac arrhythmias when little or no information regarding previous digitalization is available. (The determination of serum digitalis levels is discussed in detail later in this chapter.)

The most common manifestations of digitalis intoxication are gastrointestinal disturbances, various cardiac arrhythmias, aggravation of pre-existing congestive heart failure or the development of new congestive heart failure, neurologic disturbances, and visual disturbances.[2] Common and uncommon manifestations of digitalis intoxication are listed in Table 18–1.

II. GASTROINTESTINAL SYMPTOMS

Anorexia is often the earliest sign of digitalis intoxication, and it is usually followed by nausea and vomiting in 2 or 3 days if digitalization is continued. The nausea and vomiting are considered to be central rather than gastric in origin.

Diarrhea is a rather uncommon manifestation of digitalis intoxication, and constipation and abdominal pain have also been reported rarely. Gastrointestinal symptoms are often not clearly evident in elderly patients, probably being masked by the severity

Table 18-1. Manifestations of Digitalis Intoxication

Symptoms	Common	Uncommon
Gastro-intestinal	Anorexia, nausea, vomiting	Abdominal pain, constipation, diarrhea, hemorrhage
Cardiac	Worsening of congestive heart failure, ventricular premature contraction, paroxysmal atrial tachycardia with block, nonparoxysmal AV junctional tachycardia, AV block, sinus bradycardia	Atrial fibrillation, atrial flutter, ventricular tachycardia, ventricular flutter, sinus arrest, SA block, atrial premature contraction, AV junctional premature contraction
Visual	Color vision (green or yellow) with halos	Blurring or shimmering vision, scotoma, micropsia or macropsia, amblyopia
Neurologic	Fatigue, headache, insomnia, malaise, confusion, vertigo, depression	Neuralgia, convulsions, paresthesia, delirium, psychosis
Nonspecific	—	Allergic reaction, idiosyncrasy, thrombocytopenia, gynecomastia

of the congestive heart failure and cerebral insufficiency. It is well documented that most of the purified glycosides produce nausea and vomiting much less frequently than does digitalis leaf. Thus digitalis-induced arrhythmias are frequently the earliest manifestation of digitalis intoxication with the purified glycosides. When nausea and vomiting develop, and the possibilities of overdigitalization and underdigitalization are almost equal, digitalis should be discontinued immediately and the patient should be re-evaluated.

III. VISUAL AND NEUROLOGIC MANIFESTATIONS

Green or yellow color vision with colored halos has for many years been considered a pathognomonic feature of digitalis intoxication.[2] Other visual disturbances include scotoma, blurring, shimmering vision, and, less commonly, micropsia and temporary or permanent amblyopia.[2] Those visual manifestations may easily go unrecognized unless the physician asks specifically about them.

Cardiac glycosides may produce various neurologic symptoms, including headache, fatigue, lassitude, insomnia, malaise, depression, confusion, delirium, and vertigo and, less commonly, convulsions, neuralgias, especially trigeminal neuralgia and paresthesia. Visual and neurologic manifestations usually develop later than gastrointestinal symptoms or cardiac arrhythmias, and the symptoms just mentioned (except the color vision disturbances) are less specific for digitalis intoxication than are the gastrointestinal manifestations and the arrhythmias. Furthermore, neurologic symptoms are often difficult to evaluate in elderly people because those symptoms may be due to many other conditions, such as cerebrovascular accidents and chronic brain syndrome.

IV. RARE MANIFESTATIONS

Allergic manifestations, such as urticaria and eosinophilia, and idiosyncrasy are *not* true manifestations of digitalis intoxication.[2,5] Similarly, unilateral or bilateral gynecomastia that develops during digitalis therapy does not seem to be a manifestation of digitalis intoxication although some investigators consider it to be so. Those investigators have seen several patients who have shown no other toxic manifestations after the development of gynecomastia in spite of continued digitalis therapy.[2] Therefore gynecomastia due to an estrogen-like activity of digitalis is most likely *not* a toxic manifestation.[6] Furthermore, digitalis-induced gynecomastia seems to be duration-dependent rather than dosage-dependent because it usually develops when patients receive cardiac glycosides for more than 2 years.

A rare occurrence of digitoxin-induced thrombocytopenia has been reported, and it was considered to be a specific sensitivity action to digitoxin bound to the gamma globulin fraction of the serum.[7]

V. CARDIAC MANIFESTATIONS

The two major cardiac manifestations of digitalis intoxication are alteration of contractility and digitalis-induced arrhythmias. They often occur simultaneously.[2]

A. Alteration of Contractility

A worsening of pre-existing congestive heart failure or the development of new heart failure during digitalization is a not uncommon manifestation of digitalis intoxication.[2,5] Indeed, intractable or refractory congestive heart failure is frequently due to digitalis intoxication, a relationship that may be much more common than is recognized. Regardless of the fundamental mechanism involved, all patients with intractable congestive heart failure should be carefully re-evaluated for possible digitalis intoxication.

B. Digitalis-Induced Cardiac Arrhythmias

Although cardiac glycosides are often essential to the treatment of most supraventricular tachyarrhythmias, they may produce almost every known type of cardiac arrhythmias by altering impulse formation or conduction or both.[2] Recognition of digitalis-induced arrhythmias is extremely important because various cardiac arrhythmias may be not only the earliest but also the only sign of digitalis intoxication. The use of purified glycosides has led to an increased incidence of cardiac arrhythmias without other symptoms of intoxication. Furthermore, hypokalemia induced by the frequent use of potent diuretics predisposes the patient to the development of digitalis-induced cardiac arrhythmias.[2]

It has been estimated that some form of cardiac arrhythmias occurs in 80 to 90% of patients who have digitalis intoxication.[2,8] Various combinations of cardiac arrhythmias are commonly observed in patients who have advanced digitalis intoxication; it is not uncommon for cardiac arrhythmias to change from one type to another in the same ECG tracing.[2] Life-threatening cardiac arrhythmias often develop following ingestion of large amounts of cardiac glycosides accidentally or as a suicide attempt.

It should be emphasized that the classic digitalis effect (S-T segment and T-wave changes) in the ECG during digitalis therapy is completely unrelated to digitalis intoxication.[2,8] The digitalis effect in the ECG may be absent in about two-thirds of the cases of digitalis toxicity, and, by the same token, striking S-T segment and T-wave changes are frequently observed in the absence of any evidence of digitalis intoxication. Other ECG findings during digitalis therapy, such as a shortening of the Q-T interval, increased amplitude of the U waves, and peaking of the terminal portion of the T waves, also are not indicative of digitalis toxicity.[2]

Ventricular bigeminy or trigeminy is probably the most common digitalis-induced cardiac arrhythmia. Almost equally common are AV junctional arrhythmias, especially in the presence of pre-existing atrial fibrillation.[2]

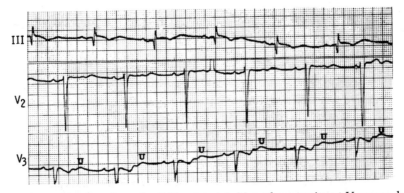

FIG. 18–1. Sinus bradycardia (49 beats/min). Note the prominent U waves due to hypokalemia.

Almost all types of cardiac arrhythmias may be induced by digitalis, but some arrhythmias do not seem to be related to cardiac glycosides. Nondigitalis-induced cardiac arrhythmias include Mobitz type II AV block, parasystole, nonparoxysmal ventricular (idioventricular) tachycardia or parasystolic ventricular tachycardia, bilateral bundle branch block of varying degree, sinus tachycardia, and paroxysmal AV junctional tachycardia.

1. Disturbances of sinus impulse formation and conduction. Minor toxic effects of digitalis may induce sinus bradycardia (Fig. 18–1), which may lead to more serious arrhythmias, such as sinus arrest and sinoatrial (SA) block if digitalization continues. A sudden reduction of the heart rate to below 50 beats/min in an adult during digitalization should raise the suspicion of digitalis intoxication (Fig. 18–1). A pulse rate below 100/min in an infant has the same clinical significance. SA block with or without the Wenckebach phenomenon is not uncommon in digitalis intoxication, especially in children.[2] Indeed, digitalis may be the most common cause of SA block. Sinus tachycardia does not seem to be induced by digitalis. It should be noted, however, that some patients who have congestive heart failure may have persisting sinus tachycardia even after full digitalization. That happens when the congestive heart failure is associated with other diseases, such as chronic pulmonary diseases, hyperthyroidism obesity, and anemia.

   Spontaneous sinus bradycardia, sinus arrest, or SA block, particularly in elderly people, is often due to the sick sinus syndrome (Chapter 11).

2. Atrial arrhythmias. It is well documented that various atrial tachyarrhythmias may be produced by digitalis, even

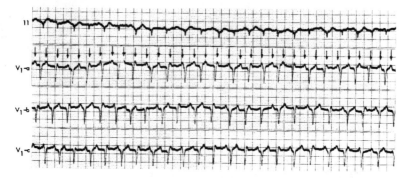

FIG. 18–2. Leads V_1-a, b, and c are continuous. The arrows indicate P waves. The rhythm is atrial tachycardia (atrial rate: 210 beats/min) with varying degrees of Wenckebach AV block (ventricular rate: 145 to 165 beats/min).

though digitalis is often the drug of choice in the treatment of most atrial tachyarrhythmias.

a) Atrial tachycardia. Atrial tachycardia is the most common digitalis-induced atrial arrhythmia, and it is frequently associated with varying degrees of AV block (Fig. 18–2).[2,9] The condition is called paroxysmal atrial tachycardia (PAT) with block. Although the frequent occurrence of digitalis-induced PAT with block is often emphasized, it actually accounts for only about 10% of digitalis-induced cardiac arrhythmias.[2]

It has been said that carotid sinus stimulation frequently terminates PAT with block not due to digitalis intoxication but is ineffective when digitalis is the cause.[8] The danger, however, of applying carotid sinus stimulation to patients with suspected digitalis intoxication cannot be over-emphasized. Some patients have died from ventricular fibrillation during or after carotid sinus stimulation.[10,11] All of those patients had been critically ill and had received cardiac glycosides. Based on those observations, carotid sinus stimulation should be avoided if at all possible in patients who are taking even small amounts of digitalis.

As for the fundamental mechanism responsible for the production of atrial tachycardia, the refractory period of the atrial musculature is markedly shortened by an indirect vagal stimulating action of digitalis. Thus increased conductivity within the atrial muscle can produce various atrial tachyarrhythmias. A combination of the depressive effect on the AV conduction and the shortening effect on the atrial refractory period results in atrial tachycardia with varying degrees of AV block.[2]

b) Atrial fibrillation or flutter. Atrial fibrillation or flutter

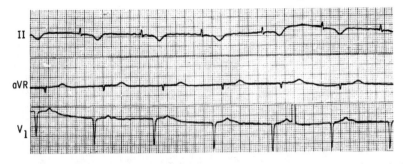

FIG. 18–3. Atrial fibrillation with AV junctional escape rhythm (46 beats/min) due to complete AV block.

may be produced by digitalis, but its occurrence is very rare indeed. It is not clear why digitalis-induced atrial fibrillation or flutter is so rare in comparison with atrial tachycardia.

    c) Atrial premature contractions. Although atrial premature contractions are not as common as ventricular ones, when they do occur the ectopic P waves are frequently not conducted to the ventricles (nonconducted or blocked atrial premature contractions) in spite of relatively long coupling intervals. The combination of impaired AV conduction and the increased excitability in the atria results in frequent nonconducted atrial premature contractions.

3. AV junctional arrhythmias. As mentioned previously, the incidence of various AV junctional arrhythmias in digitalis intoxication is probably as high as the incidence of ventricular premature contractions.[2] Digitalis induces various AV junctional arrhythmias, due either to passive impulse formation resulting in AV junctional escape rhythm (Fig. 18–3) or to enhancement of AV junctional impulse formation resulting in nonparoxysmal AV junctional tachycardia (Fig. 18–4).

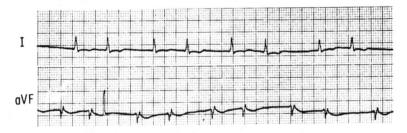

FIG. 18–4. Nonparoxysmal AV junctional tachycardia with 3:2 Wenckebach exit block in the presence of atrial fibrillation, producing complete AV dissociation.

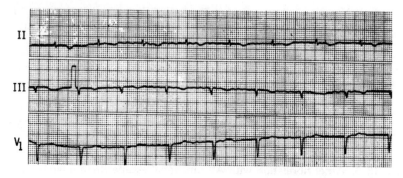

FIG. 18–5. Nonparoxysmal AV junctional tachycardia (68 beats/min) in the presence of atrial fibrillation producing complete AV dissociation.

a) Nonparoxysmal AV junctional tachycardia. Nonparoxysmal AV junctional tachycardia is probably the most common digitalis-induced cardiac arrhythmia, particularly in the presence of underlying atrial fibrillation (Fig. 18–4). For that reason digitalis intoxication should be considered as the first probable cause when one is dealing with unexplainable nonparoxysmal AV junctional tachycardia. It should be emphasized that paroxysmal AV junctional tachycardia is *not* observed in patients who have digitalis intoxication.

In advanced digitalis intoxication, exit block of varying degree may develop around the AV junctional pacemaker, and the ventricular cycle may become slower or irregular. When the exit block is Wenckebach type, the ventricular cycle may show regular irregularity (Fig. 18–5). Ventricular tachycardia may be closely simulated by AV junctional tachycardia with aberrant ventricular conduction, especially in the presence of pre-existing atrial fibrillation. On rare occasions, double AV junctional rhythm or tachycardia may be produced by digitalis; the phenomenon is a rare form of AV dissociation (Fig. 18–6). It should be emphasized that the basic rhythm is frequently atrial fibrillation when digitalis-induced AV junctional arrhythmias develop (Figs. 18–4 and 18–5). At times, the atrial mechanism may be atrial flutter or tachycardia in the presence of AV junctional tachycardia (Fig. 18–7), leading to double supraventricular tachycardia.

b) AV junctional escape rhythm. AV junctional escape rhythm is much less common than nonparoxysmal AV junctional tachycardia in digitalis intoxication. Again, the underlying rhythm is often atrial fibrillation, and the electrophysiologic mechanism that produces AV junctional

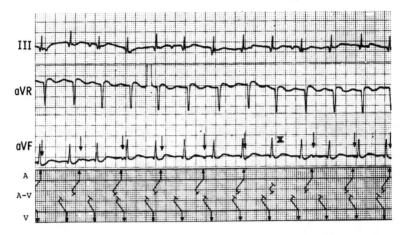

FIG. 18–6. Double AV junctional tachycardia. One of the AV junctional tachycardias (75 beats/min) controls the atria in a retrograde fashion (indicated by
arrows), whereas another AV junctional tachycardia activating the ventricles
produces a faster rate (100 beats/min). Retrograde block is most likely responsible
for the absence of a P wave in lead aVF (marked X).

escape rhythm is usually high-degree (advanced) or complete AV block (AV nodal block, Fig. 18–3).
4. AV conduction disturbances. Digitalis may produce various
degrees of AV block resulting from both the direct and indirect actions of the drug.[2] Those actions are, needless to say,

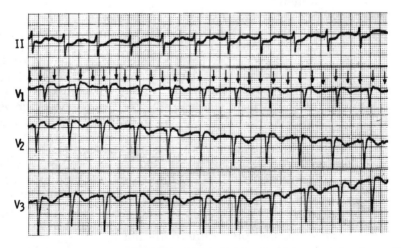

FIG. 18–7. The arrows indicate atrial activity. The rhythm is atrial tachycardia
(atrial rate: 220 to 240 beats/min) with nonparoxysmal AV junctional tachycardia
(84 beats/min), producing complete AV dissociation (double supraventricular
tachycardia).

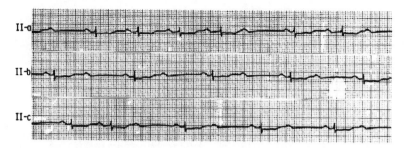

FIG. 18–8. Leads II-a, b, and c are *not* continuous. The tracing shows sinus rhythm (atrial rate: 66 beats/min) with 2:1 AV block and varying degrees of intermittent Wenckebach AV block.

essential to the management of various supraventricular tachyarrhythmias, especially atrial fibrillation. The degree of AV block in digitalis intoxication depends largely on the dosage of the drug, underlying heart disease, pre-existing AV conduction disturbances, and electrolyte imbalance.

a) First-degree AV block. Although first-degree AV block is one of the earliest manifestations of digitalis intoxication, some investigators do not include it among the toxic manifestations of the drug. Digitalis-induced second- or higher-degree AV block is, however, often followed by first-degree AV block when digitalis is stopped. Therefore, first-degree AV block during digitalization should definitely be considered a manifestation of digitalis intoxication.

b) Second-degree AV block. The average incidence of second-degree AV block in different series is estimated to be 11%.[2,8] Among second-degree AV blocks, Wenckebach (Mobitz type I) AV block is more common than is 2:1 AV block. On the other hand, Mobitz type II AV block has not been reported as a manifestation of digitalis intoxication. It is common to observe that Wenckebach AV block and 2:1 AV block often coexists in the same ECG tracing (Fig. 18–8).

c) High-degree or complete AV block. High-degree (advanced) or complete AV block is very common in digitalis intoxication when the underlying rhythm is atrial fibrillation. It has been said that digitalis intoxication is the second most common cause of complete AV block.[2]

5. Ventricular arrhythmias

a) Ventricular premature contractions
Ventricular premature contractions, particularly ones that are multifocal in origin, are the most common and often the earliest manifestation of digitalis intoxication in adults. The incidence has been reported to be approxi-

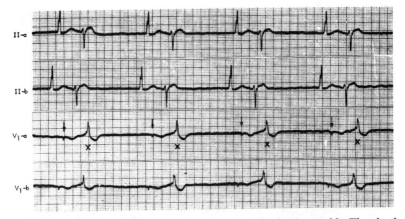

FIG. 18–9. Leads II-a and b are continuous, as are leads V_1-a and b. The rhythm is atrial fibrillation with AV junctional escape rhythm (indicated by arrows) due to complete AV block and ventricular bigeminy (marked X).

mately 50% of all digitalis-induced arrhythmias. It has been known for many years that ventricular bigeminy (Fig. 18–9) is a hallmark of digitalis-induced arrhythmia.[2,8] The diagnostic probability of digitalis intoxication is 100% when ventricular bigeminy coexists with nonparoxysmal AV junctional tachycardia or AV block, especially in the presence of atrial fibrillation (Fig. 18–9).

In children and in healthy adults, supraventricular arrhythmias and AV conduction disturbances are more common than are ventricular premature contractions.[2,8] Ventricular bigeminy or trigeminy induced by digitalis occurs frequently in the presence of a diseased myocardium, particularly in the aged. Ventricular premature contractions may originate from a single focus, or they may be multifocal. Multifocal ventricular premature contractions are more pathognomonic for digitalis intoxication than are unifocal ones.

b) Ventricular tachycardia and fibrillation. When ventricular premature contractions are frequent, particularly multifocal or bidirectional ones, ventricular tachycardia may develop, producing unidirectional or bidirectional tachycardia or even ventricular fibrillation. The average incidence of ventricular tachycardia has been estimated to be 10% of all digitalis-induced arrhythmias.[2,8] If ventricular tachycardia persists, the development of ventricular fibrillation and sudden death is always a possibility. The mortality rate of patients with digitalis-induced ventricular tachycardia is extremely high (68 to 100%).

Bidirectional ventricular tachycardia (Fig. 18–10) is

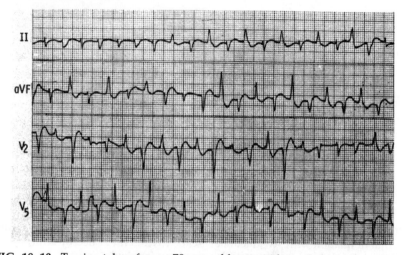

FIG. 18–10. Tracing taken from a 70-year-old man with cor-Pulmonale and thyrotoxicosis who died soon after this ECG was recorded. The serum digoxin level was more than 10 ng/ml. The rhythm is atrial fibrillation with bidirectional ventricular tachycardia (176 beats/min), producing complete AV dissociation.

considered more pathognomonic for digitalis intoxication than is the unidirectional entity.[2] Bidirectional ventricular tachycardia is more common in advanced heart disease, and frequently the basic atrial mechanism is atrial fibrillation, flutter, or tachycardia (Fig. 18–10).

It should be emphasized that nonparoxysmal ventricular (idioventricular) tachycardia (accelerated ventricular rhythm) and parasystolic ventricular tachycardia are *not* due to digitalis intoxication.

Except for idioventricular rhythm, the mechanism of ventricular tachycardia or fibrillation is most likely similar to that responsible for the production of ventricular premature contractions. Enhancement of automaticity is probably responsible for most digitalis-induced ventricular arrhythmias.

VI. DETERMINATION OF SERUM DIGITALIS LEVELS BY RADIO-IMMUNOASSAY

In the past 20 to 25 years, various methods of determining the levels of serum cardiac glycosides in order to assess an optimal therapeutic dosage and to diagnose digitalis intoxication with accuracy have been proposed.[3,4] The radioimmunoassay method most commonly used at present was first employed by Oliver and his coworkers to determine serum digitoxin levels.[12] Later, Smith and his co-workers developed a radioimmunoassay method for measuring serum digoxin levels.[3]

The clinical importance of serum cardiac glycoside levels rests in the reasonably close correlation between blood content and tissue content of digitalis. The blood levels reflect total body and myocardial concentrations.[4] That relationship was first noted by Doherty and his co-workers, who observed a relatively constant ratio between blood and myocardial levels of digoxin in animals as well as in man.[4]

At present, it is generally agreed that patients who have unequivocal digitalis intoxication have significantly higher serum or plasma levels of digoxin or digitoxin than have nonintoxicated patients. Nevertheless, substantial overlap exists between toxic and nontoxic serum or plasma cardiac glycoside levels, particularly in patients suffering from intractable congestive heart failure or various complex arrhythmias. As has been emphasized repeatedly, the dosage of digitalis varies not only from patient to patient but also from time to time in the same patient. Similarly, toxic and nontoxic serum or plasma digitalis levels may differ from patient to patient because of various modifying factors, including electrolyte imbalance, thyroid disease, renal disease, acute or chronic lung disease, and, particularly, the nature and severity of the underlying heart disease.

In a prospective study by Beller and his co-workers of 931 consecutively studied patients with digitalis intoxication, serum concentrations of digoxin and digitoxin in intoxicated patients were 2.3 ±1.6 ng/ml and 34 ±18 ng/ml, respectively.[13] On the other hand, serum concentrations of digoxin and digitoxin in nonintoxicated patients were 1 ±0.5 ng/ml and 20 ±11 ng/ml, respectively, in the same study. Clearly, the two groups have a significant overlap of values.

In general, serum digoxin levels of 2 ng/ml or below and serum digitoxin levels of 20 ng/ml or below are considered nontoxic, even though intoxicated patients may have serum levels below those values.[3,4,12,13] Very low serum cardiac glycoside concentrations (digoxin levels below 0.4 ng/ml or digitoxin levels below 10 ng/ml) usually indicate underdigitalization.[3,4,12,13] Such low values are, as a rule, not observed among intoxicated patients.

Remember that the serum digoxin level often rises when quinidine is given together so that digoxin toxicity frequently occurs under this circumstance. The serum digitoxin value, however, is *not* altered by the simultaneous administration of quinidine.

The radioimmunoassay methods are extremely valuable when the serum cardiac glycoside levels are evaluated in conjunction with the total clinical picture and ECG findings. Determination of the serum digitalis level is useful when little or no information is available about the patient's previous use of digitalis. Once the serum digitalis level in such a patient is known, the subsequent additional digitalis dosage may be determined much more accurately. Determination of serum digitalis levels is also valuable in patients in whom various modifying factors dictate the daily regulation of the digitalis dosage. Another use of the determination of serum digitalis levels is in the assessment of underdigitalization, which may be difficult or even impossible to ascertain clinically or electrocardiographically, especially in the presence of sinus rhythm.

The most important use of the determination of serum digoxin or digitoxin levels by radioimmunoassay methods is in establishing the optimal dosage for a patient. It is hoped that those methods may enable many physicians to prescribe cardiac glycosides more effectively and more appropriately so that the risk of digitalis intoxication can be minimized or even eliminated.

VII. DETERMINATION OF SALIVA ELECTROLYTES

The electrolyte content of the saliva is closely related to digitalis intoxication. Wotman and his co-workers demonstrated that patients who have digitalis intoxication have disproportionately high concentrations of potassium and calcium in their saliva.[14] Intoxicated and nonintoxicated groups overlapped a little although mean values of saliva potassium and calcium were significantly higher in the group with digitalis intoxication. Further clinical evaluation is needed to assess the value of the saliva test.

Evaluation of the total clinical condition of each patient during digitalis therapy is essential; the results of any single laboratory test must not be used as the basis for diagnosis or treatment.

VIII. MANAGEMENT OF DIGITALIS INTOXICATION (See also Table 18–2)

Various drugs have been tried in the treatment of digitalis intoxication with varying success; phenytoin and potassium have proved the most effective in terminating various digitalis-induced tachyarrhythmias. In recent years, digoxin-specific Fab antibody fragments have been used for life-threatening digitalis intoxication with a very favorable result (will be discussed later in this Chapter).

The most important treatment for digitalis intoxication is immediate withdrawal of the drug, not merely a reduction in dosage.[2] Most patients with mild digitalis intoxication (showing such effects as sinus bradycardia, first-degree AV block, and occasional ventricular premature contractions) can recover from digitalis intoxication if the drug is discontinued for several days. Generally, in patients who have digitalis intoxication, emotional stress and physical activity should be restricted, and all other factors that may aggravate the intoxication should be eliminated. Any patient who has advanced digitalis intoxication, particularly serious cardiac arrhythmias, should be treated in a cardiac care unit or a room similarly equipped. Various drugs can be given orally, intramuscularly, or IV, depending on the clinical situations.

A. Potassium

Potassium is one of the most effective drugs for abolishing various atrial and ventricular tachyarrhythmias in digitalis intoxication.[2,15]

1. Administration and dosage. The amount of potassium to be administered depends on the severity of the intoxication,

Table 18–2. Treatment of Digitalis Intoxication

Drugs and Other Methods	Mild Intoxication	Severe Intoxication	Contra-indications
		IMMEDIATE WITHDRAWAL OF DIGITALIS!	
Potassium	1–2 g KCl q̄ 4 hr	40–60 mEq/liter KCl in 500 ml 5% D/W IV injection (2–3 hr period) under ECG monitor and periodic serum K⁺ determination	Hyperkalemia, uremia, second- and third-degree AV block, SA block
Phenytoin (Dilantin)	100 mg tid or qid by mouth	125–250 mg IV injection (2–3 min period) under ECG monitor. Same dosage may be repeated q̄ 5–10 min.	Second- and third-degree AV block, SA block, marked sinus bradycardia
Lidocaine (Xylocaine)	—	1 mg/kg body wt. IV injection q̄ 20 min. Maximum dose: 750 mg	Similar to diphenylhydantoin (see above)
Propranolol (Inderal)	10–30 mg tid or qid before meals and at bedtime	1–3 mg slow IV injection (not to exceed 1 mg/min) under ECG monitor. Second dose may be repeated after 2 min. Additional medication should be withheld for at least 4 hr.	Bronchial asthma, allergic rhinitis, marked sinus bradycardia, SA block, second- and third-degree AV block, cardiogenic shock, heart failure, pulmonary hypertension
Procainamide (Pronestyl)	250–500 mg q̄ 3–4 hr by mouth	50–100 mg q 2–4 min slow IV injection or 1 g in 200 ml 5% D/W IV drip (30–60-min period) under ECG monitor. Maximum dose: 2 g	Similar to phenytoin (see above)
Quinidine	300–400 mg qid by mouth	0.6 g in 200 ml 5% D/W IV drip (30–60 min period) under ECG monitor	Similar to phenytoin (see above)
Digoxin-specific Fab antibody fragments	Should be used only for life-threatening digitalis intoxication (see text)		
Magnesium sulfate	Slow (1 ml/min) IV infusion (20 ml of 20% solution) under continuous ECG monitoring		
Sodium EDTA	Not recommended for clinical use		
Direct current countershock	Not recommended except as a last resort after all available measures have been exhausted		
Artificial pacemaker	Temporary demand pacemaker is indicated for third-degree AV block and occasionally for second-degree AV block or SA block		

the degree of suspected potassium deficiency in the myocardium, and the response to potassium therapy. Potassium in the form of potassium chloride may be administered orally in doses of 20 to 80 mEq/L/day or by a slow IV infusion in doses of 40 or 60 mEq/L over a 2 to 3 hour period initially. Intravenous administration is preferred because the exact amount received by the patient can be controlled and the drug can be discontinued at any time.[2] Oral administration is widely used for milder cases of digitalis intoxication when hypokalemia is suspected or is known to be present. During the IV administration of potassium, continuous ECG monitoring is essential to prevent hyperkalemia or cardiac arrhythmia.

2. Precautions and contraindications. Potassium is absolutely contraindicated in the presence of renal failure and hyperkalemia. Potassium is also relatively contraindicated in the presence of second-degree or complete AV block unless the serum potassium level is very low. Frequent determination of the serum potassium level is also indicated.

   Needless to say, potassium is most effective when a significant degree of hypokalemia is present (Fig. 18–1).

B. Phenytoin (Dilantin)

   Clinical investigations have demonstrated that phenytoin is effective in treating digitalis-induced arrhythmias, including paroxysmal atrial tachycardia, AV junctional rhythm, wandering atrial pacemaker, ventricular bigeminy, multifocal ventricular premature contractions and AV junctional or ventricular tachycardia (Fig. 18–11).

1. Administration and dosage. Most patients respond in 3 seconds to 5 minutes to the IV administration of phenytoin. The duration of response varies from 5 minutes to 4 to 6 hours. The initial IV dose is 125 to 250 mg for 1 to 3 minutes given under ECG monitoring. The same dose may be repeated every 5 to 10 minutes until the effect is established.

   After conversion to sinus rhythm or after digitalis-induced arrhythmias have been terminated, an oral maintenance dosage (200 to 400 mg) given in divided doses is sufficient.

2. Side effects and toxicity. Toxic manifestations or side effects of phenytoin include respiratory arrest, skin reaction (urticaria, purpura), drowsiness, depression, nervousness, arthralgia, gingival hyperplasia, transient eosinophilia, and transient hypotension. Those manifestations are rare and usually not serious.

3. Prophylactic value in post-cardioversion arrhythmias. It has been shown that phenytoin is of prophylactic value before direct current shock in a digitalized patient. The drug is capable of preventing arrhythmias induced by cardioversion by increasing the threshold of the excitability of the heart by counteracting the electrophysiologic actions of digitalis.[2]

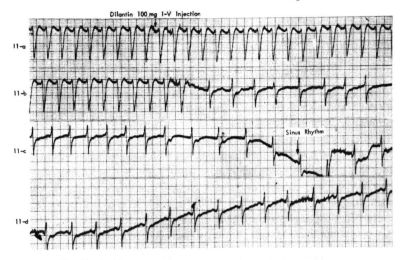

FIG. 18–11. Leads II-a, b, c, and d are continuous. Ventricular tachycardia (155 beats/min) has been converted to sinus rhythm by the IV administration of 100 mg of phenytoin.

Phenytoin is probably the safest and most effective drug for the treatment of all types of digitalis-induced tachyarrhythmias.

C. Beta-Adrenergic Blocking Drugs

Propranolol is the most commonly used beta-adrenergic blocking drug.[18,19]

1. Administration and dosage. The usual IV dose of propanolol is 1 to 3 mg given under continuous ECG monitoring. The drug should be administered slowly, at a rate not exceeding 1 mg (1 ml)/min. Sufficient time should be allowed to enable a slow circulation to carry the drug to its site of action. A second dose, if needed, may be repeated after 2 minutes. Additional medication should be withheld for at least 4 hours. Propranolol may be given orally as soon as cardiac arrhythmias are abolished or are markedly improved.[18,19] Intravenous atropine (0.5 to 1 mg) may be needed if marked bradycardia occurs. In nonurgent situations, propranolol may be given orally in doses of 10 to 30 mg, 3 to 4 times a day, before meals and at bedtime. The same dosage is also recommended for long-term use and for prophylaxis.

2. Precautions and contraindications. Propranolol is probably contraindicated for patients who have bronchial asthma and allergic rhinitis (especially during the pollen season), marked sinus bradycardia, second- or third-degree AV block, SA block, sinus arrest, cardiogenic shock, and significant congestive heart failure.[18,19] The drug is also contraindicated in patients receiving anesthetics that produce myocardial

depression, such as chloroform and ether. Patients receiving adrenergic-augmenting psychotropic drugs (including MAO inhibitors) also should not receive the drug. Propranolol may be given with caution after the 2-week withdrawal period from such drugs. It should be emphasized that ECG monitoring is mandatory during the IV administration of propranolol. In our experience, propranolol has not been as effective as potassium or phenytoin for the treatment of digitalis intoxication.

3. Side effects and toxicity. The most common side effect of propranolol is slowing of the sinus rate. At times, propranolol may produce marked sinus bradycardia. Other untoward effects include production or aggravation of congestive heart failure, bronchial asthma, and hypotension. It has been emphasized that cardiopulmonary resuscitation is often difficult in patients who are receiving large amounts of propranolol, particularly during major cardiac surgery. Thus it is advised that the drug be discontinued or the dosage be significantly reduced at least a few days before surgery as the clinical circumstance permits.

D. Procainamide (Pronestyl) and Quinidine

Procainamide and quinidine may be effective in abolishing supraventricular and ventricular tachyarrhythmias induced by digitalis.[2] Procainamide may be used if potassium, phenytoin, and propranolol are ineffective or contraindicated. Quinidine has been less widely used because of the frequent occurrence of hypotension during parenteral administration. Its effect is unpredictable and often hazardous. In addition, the use of quinidine is often discouraged by the fact that the serum digoxin level may be further increased when quinidine is administered so that the clinical situation may become even more deteriorated.

1. Administration and dosage. Procainamide may be given IV in a slow drip not exceeding 50 to 100 mg every 2 to 4 minutes, or orally in a dose of 250 to 500 mg every 2 to 4 hours. The usual dosage of quinidine is 0.3 to 0.4 gm every 6 hours orally. Parenteral administration of quinidine is seldom used at present because it has significant side effects.

2. Precautions and contraindications. During the parenteral administration of either procainamide or quinidine, ECG monitoring and frequent blood pressure determinations are indicated. A vasopressor drug should be readily available.

3. Side effects and toxicity. The therapeutic effects of quinidine and procainamide include prolongation of the Q-T interval, widening and notching of the P waves, flattening or inversion of the T waves, and depression of S-T segments. If patients exhibit toxic manifestations of those drugs, the ECG shows varying degrees of AV block, progressive intra-atrial

and intraventricular block, and atrial standstill. In severe cases, ventricular fibrillation or tachycardia may develop.

The most serious side effect of quinidine is the drug-induced torsade de pointes (atypical or multiformed ventricular tachycardia) which may be followed by ventricular fibrillation or even sudden death. Torsade de pointes induced by procainamide is only rarely observed (Chapter 12).

The lupus erythematosus-like syndrome that is induced by procainamide is relatively common and is well known. Both procainamide and quinidine are contraindicated in the presence of AV or intraventricular block.

E. Lidocaine (Xylocaine)

Like procainamide, the anti-arrhythmic mechanism of lidocaine is related to the drug's ability to raise the diastolic stimulation threshold of the ventricles.[20,21] Lidocaine penetrates the tissues more rapidly than does procaine or procainamide, but its action is often transient. Lidocaine may be effective for the treatment of digitalis-induced ventricular arrhythmias.[20,21]

1. Administration and dosage. Lidocaine may be given in doses of 1 to 2 mg/kg IV for 1 to 2 minutes. The same dose may be repeated at 20-minute intervals if needed. A constant IV drip is often necessary following the administration of a direct IV bolus of lidocaine because the duration of the anti-arrhythmic effect is relatively brief (10 to 20 minutes). Although most adult patients require 75 to 150 mg of the drug, as much as 750 mg of lidocaine has been safely used in anesthetized patients during the first hour of administration.

2. Side effects and toxicity. The side effects of lidocaine include hypotension, depression of the central nervous system, and convulsions.[20,21]

3. Precautions and contraindications. Lidocaine is contraindicated in the presence of AV block, SA block, intraventricular block, and hypotension. The drug is, of course, contraindicated in patients who show hypersensitive or idiosyncratic reactions.

F. Chelating Agents

Sodium EDTA (ethylenediaminotetraacetate) is occasionally of value in the treatment of digitalis-induced ventricular arrhythmias and AV block.[22,23] The chief advantage of the drug is its rapid onset of action; its disadvantages include its transient effect and the hypotension and renal damage that occasionally follow large doses. Chelating drugs may be used when potassium and phenytoin are contraindicated or ineffective. In general, chelating drugs are not recommended for clinical use because many superior drugs are now available.

G. Magnesium Sulfate

Clinical and experimental investigations have shown that

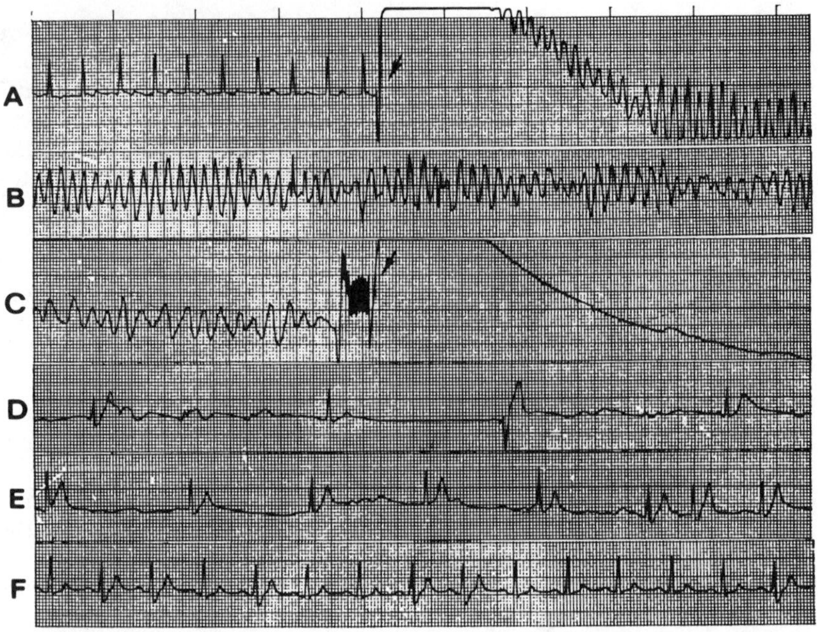

FIG. 18–12. The rhythm strips A, B, C, D, E, and F are continuous. Direct current shock is applied for atrial fibrillation, but ventricular fibrillation is provoked by the procedure (arrow in strip A). Direct current shock-induced ventricular fibrillation is successfully terminated by the second application of direct current shock (arrow in strip C). Note that a long period of slow and unstable cardiac rhythm follows the second direct current shock until a stable sinus rhythm is restored (strip F). It is easy to recognize intermittent right bundle branch block during sinus rhythm (strip F).

hypomagnesemia predisposes one to digitalis intoxication. Therefore, magnesium sulfate should be administered when digitalis intoxication is associated with hypomagnesemia.[24,25] The drug may be given by slow (1 ml/min) IV infusion (20 ml of a 20% solution) under continuous ECG monitoring.

Clinically, hypomagnesemia and hypokalemia often coexist, and hypomagnesemia is frequently encountered in patients who have alcoholic cardiomyopathy.

H. Carotid Sinus Stimulation

Although carotid sinus stimulation has been frequently used in the differential diagnosis of various tachyarrhythmias (Chapter 8), including those that are digitalis induced, the procedure should be avoided in patients who have digitalis intoxication. Carotid sinus stimulation in the presence of digitalis intoxication may induce more serious cardiac arrhythmias, particularly ventricular fibrillation, ventricular standstill, and even death.

I. Direct Current Shock

Cardioversion should not be attempted on patients who have suspected or proved digitalis-induced arrhythmias because the procedure frequently induces more serious and irreversible arrhythmias, such as ventricular tachycardia or fibrillation (Fig. 18–12).[2,26] If cardioversion is definitely needed, the prophylactic administration of phenytoin or potassium may prevent the occurrence of serious arrhythmias. It is essential to discontinue cardiac glycosides before cardioversion. If a short-acting preparation has been given, the procedure should be postponed for at least 24 to 48 hours; if long-acting preparations have been used, the procedure should be delayed for at least 3 to 5 days.

In general, when treating the digitalis-induced tachyarrhythmias, cardioversion should be attempted only as a last resort, after all other available measures have failed.[2]

J. Artificial Pacemakers

The primary indication for an artificial pacemaker is the sick sinus syndrome (Chapter 11) and AV block associated with the Adams-Stokes syndrome. Although digitalis intoxication is reported to be the second most common cause of complete AV block, the Adams-Stokes syndrome as a manifestation of digitalis overdose has been found to be rare because the ventricular rate in digitalis-induced complete AV block tends to be faster than that in complete AV block due to other causes.[2] The main reason is that digitalis-induced AV block is a block in the AV node (intranodal block), so that the escape pacemaker is located in the AV junction, *not* in the infranodal areas. Digitalis-induced AV block is usually reversible. Therefore, simple withdrawal of digitalis is often sufficient treatment. If the underlying rhythm is atrial fibrillation, however, the incidence of Adams-Stokes seizures increases. When the Adams-Stokes syndrome develops as a result of digitalis intoxication, use of a temporary demand pacemaker is quite suitable because the AV block induced by digitalis is often transient and intermittent (Fig. 18–13). The use of an artificial pacemaker with a fixed-rate is not recommended because of the danger of provoking a pacemaker-induced parasystolic rhythm that competes with the patient's own basic rhythm or ectopic rhythm, resulting in ventricular tachycardia or fibrillation. Implantation of a permanent pacemaker for the treatment of digitalis-induced AV block is rarely called for unless there are other coexisting causes of AV block.

K. Digoxin-Specific Fab Antibody Fragments

Recently, digoxin-specific Fab antibody fragments have been used in the treatment of life-threatening digitalis intoxication with favorable clinical results.

According to a final report of a multicenter study, 150 cases with life-threatening digitalis intoxication were treated with digoxin-specific antibody fragments (Fab) purified from immunoglobulin-G produced in sheep.[27] The dose of Fab fragments

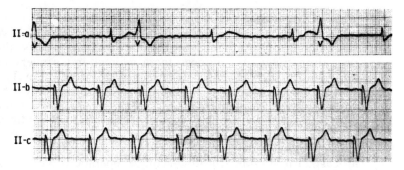

FIG. 18–13. Leads II-b and c are continuous. A temporary demand pacemaker was inserted (leads II-b and c) for the treatment of symptomatic high-degree AV block in the presence of atrial fibrillation and frequent ventricular premature contractions (marked V) shown in lead II-a.

was equal to the amount of digoxin or digitoxin in the patient's body as estimated from medical history or serum digoxin or digitoxin levels. In this study, 75 patients (50%) were receiving long-term digitalis therapy, 15 (10%) had ingested large amounts of digitalis accidentally, and 59 (39%) had ingested digitalis (overdose) as suicide attempts. In this report, 80% of the patients had resolution of all signs and symptoms of digitalis intoxication, 10% improved, and 10% revealed no response. The median time to initial response was 19 minutes, and 75% of the patients demonstrated some evidence of a response within 60 minutes.

Adverse reactions were observed in 14 patients in this study, and the most common side effects included rapid development of hypokalemia and exacerbation of CHF. No allergic reactions were observed. It can be said that the efficacy of digoxin-specific Fab antibody fragments in the treatment of life-threatening digitalis intoxication is very favorable (at least 90% of patients).

IX. SUMMARY

1. Once a patient develops digitalis intoxication, digitalis is no longer beneficial, even in the presence of congestive heart failure.

2. The most important therapeutic approach to digitalis intoxication is immediate withdrawal of the drug, not simply reduction of the dosage.

3. Almost every known type of cardiac arrhythmia may be induced by digitalis. The most common digitalis-induced arrhythmias are ventricular premature contractions, particularly those that are multifocal in origin, and nonparoxysmal AV junctional tachycardia, especially in the presence of atrial fibrillation.

4. Mild forms of digitalis-induced arrhythmias usually disappear after the withdrawal of digitalis. Treatment of advanced and

more serious tachyarrhythmias, however, involve the use of drugs as well as the withdrawal of digitalis.

5. The most effective drugs are phenytoin (Dilantin) and potassium.

6. Digitalis-induced bradyarrhythmias usually improve after the withdrawal of digitalis. In rare cases of high-degree or complete AV block, especially when the underlying rhythm is atrial fibrillation, a temporary demand pacemaker may be required. A permanent pacemaker is almost never indicated.

7. It should be re-emphasized that the dosage of digitalis varies not only from person to person but also from time to time in the same person, depending on various modifying factors, such as the status of underlying heart disease, the presence or absence of hypokalemia and hypoxia, and the status of renal and thyroid function.

8. Determination of the serum digitalis level is extremely useful, but that value should be interpreted carefully in conjunction with the clinical background and the ECG findings.

9. The serum digoxin level often rises when quinidine is administered together so that digoxin toxicity frequently occurs under this circumstance. The serum digitoxin value, however, is *not* altered by concomitant administration of quinidine.

10. Cardiac glycosides are the most useful and essential drugs for the treatment of heart disease, but they may produce serious untoward effects and even death from digitalis intoxication.

11. The serious manifestations of digitalis intoxication can be avoided if all physicians make themselves thoroughly familiar with this most valuable drug, particularly with its toxicity.

12. Direct current shock or carotid sinus stimulation should be avoided because they may produce serious cardiac arrhythmias and even death.

13. For life-threatening digitalis intoxication, digoxin-specific Fab antibody fragments should be tried.

REFERENCES

1. Withering, W.: An Account of the Foxglove and Some of Its Medical Uses with Practical Remarks on Dropsy and Other Diseases. London, M. Swinney, 1785 (Reproduced in Med. Classics, 230, 1937).
2. Chung, E.K.: Digitalis Intoxication. Baltimore, Williams & Wilkins Co., 1969.
3. Smith, T.W., and Haber, E.: Current techniques for serum or plasma digitalis assay and their potential clinical application. Am. J. Med. Sci. *259*:301, 1970.
4. Doherty, J.E., Perkins, W.H., and Flanigan, W.J.: The distribution and concentration of tritiated digoxin in human tissues. Ann. Intern. Med. *66*:116, 1967.
5. Somylo, A.P.: The toxicology of digitalis. Am. J. Cardiol. *5*:523, 1960.
6. Navab, A., Koss, L.G., and LaDue, J.S.: Estrogen-like activity of digitalis. JAMA *194*:30, 1965.
7. Young, R.C., Nachman, R.L., and Horowitz, H.I.: Thrombocytopenia due to digitoxin. Am. J. Med. *41*:605, 1966.

8. Irons, G.V., Jr., and Orgain, E.S.: Digitalis-induced arrhythmias and their management. Prog. Cardiovasc. Dis. 8:539, 1966.
9. Lown, B., Wyatt, N.F., and Levine, H.D.: Paroxysmal atrial tachycardia with block. Circulation 21:129, 1960.
10. Alexander, S., and Ping, W.C.: Fatal ventricular fibrillation during carotid stimulation. Am. J. Cardiol. 18:289, 1966.
11. Hilal, H., and Massumi, R.: Fatal ventricular fibrillation after carotid-sinus stimulation. N. Engl. J. Med. 275:157, 1966.
12. Oliver, G.C., Jr., Parker, B.M., Brasfield, D.L., et al.: The measure of digitoxin in human serum by radioimmunoassay. J. Clin. Invest. 47:1035, 1968.
13. Beller, G.A., Smith, T.W., Abelmann, W.H., et al.: Digitalis intoxication. A prospective clinical study with serum level correlations. N. Engl. J. Med. 284:989, 1971.
14. Wotman, S., Bigger, J.T., Mandel, I.D., and Bartelstone, H.J.: Cardiologists hear about rapid saliva test for digitalis toxicity. JAMA 215:1068, 1971.
15. Lyon, A.F., and DeGraff, A.C.: Reappraisal of digitalis. X. Treatment of digitalis toxicity. Am. Heart J. 73:835, 1968.
16. Ruthen, G.C.: Antiarrhythmic drugs. IV. Diphenylhydantoin in cardiac arrhythmias. Am. Heart J. 70:275, 1965.
17. Conn, R.D.: Diphenylhydantoin sodium in cardiac arrhythmias. N. Engl. J. Med. 272:277, 1965.
18. Irons, G.V., Jr., Ginn, W.B. and Orgain, E.S.: Use of a beta adrenergic receptor blocking agent (propranolol) in the treatment of cardiac arrhythmias. Am. J. Med. 43:161, 1967.
19. Stock, J.P.P.: Beta adrenergic blocking drugs in the clinical management of cardiac arrhythmias. Am. J. Cardiol. 18:444, 1966.
20. Jewitt, D.E., Kishon, Y., and Thomas, M.: Lignocaine in the management of arrhythmias after acute myocardial infarction. Lancet 1:266, 1968.
21. Harrison, D.C., Sprouse, J.H., and Morrow, A.G.: Antiarrhythmic properties of lidocaine and procaine amide: Clinical and physiologic studies of their cardiovascular effects in man. Circulation 28:486, 1963.
22. Rosenbaum, J.L., Mason, D., and Sever, M.J.: The effect of disodium EDTA on digitalis intoxication. Am. J. Med. Sci. 240:111, 1960.
23. Cohen, B.D., Spritz, N., Lubash, G.D., and Rubin, A.L.: Use of a calcium chelating agent (Na EDTA) in cardiac arrhythmias. Circulation 19:918, 1959.
24. Seller, R.H., and Moyer, J.H.: Magnesium and digitalis toxicity. Heart Bull. 18:32, 1969.
25. Kim, Y.W., Andrews, C.E., and Ruth, W.E.: Serum magnesium and cardiac arrhythmias with special reference to digitalis intoxication. Am. J. Med. Sci. 242:87, 1961.
26. Kleiger, R., and Lown, B.: Cardioversion and digitalis. II. Clinical studies. Circulation 33:878, 1966.
27. Antman, E.M., Winger, R.L., Butler, V.P., Jr., et al.: Treatment of 150 cases of life-threatening digitalis intoxication with digoxin-specific Fab antibody fragments. Final report of multicenter study. Circulation 81:1744, 1990.

SUGGESTED READINGS

Antman, E.M., Wenger, T.L., Butler, V.P., Jr., et al.: Treatment of 150 cases of life threatening digitalis intoxication with digoxin-specific Fab antibody fragments. Circulation 81:1744, 1990.

Bodemann, H.H.: The current concept for the cardiac glycoside receptor. Clin. Cardiol. 4:223, 1981.

Bowerman, R.E., Steinmetz, E.F., Schwarten, D.E., et al.: Reversal of digitalis-induced mesenteric vasospasm by sodium nitroprusside. Arch. Int. Med. 142:403, 1982.

Burchell, H.B.: Digitalis poisoning: Historical and forensic aspects. J. Am. Coll. Cardiol. 1:506, 1983.

Bussey, H.I.: Update on the influence of quinidine and other agents on digitalis glycosides. Am. Heart J. 107:143, 1984.

Bussey, H.I., Merritt, G.J., and Hill, E.G.: The influence of rifampin on quinidine and digoxin. Arch. Int. Med. 144:1021, 1984.

Castellanos, A., Ferreiro, J., Pefkaros, K., et al.: Effects of lignocaine on bidirectional tachycardia and on digitalis-induced atrial tachycardia with block. Br. Heart J. 48:27, 1982.

Cohen, L., and Kitzes, R.: Magnesium sulfate and digitalis-toxic arrhythmias. JAMA 249:2808, 1983.

Cole, P.L., and Smith, T.W.: Use of digoxin-specific Fab fragments in the treatment of digitalis intoxication. Drug Intell. Clin. Pharm. 20:267, 1986.

Constant, J.: When and how to use digitalis in patients with congestive heart failure and sinus rhythm. Pract. Cardiol. 15:45, 1989.

Doherty, J.E.: Digoxin antibodies and digitalis intoxication. N. Engl. J. Med. 307:1398, 1982.

Eisendrath, S.J., Gershengorn, K.N. and Unger, R.: Digoxin-induced organic brain syndrome. Am. Heart J. 106:419, 1983.

Fenster, P.E., Hager, W.D., Perrier, D., et al.: Digoxin-quinidine interaction in patients with chronic renal failure. Circulation 66:1277, 1982.

Ferguson, D.W., Berg, W.J., Sanders, J.S., et al.: Sympathoinhibitory responses to digitalis glycosides in heart failure patients. Circulation 80:65, 1989.

Fleg, J.L., Gottlieb, S.H., Lakatta, E.G., et al.: Is digoxin really important in treatment of compensated heart failure? A placebo-controlled cross-over study in patients with sinus rhythm. Am. J. Med. 73:244, 1982.

Gheorghiade, M., and Beller, G.A.: Effects of discontinuing maintenance digoxin therapy in patients with ischemic heart disease and congestive heart failure in sinus rhythm. Am. J. Cardiol. 51:1243, 1983.

Gorgels, A.P.M., Beekman, H.D.M., Brugada, P., et al.: Extrastimulus-related shortening of the first postpacing interval in digitalis-induced ventricular tachycardia: observations during programmed electrical stimulation in the conscious dog. J. Am. Coll. Cardiol. 1:840, 1983.

Gradman, A.H., Cunningham, M., Harbison, M.A., et al.: Effects of oral digoxin on ventricular ectopy and its relation to left ventricular function. Am. J. Cardiol. 51:765, 1983.

Hastreiter, A.R., and Van Der Horst, R.L.: Postmorten digoxin tissue concentration and organ content in infancy and childhood. Am. J. Cardiol. 52:330, 1983.

Henion, W.A., Montondo, D., Hilal, A., et al.: Changes in red blood cell electrolyte concentrations in digitalis intoxication. Am. Heart J. 106:14, 1983.

Iesaka, Y., Aonuma, K., Gosselin, A.J., et al.: Susceptibility of infarcted canine hearts to digitalis-toxic ventricular tachycardia. J. Am. Coll. Cardiol. 2:45, 1983.

Klein, H.O., and Kaplinsky, E.: Verapamil and digoxin: their respective effects on atrial fibrillation and their interaction. Am. J. Cardiol. 50:894, 1982.

Klein, H.O., Lang, R. and Kaplinsky, E.: Verapamil-digoxin interaction: an update. Prim. Cardiol. 9:105, 1983.

Klein, H.O., Lang, R., Weiss, E., et al.: The influence of verapamil or serum digoxin concentration. Circulation 65:998, 1982.

Madsen, E.B., Gilpin, E., Henning, H., et al.: Prognostic importance of digitalis after acute myocardial infarction. J. Am. Coll. Cardiol. 3:681, 1984.

Marcus, F.I., and Fenster, P.E.: Digoxin interactions with other cardiac drugs. J. Cardiovasc. Med. 8:25, 1983.

Moss, A.J., Davis, H.T., Conard, D.L., et al.: Digitalis-associated cardiac mortality after myocardial infarction. Circulation 64:1150, 1981.

Pieroni, R.E., and Fisher, J.G.: Use of cholestyramine resin in digitoxin toxicity. JAMA 245:1939, 1981.

Smith, T.W.: Digitalis in the management of heart failure. Hosp. Pract. 3:67, 1984.

Smith, T.W.: Digitalis Glycosides. New York, Grune & Stratton, 1986.

Smith, T.W., Antman, E.M., Friedman, P.L., et al.: Digitalis glycosides: mechanisms and manifestations of toxicity, part I. Prog. in Cardiovasc. Dis. 26:413, 1984.

Smith, T.W., Butler, V.P., Jr., Haber, E., et al.: Treatment of life-threatening digitalis intoxication with digoxin-specific Fab fragments: experience in 26 cases. N. Engl. J. Med. 307:1357, 1982.

Walker, A.M., Cody, R.J., Jr., Greenblatt, D.J., and Jick, H.: Drug toxicity in patients receiving digoxin and quinidine. Am. Heart J. 105:1025, 1983.

Warner, N.J., Leahey, E.B., Jr., Hougen, T.J., et al.: Tissue digoxin concentrations during the quinidine-digoxin interaction. Am. J. Cardiol. 51:1717, 1983.

Wenger, T.L., Butler, V.P., Haber, E., and Smith, T.W.: Treatment of 63 severely digitalis-toxic patients with digoxin-specific antibody fragments. J. Am. Coll. Cardiol. 5:118A, 1985.

Wilkerson, R.D.: Acute effects of intravenous furosemide administration on serum digoxin concentration. Am. Heart J. 102:63, 1981.

Williams, J.E., Jr., Potter, R.D., and Matthew, B.: Effects of arrhythmia-producing concentrations of digitoxin on mechanical performance of cat myocardium. Am. Heart J. 105:21, 1983.

Zucker, A.R., Lacina, S.J., DasGupta, D.S., et al.: Fab fragments of digoxin-specific antibodies used to reverse ventricular fibrillation induced by digoxin ingestion in a child. Pediatric 70:468, 1982.

c h a p t e r

19

PEDIATRIC CARDIAC EMERGENCY CARE

Cheryl C. Kurer and Henry R. Wagner

While medical cardiac care's roots go back centuries, specialized care for the child with heart disease is barely half a century old. Contrary to the adult, heart problems in children are usually caused by congenital deformities. Hence, the cardiac care of these children focuses on the infant and the young child and has become surgically oriented. Cardiac emergency care, however, may become necessary in any pediatric age group and disregard underlying etiology—congenital or acquired—of cardiac disease.

This chapter on pediatric cardiac emergency care is not directed to comprehensive postoperative intensive care of the ill child. It is meant to assist primary care physicians in the emergency care of young cardiac patients. The chapter discusses the most common emergency situations and uses a step-wise approach in the management:

Step 1: Initial maneuvers
Step 2: Differential diagnosis to assess further treatment
Step 3: Emergency management

Because medication dosage is crucial in small patients, medications are given on a per kilogram body weight basis. Several drugs are used in different emergency situations and in order to avoid a repetitive description we have listed the emergency drugs and dosages alphabetically in Table 19–1. In the text, the drugs have been given a number to be referenced in the summarizing formulary.

Table 19–1. Formulary for Cardiac Emergency Drugs

No.	Drug	Route	Dose	Precaution
1	Adenosine	IV Bolus	50 mcg/kg, increase to 250 mcg/kg	
2	Atropine Sulfate	IV IM	20 mcg/kgm maximum dose 1–2 mg	
3	Bretylium Tosylate	IV IM	5–10 mg/kg/dose over 10–30 min	
4	Calcium Chloride 10%	IV	20 mg/kg, max. 1 g/dose	Central vein only
5	Digoxin	IV	Total IV Digitalizing Dose	Check heart rate and rhythm before each dose
			under 1 month—40 mcg/kg	Maximum digoxin dose 1.5 mg
			1 month–2 years—50 mcg/kg	
			older than 2 years—30 mcg/kg	
			Maintenance: ⅛ of above q 12 h	
6	Dobutamine HCl	IV Pump	2–10 mcg/kg/min	Do not mix with Bicarbonate
7	Dopamine HCl	IV Pump	1–20 mcg/kg/min	Infiltration causes necrosis
8	Epinephrine	IV IM	10 mcg/kg/min po	Infiltration causes necrosis
			(=0.1 mL of 1:10,000)/kg	Tachyarrhythmia
9	Furosemide	IV	1–2 mg/kg	
10	Hydralazine HCl	IV	1.7–3.5 mg/kg/24 hours in 4–6 doses	
11	Isoproterenol HCl	IV Bolus	10 mcg/kg	Infiltration causes necrosis
		IV Pump	0.05–3 mcg/kg/min	Tachyarrhythmia
12	Lidocaine	IV Bolus	1 mg/kg	Seizures
		IV Pump	10–50 mcg/kg/min	
13	Morphine Sulfate	IV IM	0.1–0.2 mg/kg	Respiratory depression
				Antidote: Naloxone
14	Nitroprusside Na	IV Pump	0.5–8 mcg/kg/min	Hypotension. Avoid pushes
				Cyanide poisoning
15	Phenylephrine	IV	10–100 mcg/kg/dose	
		IV Pump	10–20 mcg/lg/min	
16	Phenytoin	IV	Loading 2–4 mg/kg over 5 min	Must be diluted with 0.9% NaCl
			Not to exceed 1 mg/kg/min	
17	Procainamide HCl	IV	5–15 mg/kg over 5 min	
		IV Pump	20–100 mcg/kg/min	
18	Propranolol HCl	IV	For spells: 100 mcg/kg/dose slowly	Contraindicated: asthma, heart block and heart failure
19	Prostaglandin E₁	IV Pump	100–50 mcg/kg/min	Fever, seizure, tachycardia
20	Sodium Bicarbonate	IV	1–2 mEq/kg	Check gases. Neonate:dilute 1:1
21	Verapamil	IV Bolus	0.1–0.3 mg/kg over 2 min	Not under 1 year. AV block

The chapter discusses the following emergency problems:
1. The neonate with hypoxemia
2. The neonate in shock
3. The hypercyanotic spell
4. Congestive heart failure
5. Acute life threatening arrhythmia
6. Cardio-respiratory arrest

The first three problems are age specific and discussed exclusively in this pediatric chapter. Management of the other problems, especially arrhythmia, is quite similar in adults and therefore is discussed in other chapters.

I. THE NEONATE WITH HYPOXEMIA

   A. Clinical Considerations:

      Hypoxemia may become evident at birth or within hours after birth. Deficient oxygen delivery in the neonate is manifested by cyanosis. A neonate with a hemoglobin of 18 g percent, a PO_2 of 65 mmHg, and an arterial saturation of 92% (average values at birth) carries approximately 1.5 g of desaturated hemoglobin per 100 ml of blood across the arterioles and capillaries. If the amount of desaturated hemoglobin in these compartments is increased to 4 to 5 g percent (which usually happens when the arterial saturation decreases to 75% or the PO_2 to 45 mmHg) cyanosis, signaling inadequate oxygenation, becomes evident.

      Because the recognition of cyanosis depends on the total amount of hemoglobin as well as the amount of reduced hemoglobin, cyanosis can be exaggerated by a high hemoglobin (polycythemia of the newborn) or it can be masked by anemia.

      The presence of fetal hemoglobin in the neonate shifts the oxyhemoglobin dissociation curve to the left (i.e., at a given PO_2, oxygen saturation is higher), and therefore cyanosis may be less evident in the neonate in spite of a lowered oxygen tension.

      Inadequate oxygenation signaled by cyanosis becomes an emergency situation when it leads to acidosis which can occur rapidly.

   B. Step 1: Initial Emergency Maneuvers:
     1. Laboratory verification of deficient oxygenation: Take arterial blood gas. Arterial PO_2 in room air in a normal neonate is above 60 mmHg and oxygen saturation above 92%. Acidosis, temperature, and CO_2 retention may change that value.
     2. If respiratory effort is very poor and cyanosis intense, artificial airway and ventilation may be indicated.
     3. Obtain chest x-ray, especially to rule out such noncardiac causes as pneumothorax, diaphragmatic hernia, agenesis of lung, pneumonia, and respiratory distress syndrome.

C. Step 2: Differential Diagnosis of Inadequate Oxygenation:
   1. Pulmonary:
      a) Impaired ventilation: depressed respiration, airway obstruction, meconium aspiration, restrictive lung problems, neuromuscular defect.
      b) Impaired diffusion: hyaline membrane disease, loss of lung tissue, pulmonary infection.
   2. Cardiac:
      The deranged anatomy leads to the inability of the systemic venous return to enter the pulmonary circulation. This leads to massive right-to-left shunting at the atrial, ventricular, or ductal level. List of most frequent lesions, see below.
   3. Pseudo-cardiac:
      Persistent pulmonary hypertension of the neonate or "persistent fetal circulation."
   4. Others:
      High altitude, methemoglobinemia, circulatory disturbances (septicemia, hypoglycemia).

   History, examination, x-ray and hyperoxia test will help in the above differential diagnosis. A history of fetal distress, aspiration, a low Apgar score, evidence of respiratory insufficiency or a PO_2 of 100 mmHg or above by the hyperoxia test suggest pulmonary etiology. A history of aspiration and differential cyanosis between arms and legs is usually found in pulmonary hypertension of the neonate. Maternal diabetes, presence of a heart murmur, signs of heart failure, differential cyanosis, a large heart on x-ray and a low PO_2 below 100 mmHg in spite of high inspired oxygen concentrations (positive hyperoxia test, see below) will signal cardiac disease.

   If cardiac disease is suspected, obtain an electrocardiogram (look for right or left ventricular hypertrophy, absence of anterior forces, disease specific frontal QRS axis), a 2-dimensional echocardiogram, and a color Doppler.

   A cursory echocardiogram can frequently pinpoint the underlying lesion rapidly and a comprehensive echocardiogram may be deferred until after emergency treatment is given. Specifically, look for the tricuspid valve, size of the right ventricle, the right ventricular outflow tract, the pulmonary valve, interrelationship of pulmonary and aortic valves, pulmonary artery size, pulmonary artery branches, the patency of the ductus arteriosus, and its shunt direction.

   If a cardiac defect exists, evaluate whether pulmonary circulation is maintained through patency of the ductus arteriosus. The most frequent congenital cardiac lesions leading to these situations are:
   1. Pulmonary stenosis or pulmonary atresia
      a) With intact ventricular septum (hypoplastic right ventricle)
      b) With ventricular septal defect (tetralogy of Fallot)

   c) With single ventricle
   2. Tricuspid atresia with normally related great arteries
   3. Transpositions of the great arteries with poor mixing
   4. Ebstein's anomaly
D. Step 3: Emergency Management:
   1. Perform a hyperoxia test. While neonate is breathing room air, obtain a right radial artery blood gas, umbilical artery blood gas, or both. Then cover the infant's face with a mask (or through intubation) and give 100% oxygen for 10 minutes. Repeat blood gases as above. Patients with pulmonary disease are able to raise their PO_2 well above 100 mmHg. Infants with cardiac disease will retain a low PO_2 (usually below 100 mmHg). Infants with persistent fetal circulation will have variable but differential hypoxemia between arm and umbilical artery sample.
   2. If cardiac disease is proven and ductus arteriosus dependency is established use prostaglandin E_1 intravenously either through a peripheral vein or umbilical vein (formulary #19). Prostaglandin E_1 is a potent dilator of the ductus arteriosus and allows aortic blood to enter the pulmonary circulation (i.e., left to right shunting). Watch for apnea: infant may have to be ventilated especially for transport cases. Other side effects of prostaglandin E_1 are fever, restlessness, or seizures. Infants with transposition of the great arteries and poor mixing may need a balloon septostomy in order to profit from prostaglandin E_1 infusion. For patients with Ebstein's anomaly, prostaglandin E_1 may aggravate pulmonary and tricuspid valve regurgitation and exaggerate hypoxemia. Prostaglandin E_1 is usually effective during the first 7 to 10 days of life.
   3. Correct metabolic acidosis with sodium bicarbonate (formulary #20).
   4. It is usually satisfactory to place these infants in 40% oxygen because higher concentrations are of limited value.
   5. Place umbilical arterial line in order to monitor oxygen tension and saturation.
   6. Refer patient to the pediatric cardiac center
II. THE NEONATE IN SHOCK
   A. Clinical Considerations:
      A specific shock syndrome exists in neonates with certain types of congenital cardiac defects, when patency of the ductus arteriosus is necessary to sustain adequate systemic blood flow and blood pressure. If the ductus arteriosus starts to constrict, this helping mechanism fails and shock symptoms become evident. This usually occurs in the first week of life.
      Shock criteria are comparable to adults—a syndrome of poor circulatory perfusion manifested by hypotension, systolic blood pressure of less than 50 mmHg, pale gray or ashen color, cold

clammy extremities, weak pulses, absent urinary flow, respiratory distress, poor ventilatory effort, and acidosis.
B. Step 1: Initial Emergency Maneuvers:
 1. Check for above criteria especially quality of pulses
 2. Monitor electrocardiogram
 3. Perform cardiopulmonary resuscitation if indicated
 4. Establish vascular access
 5. Obtain complete blood count, blood sugar, electrolytes, and blood gases
 6. Perform echocardiogram
C. Step 2: Differential Diagnosis:
 1. Cardiogenic shock (most frequent type of shock in neonates): congenital heart disease, arrhythmia, neonatal myocarditis
 2. Hypovolemic shock: perinatal blood loss, twin to twin transfusion
 3. Septic shock: perinatal infection leads to perfusion failure due to expansion of resistance vessels
 4. Endocrine problem: salt loss, adrenal insufficiency
Use tools for above differential diagnosis and to check for heart disease. Cardiac disease is indicated by examination (marked tachycardia or bradycardia, heart murmur, prominent gallop rhythm, absent or weak femoral or dorsalis pedis pulses, large liver, skin color usually ashened or only mildly cyanotic). X-ray usually shows large heart and congested lungs. Electrocardiogram: Look for severe right ventricular hypertrophy, absent left ventricular forces, evidence of paroxysmal tachycardia. Echocardiogram to define diagnosis: specifically look for left ventricular size (small or dilated), absence or stenosis of mitral or aortic valve, aortic arch patency, patent ductus arteriosus and its right-to-left shunt direction.

If a cardiac defect exists, evaluate if lesion is dependent upon patency of ductus arteriosus such as:
 a) Hypoplastic left heart syndrome (small left ventricle with aortic atresia) or variant of hypoplastic left heart syndrome
 b) Coarctation syndrome: pre-ductal or juxta-ductal narrowing of aorta (may have large hypocontractile left ventricle) or interruption of aortic arch
D. Step 3: Emergency Management:
 1. If shock is due to arrhythmia, see paragraph on life threatening arrhythmia
 2. If congenital heart disease is of one of the above types necessitating patency of the ductus arteriosus for systemic blood flow, use prostaglandin E_1 intravenously (formulary #19) through peripheral or umbilical vein. Prostaglandin E_1 is a potent dilator of the ductus arteriosus and allows pulmonary blood to enter the aorta (i.e., right to left shunting).
 3. Neonate may need intubation if CO_2 retention is present or if apnea from prostaglandin occurs. In order to avoid pul-

monary vascular dilatation and subsequent pulmonary congestion, do not over-ventilate infant. Keep pH at 7.4, P_{CO_2} at 40 mmHg and P_{O_2} at 40 mmHg.

4. Circulatory support may be necessary with dopamine (formulary #7), Isoproterenol (formulary #11).
5. If shock is hypovolemic, start therapy with volume expanders.
6. If shock is septic, treat suspected infection after blood cultures and spinal fluid cultures are obtained.

III. THE HYPERCYANOTIC SPELL
   A. Clinical Considerations:

   Hypercyanotic or "blue" spells occur in neonates and young children. These patients are usually diagnosed as having cyanotic congenital heart disease with reduced pulmonary blood flow, such as tetralogy of Fallot, pulmonary atresia, or pulmonary stenosis associated with transposition of the great arteries or single ventricle.

   The reasons for the acute nature of these spells are not uniform. In many cases, spasm of the hypertrophied muscular right ventricular outflow tract leading to decreased pulmonary blood flow and increased right to left shunting may be responsible. In others, such as patients with pulmonary atresia, sudden changes in systemic vascular resistance and venous return to the heart also affecting intracardiac right to left shunting, have been suspected.

   Hypoxic spells are frequently early morning events after awakening or breakfast. Initially, these spells may be short with transient hyperpnea and increased cyanosis, or the spells may be more dramatic, leading to marked irritability, loss of consciousness, and possibly stroke or death. Episodes can occur in children with little or no cyanosis, especially if anemia is present.

   During a spell, there may be lessening of a previously heard heart murmur of pulmonary stenosis, since pulmonary blood flow through the stenotic right ventricular outflow tract is frequently reduced.

   B. Emergency Management:
     1. At home:
        a) The child should be calmed and made comfortable. Knee-chest position can be attempted but should be very gentle because any forceful maneuver may upset the child further.
        b) If the spell persists, the child should be brought to an emergency room or fire station where oxygen is available.
        c) Parents are instructed to report even mild spells immediately.
     2. In the emergency room:
        a) If the child is still unconscious or in distress, an intra-

venous line should be established immediately and 100% oxygen given.

b) The drugs of choice are phenylephrine intravenously, (see formulary #15), morphine (formulary #13), and propranolol (formulary #18). In pulmonary atresia, do not use propranolol.

c) If the spell is considered to be prolonged or severe, arterial blood gas is obtained and metabolic acidosis should be corrected (sodium bicarbonate, formulary #20).

d) The occurrence of hypoxic spells in the setting of a specific cyanotic heart condition should be considered as indication for surgical help, either palliative or corrective. If this is not feasible, correction of anemia with blood transfusion or oral iron therapy may be helpful. Long-term treatment with propranolol (Inderal) has been advocated, but should be considered secondary to the surgical options.

IV. CONGESTIVE HEART FAILURE

A. Clinical Considerations:

Congestive heart failure is a clinical syndrome usually manifested by compensatory mechanisms that signal that the myocardium is unable to meet the metabolic demands of the body. Adequacy of cardiac function is maintained by heart rate, preload factors (venous return and filling pressures), myocardial contractility, and afterload factors (especially systemic vascular resistance). Disturbances of any of these factors may lead to inadequate cardiac output and signs of congestive heart failure.

Signs of left-sided heart failure are tachypnea, tachycardia, gallop rhythm, pulmonary rales, and wheezing. Signs of right-sided heart failure frequently associated with above are hepatomegaly, peripheral edema, and raised jugular venous pressure.

B. Step 1: Initial Emergency Maneuvers:

1. If congestive heart failure is extreme, the child may present in shock and may need cardiopulmonary resuscitation.
2. Establish vascular access
3. Obtain 12 lead electrocardiogram
4. Obtain blood sample for blood sugar, electrolytes, creatinine, digoxin level, and blood gas
5. Obtain chest x-ray
6. Measure arterial blood pressure and vital signs

C. Step 2: Differential Diagnosis:

Etiologic factors in the young are usually based on the type of congenital heart disease. Excessive blood volume load is usually due to a large left to right shunt, especially when associated with pulmonary hypertension in the setting of ventricular septal defects, patent ductus arteriosus, anomalous pulmonary venous connections, or regurgitation of blood through any of the heart valves.

The most frequent reasons for excessive blood pressure load in the pediatric age group are aortic stenosis or coarctation of the aorta.

Contractility of the myocardium may be reduced by inflammatory myocardial disease, fibroelastosis, or anomalous origin of the left coronary artery from the pulmonary artery. Especially in neonates, metabolic disturbances such as acidosis, low blood sugar, calcium or magnesium, as well as hypoxemia, may disturb contractility.

D. Step 3: Emergency Management:
 1. Place infant in reclining infant seat
 2. Withhold oral feeding
 3. Restrict intravenous fluid: 60 to 80 ml/k per day
 4. Digitalize patient with intravenous digoxin (formulary #5). Half of total dose given initially, followed by ¼ of total dose after 8 hours and 16 hours. Total dose varies according to patient size.
 5. Obtain rhythm strip before each subsequent dose.
 6. Use a fast acting diuretic such as furosemide intravenously (formulary #9).
 7. Patients who present in shock may initially receive dopamine (formulary #7) or dobutamine (formulary #6) or isoproterenol (formulary #11) possibly in combination with afterload reducing agents nitroprusside (formulary #14) or hydralazine (formulary #10).
 8. Watch for digitalis toxicity (atrioventricular conduction abnormality, bradycardia, ventricular ectopy, vomiting) and follow potassium levels.
 9. Maintenance therapy with digoxin (formulary #5) after 24 hours.
V. LIFE-THREATENING ARRHYTHMIAS
 A. Clinical Considerations:
  Transient arrhythmias are generally well tolerated in the pediatric population. However, sustained tachyarrhythmia may cause hemodynamic embarrassment and even death, especially in children with associated congenital heart defects. Signs and symptoms of tachycardias in the infant or young child are nonspecific and may include irritability, poor feeding or vomiting, tachypnea, diaphoresis, and pallor. When arrhythmia has been present for more than 24 to 48 hours, infants may present with poor perfusion, shock, or impending cardiovascular collapse.
  Predisposing factors for the development of supraventricular tachycardia include Wolff-Parkinson-White syndrome, congenital heart defects such as unrepaired atrial septal defects, corrected transposition of the great arteries, Ebstein's anomaly of the tricuspid valve, and mitral valve prolapse. Patients after atrial surgeries, such as the Mustard or Senning repairs for D-transposition of the great arteries, Fontan repair, and arterial

septal defect repair, are also at risk for late development of atrial arrhythmias. Sympathomimetic agents such as epinephrine, nasal decongestants, caffeine, ephedrine, and methylphenidate, even in therapeutic doses, may contribute to the development of supraventricular arrhythmias. Other risk factors include cardiomyopathy, myocarditis, cardiac tumors, chest trauma, muscular dystrophy, encephalitis, hyperthyroidism, diabetic ketoacidosis, and fever.

Predisposing risk factors for the development of ventricular tachycardia include uncorrected congenital heart defects with poor hemodynamics, postoperative repair of tetralogy of Fallot, Purkinje cell hematomas, the long QT syndrome (either congenital or acquired), cardiomyopathy, myocarditis, previous myocardial infarction, and arrhythmogenic right ventricular dysplasia. Electrolyte abnormalities, such as hyper- or hypokalemia and hypoglycemia may produce ventricular arrhythmias. Certain drugs may predispose patients to the development of ventricular ectopy, including digitalis (especially in association with hypokalemia or myocarditis), type Ia antiarrhythmic agents (procainamide, quinidine), phenothiazines, sympathomimetic agents, caffeine, nicotine and anesthetic agents, such as cyclopropane and fluothane.

Bradyarrhythmias, in isolation or associated with the sick sinus syndrome, may cause low output states, syncope, and sudden death. Young infants with bradyarrhythmias may exhibit nonspecific symptoms such as tachypnea, diaphoresis with feeds, poor weight gain, and inadequate growth. Older children may complain of dizziness, exercise intolerance, or Stokes-Adams attacks.

B. Step 1: Initial Emergency Care:
   1. Assess airway, breathing, and circulation. Resuscitate if necessary. If respiratory efforts are poor, establish an artificial airway and begin ventilation.
   2. Establish vascular access.
   3. Perform a 12 lead ECG. A single or dual channel rhythm strip is not sufficient to analyze an arrhythmia appropriately and should not be relied upon unless the patient is hemodynamically compromised.
   4. Any patient in shock or impending cardiovascular collapse should receive synchronized direct current countershock (0.5 to 1.0 joules/kg) *as soon as possible.*

C. Step 2: Differential Diagnosis of Arrhythmias:
   1. Tachyarrhythmias:
      a) Supraventricular tachycardia is an abnormally fast rhythm with its origin above the bifurcation of the bundle of His. QRS morphology during the tachycardia is usually similar to the QRS morphology in normal sinus rhythm. Wide QRS complex supraventricular tachycardias are uncommon in children and may be seen in

patients with bundle branch block or an intraventricular conduction delay in sinus rhythm, atrial fibrillation, or antidromic AV reciprocating tachycardia with Wolff-Parkinson-White syndrome, and supraventricular tachycardia with aberration (rarely a sustained arrhythmia in children).

b) Ventricular tachycardia is an abnormally fast rhythm of three or more beats with its origin distal to the bifurcation of the bundle of His. The QRS duration is prolonged during the tachycardia and the QRS morphology is distinctly different from the morphology during sinus rhythm. AV dissociation with the ventricular rate faster than the atrial rate, and with intermittent fusion beats, is pathognomonic for ventricular tachycardia. However, in young children this constellation is not always seen and 1:1 ventriculo-atrial conduction may be present. Therefore, wide-complex tachycardia with a QRS morphology that differs from the morphology during sinus rhythm should be considered ventricular in origin until proven otherwise by electrophysiologic investigation, even when 1:1 ventriculo-atrial conduction is present.

2. Bradyarrhythmias:
   a) Sinus bradycardia is present when a sinus mechanism results in a heart rate that is slower than the normal range for age. This is frequently a normal variant and may be seen in well conditioned athletes. Predisposing pathologic conditions producing sinus bradycardia include hypothyroidism, increased intracranial pressure, and drugs such as β-adrenergic blocking agents.
   b) Sick sinus syndrome (also known as the tachy-brady syndrome) is a disease process that includes depression of normal sinus node function with resultant slow sinus, ectopic atrial or junctional escape rhythms alternating with periods of supraventricular tachycardia.
   c) Atrioventricular (AV) block is a failure of conduction of the atrial impulses to the ventricles. AV block may be incomplete, resulting in occasional dropped beats or complete, resulting in AV dissociation with atrial rates faster than ventricular rates. The ventricular escape rate is frequently slow, with rates less than 60 bpm. Complete AV block may be congenital (frequently with clinical or serologic evidence for systemic lupus erythematosus in the mothers of patients with structurally normal hearts, or associated with congenital heart defects. Acquired heart block may occur with myocarditis, endocarditis, collagen vascular diseases, muscle diseases, cardiac tumors, or cardiac sclerosis. Surgically acquired AV block may be an immediate postoperative problem or a late

postoperative sequela occurring months to years following open heart surgery.
D. Step 3: Emergency Management:
1. Acute management of supraventricular tachycardia
   a) Direct current countershock should be used in any
   patient who is hemodynamically compromised.
   b) If a patient is stable one of the following vagal maneuvers
   may be used.
   (1) Diving reflex. Perform by applying an ice water bag
   to the entire face for 10 to 15 seconds or by direct
   facial immersion in an ice cold water bath.
   (2) Carotid sinus massage (usually not effective in
   infants)
   (3) Valsalva maneuver. Direct abdominal pressure may
   be used in patients too young to cooperate or understand how to perform the traditional Valsalva maneuver.
   (4) Head stand
   (5) Gag reflex
   (6) Rectal stimulation
   (7) Ocular pressure. CAUTION: This method may produce retinal detachment.
   c) Pharmacologic therapy may include the following drugs.
   (1) Intravenous digoxin (formulary #5). The total digi-
   talizing dose should be given rapidly over 6 to 12
   hours. Once digoxin has been given, conversion to
   sinus rhythm may be spontaneous or may be
   achieved with vagal maneuvers, even when previously unsuccessful. Digoxin is contraindicated in
   older patients with Wolff-Parkinson-White syndrome
   and a history of atrial fibrillation or flutter.
   (2) Intravenous verapamil (formulary #21). Contraindications include: infants less than one year of age,
   patients with Wolff-Parkinson-White syndrome and
   a history of atrial fibrillation or flutter, chronic beta
   blockade therapy, congestive heart failure, sick sinus
   syndrome and second or third degree AV block.
   (3) Intravenous procainamide (formulary #17). This
   drug may be especially helpful for treatment of
   arrhythmias that are refractory to direct current cardioversion, such as automatic atrial or junctional
   ectopic tachycardias and atrial flutter.
   (4) Intravenous adenosine (formulary #1). Currently an
   investigational drug in the United States, adenosine
   shows great promise for acute treatment of supraventricular tachycardia because of its rapid onset of
   action and brief elimination half life.
   (5) Intravenous propranolol (formulary #18). This drug
   may be very effective in patients with Wolff-Parkin-

son-White syndrome, but is contraindicated in patients with congestive heart failure. Extreme caution should be used in patients with a history of bronchospasm.

d) Rapid overdrive pacing may be performed by a skilled cardiologist utilizing a temporary transesophageal pacing catheter or endocardial pacing system. In patients with permanent atrial pacing systems, underdrive pacing may be performed by placing a magnet over the pacemaker generator, which puts the pacemaker in an asynchronous mode at a fixed rate. If a tachycardia does not terminate with the above pacing methods, it may be possible to pace the atria at a rate faster than the tachycardia and produce 2:1 AV nodal block thereby effectively decreasing the ventricular rate by almost half. This technique may provide hemodynamic stability while therapeutic drug levels are being achieved.

e) Following conversion to sinus rhythm, chronic therapy should be started in infants, patients with congenital heart defects (both uncorrected and surgically repaired), and older children with a history of frequent or life-threatening episodes of tachycardia.

2. Acute management of ventricular tachycardia

a) Any patient presenting in shock or impending cardiovascular collapse should receive immediate direct current countershock.

b) Intravenous lidocaine (formularly #12) should be given as a bolus to convert the more stable patient in sinus rhythm. Following conversion, a continuous infusion may be needed to maintain sinus rhythm.

c) Intravenous bretylium (formulary #3) may be effective in the acute treatment of ventricular arrhythmias, especially ventricular fibrillation.

d) Intravenous procainamide (formulary #17) and phenytoin (formulary #16) are also useful drugs for management of ventricular arrhythmias. Procainamide is contraindicated in patients with the long QT syndrome.

e) Patients with long QT syndrome may not respond to either lidocaine or direct current countershock. If these approaches are unsuccessful, intravenous propranolol should be given.

f) Predisposing factors, such as electrolyte abnormalities, should be treated when present.

g) Atrial or ventricular overdrive pacing may be a successful treatment for some patients who fail pharmacologic therapy. These procedures should be performed by a cardiologist.

3. Acute management of bradyarrhythmias. The following

therapies may be used if an immediate increase in heart rate is needed to improve cardiac output:

  a) Intravenous atropine (formulary #2)
  b) Intravenous isoproterenol (formulary #11) infusion
  c) Temporary pacing. Emergency pacing modalities include: transcutaneous pacing (which may produce cutaneous burns in children and should be used only for short periods of time), transesophageal pacing (if AV block not present), transvenous pacing, and transthoracic pacing.

VI. CARDIOPULMONARY ARREST
  A. Clinical Considerations:

Contrary to adults, cardiopulmonary arrest in infants and children is rarely a primary cardiac event. It is the end result of a string of problems leading to hypoxia and shock; such causes are injury, suffocation, smoke inhalation, sudden infant death syndrome, respiratory tract infection, acidosis, and hypercyanotic spell. Outcome of primary cardiac arrest is frequently poor, but it is better for primary respiratory arrest.

A state of compensated shock frequently precedes the arrest with signs of tachycardia, altered mental state, inadequate respiratory effort, normal central but weak peripheral pulses. This phase is followed by bradycardia, hypotension, asystole and, rarely, by ventricular dysrhythmia (uncompensated shock).

  B. Step 1: Initial Emergency Maneuvers (Basic life support)
Resuscitation skills have to be acquired in a structured course.
  1. Call for help to provide ventilation, oxygenation, and perfusion.
  2. Airway: Make sure upper airways are clear and assess respiratory effort.
  3. Breathing: Mask and bag ventilation with slightly extended neck. Intubation if inadequate ventilatory effort. Mouth-to-mouth breathing if intubation tools not available.
  4. Circulation: Cardiac massage if no pulse or pulse below 60 per minute. Compress lower sternum 60 times per minute.
  5. Place on cardiac monitor.
  6. Establish vascular access: cannulation of large vein as soon as possible (jugular or femoral vein).
  C. Step 2: Differential Diagnosis:
  1. Assessment of situation is equally important as differential diagnosis.
  2. Remember that the child may have aspirated a foreign body. Inspect pharynx. Apply back blows or Heimlich maneuver: 6 rapid subdiaphragmatic thrusts.
  3. If ventricular dysrhythmia (ventricular tachycardia or fibrillation) documented, use immediate cardioversion (see life-threatening arrhythmia).
  D. Step 3: Emergency Drugs:
  1. Oxygen in high concentration.

2. Give early epinephrine (formulary #8) for inotropic action and to increase peripheral resistance. This may be repeated in 5 minutes with double dose, intracardiac, or through endotracheal tube.
3. Atropine (formulary #2). Because bradycardia usually is not secondary to vagal response, this may be of limited value.
4. Sodium bicarbonate (formulary #20) may improve acid-base balance in blood but may produce intracellular acidosis.
5. Calcium chloride (formulary #4) counteracts elevated potassium, has inotropic action.
6. Lidocaine (formulary #12) for ventricular tachycardia and fibrillation.
7. Correct electrolyte imbalance.
8. If vascular access is not available, lidocaine, epinephrine and atropine can be given through endotracheal tube or through intra-osseous route (anterior tibia with bone marrow needle).
9. Fluid replacement in case of dehydration or blood loss: 20 ml per kilogram isotonic fluid (normal saline or Ringer's lactate). Blood transfusion if necessary.

SUGGESTED READINGS

Barkin, R.M. and Rosen, P.: A Guide to Ambulatory Care. St. Louis, C.V. Mosby Co., 1987.

Benson, D.W., Smith, W.M., Dunnigan, A., et al.: Mechanisms of regular, wide QRS tachycardia in infants and children. Am. J. Cardiol. 49:1778–1788, 1982.

Gewitz, M.H., and Vetter, V.L.: Cardiac Emergencies. In: Textbook of Pediatric Emergency Medicine, 2nd edition, G. Fleisher and S. Ludwig (eds). Baltimore, Williams & Wilkins, 1988.

Gillette, P.C., Garson, A., Crawford, F., et al.: Dysrhythmias. In Heart Disease in Infants and Adolescents, 4th ed. F.H. Adams, G.C. Emmanouilides, T.A. Riemenschneider (eds). Baltimore, Williams & Wilkins, 1989.

Gillette, P.C., Ross, B.A., Fyfe, D.A., et al.: Neonatal cardiac arrhythmias and their potential role in sudden infant death syndrome. Clin. Perinatol. 15:699–712, 1988.

Gillette, P.C., and Garson, E.D.: Pediatric Cardiac Dysrhythmias, New York, Grune & Stratton Inc., 1981.

Pascoe, D.J. and Grossman, M: Quick Reference to Pediatric Emergencies, 3rd ed. Philadelphia, J.B. Lippincott, 1984.

Reece, R.M.: Manual of Emergency Pediatrics. Philadelphia, W.B. Saunders, 1984.

Schneeweiss, A.: Drug Therapy in Infants and Children with Cardiovascular Diseases. Philadelphia, Lea & Febiger, 1986.

Selbst, S.M., and Torrey, S.B.: Pediatric Emergency Medicine for the House Officer. Baltimore, Williams & Wilkins, 1988.

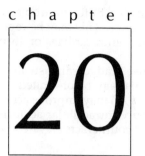

SURGICAL CARDIAC
EMERGENCY CARE

Marvin A. Bowers, III and Richard N. Edie

Conditions that acutely interfere with the ability of the heart to deliver adequately oxygenated blood constitute cardiac emergencies. These physiologic derangements usually have a mechanical or structural basis which can be corrected surgically.

I. TRAUMA
  A. Penetrating
    1. History
      a) 1897—first successful closure of a stab wound by Rehn
      b) 1943—Blalock and Ravitch suggested pericardiocentesis as a nonoperative approach for penetrating wounds of the heart
      c) The current treatment is surgical due to the failure/complications of nonoperative treatment e.g., tamponade and pseudoaneurysm
    2. Pathology
      a) One-half of people with penetrating cardiac injuries die immediately
      b) Any chamber may be affected—70% are to the ventricles
        (1) Right ventricle 35%, due to anterior position
        (2) Left ventricle, 25% of the time
        (3) Both ventricles 10%

3. Pathophysiology
   a) Acute hemopericardium and cardiac tamponade
      (1) Usually from injury to low pressure chambers (both atria or right ventricle)
      (2) 50 to 200 ml of blood contained by the normally non-distensible pericardium leads to limited diastolic expansion with resulting decreased cardiac filling, and decreased cardiac output
      (3) Immediate improvement with relief of tamponade
   b) Hypovolemic shock
      (1) Usually from wounds to high pressure chambers (left ventricle or aorta)
      (2) Higher mortality due to cerebral edema resulting from acute hypovolemic shock
4. Diagnosis
   a) High index of suspicion e.g., shock out of proportion to blood loss
   b) History and physical
   c) Stab wounds
      (1) Usual cause of cardiac tamponade
      (2) Usually clean
      (3) Minimal adjacent tissue destruction
      (4) Injury/injuries in the direct path of the stab
   d) Gun shot wounds
      (1) More likely to cause hypovolemic shock
      (2) Usually clean (except shotgun blast)
      (3) Tissue damage adjacent to the bullet tract proportional to the square of the velocity of the bullet, usually minimal with civilian weapons
      (4) Injury is not always in the "apparent path of the bullet"
      (5) Missile embolism from heart should be suspected
5. Treatment
   a) Pericardiocentesis is a life-saving measure for those patients in extremis
   b) Immediate operation, either through anterior thoracotomy or sternotomy for relief of cardiac tamponade and control of the cardiac injury
      (1) Penetrating objects in place at the time of presentation should be removed only at surgery
      (2) Opening the pericardium immediately relieves tamponade and restores proper hemodynamic mechanics
      (3) The technique of repair of myocardial injuries is dependent on the extent of the injury and pressure in the injured chamber
      (4) Autotransfusion should be used if available
      (5) Cardiopulmonary bypass (extracorporeal circulation) is rarely needed

6. Complications
   a) Of early complications, dysrhythmias are most common
   b) New postop cardiac murmurs may indicate intracardiac lesions (VSD, AV fistula, etc.) which can be repaired electively
B. Nonpenetrating Cardiac Trauma
   1. Pathology
      a) The heart is suspended by the aortic root and great veins
      b) Mechanism of injury is usually deceleration with direct sternal impact (i.e., steering column or crush)
      c) Impact on sternum causes a backward and twisting motion of the heart against the fixed spine
   2. Pathophysiology
      a) Cardiac contusion
         (1) Most frequent myocardial injury following blunt chest trauma
         (2) May have extensive cardiac damage despite little or no external findings
         (3) The right ventricle is the most commonly involved chamber
         (4) For confirming diagnosis, MUGA scan is reliable; ECG changes and enzymes are unreliable
         (5) Treatment is monitored rest and antiarrhythmic therapy
         (6) Early complications are dysrhythmias and low cardiac output
         (7) Late complications of myocardial rupture and ventricular aneurysm are rare
      b) Myocardial rupture
         (1) Myocardial rupture most frequently involves the ventricles and is associated with immediate death
         (2) 20% patients with atrial rupture may live long enough for suture repair
      c) Valvular rupture
         (1) Most frequently involves atrio-ventricular valves
         (2) Repair on an emergency basis is necessary
      d) Ventricular septal defect
         (1) Occurrence may be immediate but is usually delayed
         (2) Urgency of repair depends on the degree of hemodynamic derangement
      e) Coronary artery occlusion
         (1) Rare injury
         (2) Left anterior descending artery is most commonly involved
         (3) Once suspected, the diagnosis is made by cardiac catheterization
         (4) Immediate revascularization is indicated
      f) Transection of the descending thoracic aorta must be suspected in association with any blunt cardiac injury

II. ISCHEMIC HEART DISEASE
  A. Complications of Myocardial Infarction
    1. Cardiogenic shock
      a) Pathology
        (1) Loss of functional myocardial mass due to infarction
        (2) Requires loss of approximately 40% of left ventricle
      b) Pathophysiology
      Inadequate muscle mass to provide sufficient cardiac output to perfuse organ systems
      c) Diagnosis
        (1) Clinical: tachycardia, oliguria, hypotension, or mental confusion
        (2) Objective
          (a) Cardiac index (CI) less than 1.7 liters/minute/square meter of body surface, with a pulmonary capillary wedge pressure greater than 20 mm Hg
          (b) Systolic blood pressure of less than 80 mm Hg with adequate preload pressures
      d) Treatment
        (1) Medical
          (a) Cardiotonic agents
          (b) Afterload reduction
          (c) Intra-aortic balloon counterpulsion
        (2) Surgical
          (a) Revascularization is indicated if
            i) The above measures do not reverse the suboptimal perfusion and
            ii) If there is sufficient residual cardiac muscle
            iii) Operative mortality is high, with survival related to residual functional cardiac muscle and degree of successful revascularization
    2. Acute ventricular septal defect
      a) Pathology
        (1) Due to necrosis of infarcted ventricular septal myocardium
        (2) Usually associated with a large anterior myocardial infarction
        (3) Usually occurs in the first two weeks following acute myocardial infarction
      b) Pathophysiology
        (1) Acute large left-to-right shunt, with pulmonary artery hypertension, congestive heart failure, and, frequently, cardiogenic shock
        (2) Poorly tolerated because of associated large infarct; 25% die in the first 24 hours, 65% in 2 weeks, and over 90% in 1 year
      c) Diagnosis
        (1) Clinical
          (a) New loud holosystolic murmur best heard in the lower left sternal border

           (b) Sudden onset of congestive heart failure
      (2) Objective
           (a) Cardiac catheterization demonstrates an oxygen step-up in the right ventricle
           (b) Right ventricular hypertension
           (c) Angiogram shows ventricular septal defect
    d) Treatment
      (1) Medical
           (a) Inotropic agents
           (b) Afterload reduction
           (c) Intra-aortic balloon counterpulsion
      (2) Early surgical treatment affords better long term results as it minimizes end organ failure and sepsis
           (a) A left ventriculotomy through the infarct is used for exposure of the VSD
           (b) The defect is usually large with indistinct borders and should be closed with a prosthetic patch

  3. Mitral valve insufficiency
    a) Pathology
      (1) Transient: from papillary muscle ischemia or annular dilatation secondary to ventricular dysfunction
      (2) Permanent: due to papillary muscle infarction and rupture of chordae tendineae resulting in flail leaflet (Posterior:Anterior, 4:1)
    b) Pathophysiology
      (1) Disruption of the mitral valve support or flail leaflet causes massive acute mitral regurgitation, congestive heart failure, and cardiogenic shock
      (2) Prognosis is poor; 70% mortality in the first 24 hours, 85% mortality at 2 months
    c) Diagnosis
      (1) Clinical
           (a) New apical systolic murmur 2 to 10 days after a myocardial infarct
           (b) Left ventricular failure
      (2) Objective
           (a) Pulmonary artery catheter pressure tracings will show large mitral "v" waves
           (b) Absence of oxygen saturation step-up in right ventricle
    d) Treatment
      (1) Medical
           (a) Inotropic support
           (b) Diuretics
           (c) Afterload reducing agents
           (d) Intra-aortic balloon counterpulsation
      (2) Surgical
           (a) Immediate mitral valve repair or replacement

  4. Left ventricular rupture
    a) Pathology

(1) Due to postinfarction necrosis of the ventricular wall
(2) Usually occurs within 2 weeks of the myocardial infarction
(3) Higher probability in women and hypertensives in the seventh decade
(4) If limited by pericardial adhesions, pseudoaneurysm will develop
  b) Pathophysiology
(1) Rupture results in tamponade, profound cardiogenic shock, and usually sudden death
  c) Diagnosis
(1) Sudden right heart failure 3 to 10 days after an acute myocardial infarction with electromechanical dissociation
  d) Treatment
(1) Pericardiocentesis
(2) Emergency surgery if pericardiocentesis is successful
B. Unstable Angina Pectoris
  1. Pathology
    a) Ongoing ischemia in areas of viable myocardium
  2. Pathophysiology
    a) Left ventricular dysfunction dependent on the degree of inadequate collateral flow with resulting myocardial ischemia
  3. Diagnosis
    a) Clinical
(1) Change in the degree or pattern of pre-existing angina
(2) Angina at rest
    b) Objective
(1) ECG
(2) Exercise stress test and nuclear isotope stress test
(3) Cardiac catheterization confirms anatomy and left ventricular function
  4. Treatment
    a) Medical
(1) Nitrates
(2) Afterload reducing agents
(3) Intra-aortic balloon counterpulsion
    b) Percutaneous transluminal coronary angioplasty
    c) Coronary artery bypass
C. Failed Percutaneous Coronary Angioplasty (PTCA)
  1. Pathology
    a) Interruption of blood flow to viable myocardium
(1) Coronary artery dissection—46%
(2) Coronary artery occlusion—20%
(3) Prolonged angina—14%
(4) Coronary artery spasm—11%

    2. Pathophysiology
       a) Acute obstruction of coronary artery resulting in acute increased ischemia distal to the lesion
       b) Myocardial salvage is directly related to interval between onset of the ischemia and reperfusion
    3. Diagnosis: anatomy is confirmed by cardiac catheterization
    4. Treatment
       a) Intra-aortic balloon counterpulsation
       b) Stenting of the lesion with a perfusion coronary artery catheter to maintain distal flow (if available)
       c) Immediate surgical revascularization

III. ACUTE AORTIC DISSECTION
   A. Pathology
     1. Associated with hypertension, cystic medial necrosis and senile atherosclerosis
     2. Intimal tear of the aorta with creation of true and false lumens
       a) Two-thirds have intimal tear distal to aortic valve (Type I, II or A); one-third have the tear distal to the left subclavian artery (Type III or B)
       b) Acute occlusion of major arteries with resulting neurologic and/or ischemic symptoms
   B. Pathophysiology
     1. The most common catastrophe involving the aorta
     2. If untreated, 50% die in 48 hours, 90% die in 6 months
     3. Acute rupture with tamponade
     4. Blood in the false lumen occludes blood vessels from the aorta and/or dissects the aortic valve from its support depending on the location of the tear
     5. Type I and II or A
       a) Acute aortic insufficiency
       b) Acute myocardial ischemia caused by occlusion of right coronary artery
       c) Tamponade and/or central neurologic symptoms more frequent
     6. Type III or B
       a) Distal symptoms similar
       b) Retrograde dissection can occur
   C. Diagnosis
     1. Clinical
       a) Acute severe, tearing, substernal, interscapular pain which radiates to the back and neck
       b) Unequal distal pulses
       c) Varying neurologic signs
       d) New murmur of aortic insufficiency
       e) Signs of cardiac tamponade
     2. Objective
       a) Chest X-ray
          (1) Widened mediastinum
          (2) Abnormal aortic knob

        (3) Pleural effusion (more commonly on left)
        (4) Pleural capping
     b) ECG changes of inferior ischemia
     c) Computed tomography scan showing intimal flap
     d) Aortography
        (1) Location of tear
        (2) Aortic insufficiency
        (3) Occlusion of major arterial branches
        (4) Extent of dissection

D. Treatment
  1. Medical—initial treatment for all types of dissection
     a) Analgesics
     b) Lower blood pressure
     c) Beta blockers to reduce dP/dT
  2. Surgical—to restore flow
     a) Type I and II (A)—mandatory
     b) Type III (B)—if medical treatment fails
     c) Marfan's syndrome

IV. VALVULAR HEART DISEASE
A. Acute Insufficiency
  1. Pathology
     a) Usually involves the aortic valve from:
        (1) Dissection of the aorta
        (2) Blunt trauma
        (3) Infective endocarditis
  2. Pathophysiology
     a) Acute congestive heart failure due to volume overload on the left ventricle
     b) Acute myocardial ischemia if the regurgitation prevents sufficient coronary perfusion pressure
  3. Diagnosis
     a) Clinically:
        (1) A new aortic diastolic murmur
        (2) Widened pulse pressure may or may not be present
        (3) Congestive heart failure
     b) Objective
        (1) Echocardiography
        (2) Cardiac catheterization
  4. Treatment
     a) Acute aortic dissection and blunt trauma have been discussed previously
     b) Endocarditis
        (1) Medical
           (a) Antibiotics
           (b) Cardiotonic regimen for congestive heart failure
        (2) Surgical—valve replacement
  5. Complications
     a) Ongoing infection
     b) Persistent congestive heart failure

B. Acute Valvular Obstruction (Usually Prosthetic)
1. Pathology
   a) Formation of thrombus on a prosthetic valve
   b) Most commonly occurs on "tilting disk" valves especially without anticoagulation
2. Pathophysiology
   a) Acute obstruction by thrombus causing decreased cardiac output and shock
   b) Prevention of complete closure of leaflet causes acute valvular insufficiency with congestive heart failure
3. Diagnosis
   a) Clinical
      (1) History of low profile "tilting disk" valve prosthesis
      (2) Change in murmur or heart sounds
      (3) Symptoms of low cardiac output
   b) Objective
      (1) Echocardiography
4. Treatment: emergency valve debridement or replacement
V. CONGENITAL HEART DISEASE
   A. Cyanotic
   1. Decreased pulmonary blood flow
      a) Critical pulmonary stenosis
         (1) Surgical emergency at birth
         (2) Survival dependent on patent ductus arteriosus (PDA)
         (3) Treatment: closed valvotomy with or without systemic to pulmonary artery shunt
      b) Pulmonary atresia
         (1) Survival dependent on PDA
         (2) Valvotomy and a systemic–pulmonary arterial shunt is performed
      c) Tetralogy of Fallot
         (1) Usually presents after infancy
         (2) Treatment
            (a) Palliative: Systemic–pulmonary arterial shunt
            (b) Total correction
   2. Inadequate mixing
      Survival depends on mixing oxygenated blood with desaturated blood via an atrial septal defect (ASD), a ventricular septal defect (VSD), or patent ductus arteriosus (PDA)
      a) Transposition of great vessels (TGV)
         (1) Initial treatment is to insure mixing by balloon atrial septostomy
         (2) Definitive correction by atrial inversion (Mustard or Senning procedure) or arterial switch (Jatene)
      b) Total anomalous pulmonary venous connection (TAPVC)
         (1) Survival depends on an ASD and degree of pulmonary venous obstruction

        (2) Treatment is emergency correction for all types with connection of pulmonary veins to the left atrium

    c) Tricuspid atresia

        (1) Multiple anatomic subtypes

        (2) Initial surgical treatment depends on whether there is enough, too little, or too much pulmonary blood flow

        (3) Palliation can be attained by systemic to pulmonary artery shunt, and enlargement of inadequate atrial septal defect

        (4) Definitive therapy, by a right atrial to pulmonary artery connection (modified Fontan procedure) is usually delayed until childhood because of high pulmonary vascular resistance in infancy

B. Overcirculation with Left to Right Shunt

    1. Usually presents at 2 to 3 weeks of age, when pulmonary vascular resistance has decreased from the increased neonatal levels

    a) Patent ductus arteriosus (PDA)

        (1) Treatment

            (a) Medical—Indocin

            (b) Surgical—ligation of the PDA if medicine fails

    b) Ventricular septal defect (VSD)

        (1) Treatment—surgical closure

C. Obstructive Lesions

    1. Pathology

    a) CHF due to left ventricular obstruction

    b) May be associated with other lesions

        (1) Coarctation

            (a) Usual presentation is congestive heart failure, poor perfusion, acidosis, and oliguria

            b) Over two-thirds of patients with coarctation and congestive heart failure have associated extracardiac and intracardiac defects (most commonly VSD), with a nonoperative mortality approaching 100%

            c) Treatment is repair of the coarctation with a subclavian patch angioplasty, patch angioplasty or resection, and primary end-to-end anastomosis

        (2) Congenital aortic stenosis

            (a) Emergency balloon aortic valvuloplasty or surgical valvotomy

        (3) Hypoplastic left heart

            (a) Stabilization of flow through the ductus arteriosus with PGE 1

            (b) Creation of a nonrestrictive intra-atrial communication and single outflow tract, with a systemic to pulmonary artery shunt as a temporary source

of pulmonary blood flow for immediate palliation (Norwood procedure)

VI. CARDIAC TUMORS
  A. Primary
    1. Benign
       a) Pathology
          (1) Myxoma is the most common primary benign cardiac tumor
          (2) Usually arising in the left atrium, attached to the atrial septum via a stalk
       b) Pathophysiology
          (1) Distal emboli from the friable tumor
          (2) Obstruction of blood flow at the level of the atrio-ventricular valve (mitral valve) due to mass effect
       c) Diagnosis
          (1) Two-dimensional echocardiography
          (2) Angiocardiography
       d) Treatment: Surgical removal of the tumor and its point of attachment
    2. Malignant
       a) Pathology—sarcoma is the most common malignant primary cardiac tumor, with 3 growth patterns
          (1) Exophytic growth on myocardium
              (a) Bloody pericardial effusions
              (b) Extension into pericardium
          (2) Intramural growth
              (a) Conduction abnormalities with this growth pattern
              (b) Symptoms of congestive heart failure
          (3) Intracavitary growth
              (a) Usually broad-based stalk
              (b) Ball valve obstruction at atrioventricular level
       b) Pathophysiology
          (1) Dependent on growth pattern
          (2) Effects are due to mechanical replacement of myocardium, interruption of conduction pathways, or distal embolization
       c) Diagnosis
          (1) ECG with heart block
          (2) Echocardiogram
          (3) Chest x-ray with irregular heart borders
          (4) Cytologic evaluation of bloody pericardial fluid
       d) Treatment
          (1) Surgical excision if possible
          (2) Prognosis poor, most patients die within 1 year of diagnosis
  B. Metastatic
    1. May be from any tumor
    2. Usually asymptomatic

3. Renal cell by direct extension via the inferior vena cava to right atrium common
4. Prognosis usually related to the primary tumor characteristics

VII. SUMMARY

Conditions which produce mechanical hindrances to perfusion of the vascular system with oxygenated blood may be due to trauma, acquired disease, or congenital abnormality. If the condition poses life threatening hemodynamic instability, emergency surgical intervention is necessary in order to restore normal functional cardiac hemodynamics.

SUGGESTED READINGS

Benfield, J.R.: Chest Trauma in Critical Surgical Illness, James D. Hardy, M.D. (Ed.). Philadelphia, W.B. Saunders, 1980, pp. 135–163.

Cohn, L.H.: Surgical management of acute and chronic cardiac mechanical complications due to myocardial infarction. Am. Heart J. *102*:1049, 1981.

Cowley, M.J., Dorros, G., Kelsey, S.F., et al: Emergency coronary bypass surgery after coronary angioplasty: The National Heart, Lung and Blood Institute's percutaneous transluminal coronary angioplasty registry experience. Am. J. Cardiol, *53*:220, 1984.

Holmes, D.R. Jr., Davis, K., Gersh, B.J., et al.: Risk factor profiles of patients with sudden cardiac death and death from other cardiac causes: A report from the coronary artery surgery study (CASS). J. Am. Coll. Cardiol. *13*:524, 1989.

Lauer, M.S., Eagle, K.A., Buckley, M.J. and DeSanctis, R.W.: Atrial fibrillation following coronary artery bypass surgery. Prog. Cardiovas. Dis. *31*:367, 1989.

Page, P.L., Cardinal, R., Shenasa, M., et al.: Surgical treatment of ventricular tachycardia: Regional cryoablation guided by computerized epicardial and endocardial mapping. Circulation *80*:I–124, 1989.

Parr, G.V.S., Pae, W.E., Jr., Pierce, W.S., Zelis, R.: Cardiogenic shock due to ventricular rupture: A surgical approach. J. Thorac. Cardiovas. Surg. *82*:889, 1981.

Parsonnet, V., Fisch, D., Gielchinsky, I., et al: Emergency operation after failed angioplasty. J. Thorac. Cardiovas. Surg. *96*:198, 1988.

Pierce, W.S., Pae, W.E., Myers, J.L. and Waldhausen, J.A.: Cardiac Surgery: A glimpse into the future. J. Am. Coll. Cardiol. *14*:265, 1989.

Richenbacher, W.E., Myers, J.L. and Waldhausen, J.A.: Current status of cardiac surgery: A 40 year review. J. Am. Coll. Cardiol. *14*:535, 1989.

Sade, R.M.: Tricuspid atresia. *In*: Gibbon's Surgery of the Chest, 4th ed. David C. Sabiston, Jr. and Frank C. Spencer (eds.). Philadelphia, W.B. Saunders, 1983, 1186–1203.

Talley, J.D., Jones, E.L., Weintraub, W.S. and King, S.B., III: Coronary artery bypass surgery after failed elective percutaneous transluminal coronary angioplasty. Circulation *79*:I–126, 1989.

Wilson, J.M., Dunn, E.J., Wright, C.B., et al: The cost of simultaneous surgical standby for percutaneous transluminal coronary angioplasty. J. Thorac. Cardiovas. Surg. *91*:362, 1986.

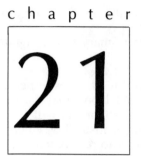

NURSING ASPECTS OF CARDIAC EMERGENCY CARE

Michael P. Savage, Edward K. Chung and Martha I. Spence

I. GENERAL CONSIDERATIONS

The nurse is frequently the first line of defense in the management of cardiac emergencies. Her ability to make critical judgments—by correlating pathophysiology with presenting signs and symptoms—may significantly affect the course of an illness. Knowledge of the mechanism of action and toxic effects of cardiovascular drugs, skill in handling emergency equipment, and skill in performing cardiopulmonary resuscitation are prerequisites to the pursuit of logical and appropriate lines of action.

Cardiac emergencies are classified in this chapter as disturbances either of electrical function or of mechanical function. Both types are closely interrelated. Serious cardiac arrhythmias are often preceded by mechanical failure, and vice versa. Two vascular emergencies, pulmonary embolism and hypertensive crisis, are also reviewed. The preventive aspects of nursing management, as well as the principles and rationale for crisis intervention, are discussed in each section. The rationale for drug therapy is emphasized.

There should be full cooperation between nursing staff and physicians when dealing with any cardiac emergency. Any nurse working in the setting of cardiac emergency should be ready to assist cardiologists or cardiac surgeons whenever such emergency care is needed.

A. The Basis For Nursing Action

Cardiac emergencies occur when the heart fails to deliver adequate oxygen to peripheral tissues. Inadequate cardiac output can be recognized by the following cardinal manifestations:

1. Changes in sensorium—restlessness, confusion, loss of consciousness.
2. Cool, clammy, or dusky skin.
3. Decreased urinary output.
4. Tachycardia (usually sinus tachycardia).
5. Hypotension.

The sensorium changes are a manifestation of hypoperfusion of the brain, with resultant tissue hypoxia. Skin color and temperature change as the body attempts to compensate for the falling cardiac output by shunting blood to more critical areas, and as arterial oxygen tension falls. Urinary output decreases as the renal blood flow is reduced. Sinus tachycardia typically occurs as compensation for the reduced cardiac output and hypotension.

A cardiac emergency may be averted if the nurse is skilled in assessing the early signs and symptoms of compromised cardiac function. The variables that maintain the integrity of the cardiovascular system are the four determinants of cardiac output:

1. The heart rate and rhythm.
2. The venous blood volume (the preload).
3. The arterial vascular tone (peripheral vascular resistance—the afterload).
4. The inotropic (contractile) state of the myocardium.

Assessment of those four determinants in the light of their effects on the myocardial oxygen demand often enables the nurse to avert a crisis or to determine the most appropriate line of action when a crisis occurs.

Emergencies related to disturbances in each of the four determinants of cardiac output are discussed in the following paragraphs. The pathophysiologic and therapeutic aspects of specific cardiac emergencies are reviewed in order to provide guidelines for effective nursing management.

II. CARDIAC EMERGENCIES DUE TO ELECTRICAL DYSFUNCTION (See also Chapters 10, 12 and 13)

Generally, cardiac arrhythmias occur as a result of disturbances in automaticity or conduction. Automaticity is the ability of the heart to initiate or generate electrical activity. Enhanced automaticity can result in tachyarrhythmias originating from any area of the heart. Tachyarrhythmias also occur as a result of altered or nonuniform conduction. Ventricular tachycardia, for example, may result from unidirectional block in a Purkinje fiber as a result of ischemia. On finding a single pathway refractory, the impulse proceeds initially to depolarize normal tissue and then re-enters the previously refractory tissue, producing an ectopic beat. Once established, such a circuit can result in the generation of a re-entry tachycardia.

Tachyarrhythmias are clinically significant because:

1. They may result in a symptomatic fall in cardiac output.
2. They decrease the time allowing for coronary artery filling.
3. They increase myocardial oxygen consumption (MVO_2).

Depressed automaticity or conduction results in bradyarrhythmias. When automaticity is depressed, the rate of discharge from automatic centers decreases and slow heart rates occur. When conduction is slowed in any part of the conduction system, the transmission of a cardiac impulse may be delayed or blocked. Bradyarrhythmias are clinically significant when:

1. They are slower than 40 beats/min.
2. They result in a symptomatic fall in cardiac output.
3. They allow a breakthrough of serious tachyarrhythmias.

When a patient presents with various cardiac arrhythmias, the nurse should mentally review a list of possible causative factors. The review helps her to decide on a line of action. In recent years, one of the very important causes in the production of various cardiac arrhythmias is cocaine. Thus, this factor should always be considered when any cardiac arrhythmia is found in suspected patients, especially young individuals. The following is a list of possible causative factors:

1. Myocardial ischemia or acute myocardial infarction.
2. Heart failure.
3. Pericarditis, myocarditis, or bacterial endocarditis.
4. Acute and chronic pulmonary disease.
5. Metabolic disturbances (electrolyte imbalance, acid-base alterations, hypoxia).
6. Potentially arrhythmogenic drugs.
7. Alterations in parasympathetic tone (vasovagal reaction) or sympathetic tone (stress-induced catecholamine excess).
8. Surgical trauma.
9. Wolff-Parkinson-White (WPW) syndrome.

A. Supraventricular Tachyarrhythmias

Supraventricular arrhythmias are arrhythmias that arise above the ventricles; that is, in the sinus, atrial, or AV junctional tissue. Supraventricular ectopic tachyarrhythmias are clinically significant when they:

1. Produce significant symptoms or a very rapid rate (more than 160 beats/min).
2. Result in a symptomatic fall in cardiac output.
3. Cause heart failure or aggravate preexisting heart failure.
4. Precipitate angina pectoris.

The most serious of these effects is the symptomatic fall in cardiac output. The persistent supraventricular tachyarrhythmias should alert the nurse or physician to look for evidence of heart failure (i.e., pathologic gallops, rales, a rising central venous pressure, and a positive fluid balance). Digitalis intoxication (Chapter 18) should be ruled out when certain supraventricular tachycardias occur; for example, nonparoxysmal AV junctional tachycardia, atrial tachycardia with varying degrees of AV block (so-called PAT with block). Drugs that have a positive chronotropic effect (e.g., beta-adrenergics) should also be considered as possible causative agents.

The initial therapy for supraventricular tachyarrhythmias is directed toward decreasing the ventricular rate. The subsequent therapy is directed toward depressing atrial or AV junctional automaticity, with possible conversion to sinus rhythm and correcting the underlying cause, such as heart failure or digitalis intoxication.

1. Pharmacologic management of supraventricular tachyarrhythmias. The drugs capable of slowing the ventricular rate are the beta-adrenergic blocking drugs (such as propranolol), digitalis glycosides, and calcium channel-blocking agents (such as verapamil). The common feature shared by all these drugs is the ability to slow conduction in AV nodal tissue.

2. Propranolol (Inderal). Propranolol is the prototypical beta-blocker available for clinical use. Propranolol decreases the heart rate (negative chronotropic effect), depresses AV conduction (negative dromotropic effect), depresses contractility (negative inotropic effect), and depresses atrial and ventricular automaticity.

   a) What Nurses Should Know/Do About Propranolol Therapy
      (1) Atropine sulfate and isoproterenol should be available for IV use to counteract a serious bradycardia.
      (2) The drugs should be given slowly IV, 1.0 mg at 5 min intervals (not to exceed 0.15 mg/kg total dose).
      (3) Monitor for signs of a therapeutic effect (slowing of the heart rate).
      (4) Observe the patient for rales, wheezing, and hypotension during administration (because of negative inotropic effects and bronchoconstriction).
      (5) Contraindications include second- or third-degree AV block, congestive heart failure, and asthma.

3. Digitalis. The digitalis glycosides slow the ventricular rate in supraventricular tachyarrhythmias by depressing AV conduction.

   Excessive levels of digitalis enhance automaticity in various cardiac tissues. As a result, paroxysmal atrial tachycardia with varying AV block, nonparoxysmal AV junctional tachycardias, and ventricular arrhythmias commonly occur (Chapter 18). The rule to remember is that virtually any arrhythmia can be induced by digitalis toxicity.

   Because digoxin is primarily excreted through the kidneys, special care in dosage is required in the presence of renal impairment.

a) What Nurses Should Know/Do About Digitalis Therapy
  (1) Observe the patient for effects of digoxin:
    (a) Slowing of the ventricular rate.
    (b) Development of new tachyarrhythmias.
    (c) Improvement in heart failure.
  (2) Determine the serum potassium and BUN levels.
  (3) The potential for digitalis-induced arrhythmias is enhanced by hypokalemia and by acute myocardial infarction.
  (4) Observe the patient for symptoms of intoxication—anorexia, nausea, and vomiting.
  (5) Phenytoin or lidocaine may be used to manage digitalis-induced tachyarrhythmias.
  (6) Digoxin causes vasoconstriction when it is given IV as a bolus.
  (7) Except as a last resort, direct current shock is contraindicated in the presence of digitalis intoxication because of potential ventricular tachyarrhythmias.
  (8) Determine the serum digoxin level when digitalis toxicity is suspected (see Chapter 19).
  (9) Digitalis is contraindicated for various tachyarrhythmias with anomalous conduction in WPW syndrome because the drug enhances the conduction via an accessory pathway so that the clinical situation further deteriorates and even sudden death may occur (see Chapter 9).
4. Verapamil. In 1981, verapamil became the first calcium-channel blocker to be approved for clinical use in the United States. Because of its potent slowing of AV conduction, it has become the drug of choice for treatment of re-entrant supraventricular tachycardia. In addition, its vasodilator effects as well as its negative chronotropic and inotropic effects make it a modest antianginal agent.
  a) What Nurses Should Know/Do About Verapamil Therapy
    (1) Intravenous verapamil should be given slowly in 5 to 10 mg doses over 2 min.
    (2) Monitor for signs of therapeutic response (slowing of ventricular rate or conversion to sinus rhythm).
    (3) Observe the patient for rales and hypotension (because of negative inotropic and vasodilator effects).
    (4) Contraindications include sick sinus syndrome, second- or third-degree AV block, and congestive heart failure.
    (5) Intravenous verapamil should *not* be given concomitantly with IV propranolol (because both have depressant effects on AV conduction and myocardial contractility).

(6) Verapamil is also contraindicated for various supraventricular tachyarrhythmias with anomalous conduction in WPW syndrome because the drug often enhances the conduction via an accessory pathway leading to further deterioration of the clinical circumstance.

5. Electrical Management—Cardioversion (See also Chapter 13). Cardioversion, the electrical management of tachyarrhythmias, is often effective in terminating atrial tachycardia, atrial flutter, atrial fibrillation, and ventricular tachycardia.

Cardioversion is the delivery of an electrical charge to the myocardium which is synchronized to the patient's QRS deflection. The equipment needed for cardioversion is a power generator, paddles, and a monitor with an ECG printout. A good quality ECG should be obtained before cardioversion is attempted, and the machine should be checked for synchronization. The patient should be in the supine position for delivery of the direct current shock.

Cardioversion is often followed by a brief period of electrical instability. The following factors enhance electrical instability, and they should be taken into consideration prior to cardioversion:
1. Hypokalemia.
2. Hypoxia.
3. Digitalization.
4. Acid-base imbalance.

Problems in premedication may occur with cardioversion. Commonly, drugs such as diazepam and sodium methohexital are used IV. On some occasions, these drugs may cause hypoventilation and respiratory depression.

The nursing measures to prevent postcardioversion respiratory complications include:
1. Watching for hypoventilation.
2. Having an airway, oxygen, and ambu at the bedside.
3. Removing the patient's dentures to prevent airway obstruction.
4. Encouraging coughing and deep breathing.

Cardioversion should be documented by ECG monitoring. Transient arrhythmias may occur immediately after the electric charge is delivered. Anti-arrhythmic drugs should be available. Failure to convert the arrhythmia may be related to hypoxia, acidosis or alkalosis, or drug intoxication.

a) What Nurses Should Know/Do About Cardioversion
(1) Explain the procedure to the patient.
(2) Connect the patient to a monitor and, with the patient supine, obtain a good quality ECG tracing.
(3) Secure a patent IV line.

    (4) Check the cardioverter and the ECG machine for proper grounding and synchronization.

    (5) Remove the patient's dentures.

    (6) Have resuscitation equipment (airway, oxygen, ambu, and crashcart) at the patient's bedside.

    (7) Have available all the commonly used cardiac emergency drugs (e.g., lidocaine, atropine sulfate, epinephrine, and isoproterenol).

    (8) Check the patient's serum potassium and blood gases levels; find out whether the patient has been taking digitalis.

    (9) Have premedications available.

    (10) Charge the machine, apply the conductive paste, and deliver the charge as ordered.

    (11) Make sure that no one is in contact with the bed or the patient.

    (12) Monitor the ECG for postcardioversion rhythm.

    (13) Observe the patient for hypoventilation and initiate respiratory supportive measures as indicated.

    (14) Observe the patient for any new cardiac arrhythmias, especially during the first hour.

    (15) Observe the patient for clinical manifestations of thromboembolic phenomena postcardioversion, especially in patients with atrial fibrillation.

  b) What Nurses Should Know/Do About Supraventricular Tachyarrhythmias

    (1) Anticipate the need for digoxin, propranolol, or verapamil.

    (2) Observe the patient for evidence of heart failure (e.g., gallops, rales, dyspnea, and distended neck veins).

    (3) Rule out drugs that could cause arrhythmias.

    (4) If medication is indicated, observe the patient for therapeutic and adverse effects (especially with IV administration).

    (5) Reduce the peripheral demands for oxygen by maintaining a calm environment for the patient.

    (6) Remember that oxygen is often indicated.

    (7) When WPW syndrome is considered to be the underlying disorder, digoxin or verapamil should be avoided (discussed previously, and see also Chapter 9).

B. Ventricular Arrhythmias

    Ventricular arrhythmias may occur as a manifestation of increased automaticity or altered conduction in the ventricles. The ventricular premature contraction (VPC) is the earliest sign of electrical instability in the ventricles. Ventricular premature contractions are easily recognizable, and they are harbingers of the most serious ventricular arrhythmias—ventricular tachycardia and ventricular fibrillation.

Ventricular arrhythmias are clinically significant because:
1. They often result in a symptomatic fall in cardiac output.
2. They may result in ventricular fibrillation and sudden death.

   Isolated VPCs are well tolerated in most clinical settings and can be seen in normal hearts. Treatment of VPCs, however, is mandatory in the presence of acute myocardial infarction because of the risk of ventricular fibrillation.

1. Ventricular Tachycardia. The term ventricular tachycardia is used when six or more VPCs occur consecutively at a rate greater than 100 beats/min. Accelerated idioventricular rhythm (slow ventricular tachycardia or nonparoxysmal ventricular tachycardia) occurs when the ventricular rate is 60 to 130 beats/min. This rhythm is most commonly seen during the first 24 to 72 hours of acute myocardial infarction. Accelerated idioventricular rhythm is usually benign and transient; anti-arrhythmic therapy is generally not indicated. Paroxysmal (ordinary) ventricular tachycardia, on the other hand, is a more rapid malignant arrhythmia. Therapy is directed toward depressing the ectopic ventricular focus through pharmacologic intervention or electrical countershock. The term, "nonsustained" VT is used when VT lasts for 29 seconds or less. On the other hand, the term, "sustained" VT is applied when VT lasts more than 29 seconds.

2. Ventricular Fibrillation. Ventricular fibrillation represents chaotic electrical activity in the ventricles with characteristic ECG features. Mechanical action is likewise disorganized and wholly inadequate, resulting in clinical death. Ventricular fibrillation may appear as rapid, high-amplitude waves or slow, low-amplitude waves. Primary ventricular fibrillation occurs in acute cardiac disease, and it shows rapid high-amplitude waves. This form of ventricular fibrillation is easily terminated. Secondary ventricular fibrillation represents a more chaotic waveform that is slow and low in amplitude and is seen in prolonged anoxic and depressive states of cardiac muscle (prolonged shock and congestive heart failure). The prognosis is extremely poor in secondary ventricular fibrillation.

3. Pharmacologic Management of Ventricular Tachyarrhythmias.

   Anti-arrhythmic drugs act by altering the abnormal automaticity and intraventricular conduction responsible for ventricular tachyarrhythmias. Lidocaine and procainamide are the agents most useful for the emergency treatment of malignant ventricular arrhythmias. Intravenous bretylium has become available for recurrent ventricular tachycardia and fibrillation. In certain cases of refractory ventricular tachycardia (especially in cases of torsade de pointes), artificial overdrive ventricular pacing may be effective.

There are many new antiarrhythmic drugs available, and some agents are still under investigations. New antiarrhythmic agents have been described in detail elsewhere (see Chapter 13).

a) What Nurses Should Know/Do About Lidocaine (Xylocaine) Therapy

(1) Anticipate the need for lidocaine in acute ventricular arrhythmias.

(2) Lidocaine is usually given IV as an initial bolus of 50 to 100 mg.

(3) A continuous IV infusion of lidocaine is titrated to achieve the therapeutic response. It is best administered with an infusion pump to avoid accidental administration of toxic doses. The usual infusion dosage is 2 to 4 mg/min.

(4) Observe the patient for hypotension when lidocaine is given IV.

(5) Signs of central nervous system depression or stimulation can occur with lidocaine intoxication—excitement, twitching, irritability, nervousness, tremor, convulsions, or lethargy.

(6) Slower infusion rates should be used in the elderly and in patients who have liver disease and congestive heart failure because of reduced hepatic metabolism.

b) What Nurses Should Know/Do About Procainamide (Pronestyl) Therapy

(1) Anticipate the need for procainamide when the patient fails to respond to lidocaine.

(2) Give the drug slowly IV and watch for hypotension (it is a peripheral vasodilator); the usual dosage is a 100-mg bolus every 5 min until the arrhythmia is suppressed or a maximum dose of 1 gm is given.

(3) Watch for QRS widening with IV administration (the drug slows intraventricular conduction).

(4) *Note:* The cardiac output may decrease because of the drug's depressant effects on contractility.

(5) Patients with liver or kidney disease receiving normal doses should be observed for signs of intoxication because of drug accumulation.

c) What Nurses Should Know/Do About Bretylium (Bretylol) Therapy

(1) Bretylium should be given in 5 to 10 mg/kg doses by slow IV infusion.

(2) Hypotension commonly occurs (due to peripheral adrenergic blockade).

(3) Immediately following injection, transient hypertension or worsening of arrhythmias may occur (due to initial norepinephrine release from adjacent nerve terminals).

       (4) *Note:* Peak anti-arrhythmic action may not occur until 20 min or more following administration.

       (5) Doses should be reduced in patients who have renal insufficiency.

  4. Electrical Management—Cardioversion and Defibrillation

      Cardioversion is indicated in ventricular tachycardia if the patient loses consciousness or is unresponsive to drugs.

      Defibrillation is the delivery of a non-synchronized high-intensity electrical charge to the myocardium. The charge completely depolarizes the myocardium and thus interrupts ventricular fibrillation.

      When ventricular fibrillation (VF) recurs in spite of all available antiarrhythmic drug therapy, especially in patients with advanced CAD and cardiomyopathies, the use of an automatic implantable cardioverter-defibrillator (AICD) should be strongly considered (see Chapter 13).

    a) What Nurses Should Know/Do About Ventricular Arrhythmias

      (1) Evaluate the possible causes of the ventricular arrhythmias:

        (a) Myocardial ischemia or infarction.

        (b) Heart failure or cardiogenic shock.

        (c) Pre-existing or underlying bradycardia.

        (d) Arrhythmogenic drugs.

        (e) Stress-induced catecholamine excess.

        (f) Metabolic cause (electrolyte and acid-base disturbance, hypoxia).

      (2) Have a cardioverter (defibrillator), ambu bag, and oxygen available:

        (a) Initiate countershock as indicated.

        (b) Institute measures as indicated to prevent the recurrence of the arrhythmia.

        (c) Have an IV infusion of lidocaine secured and started.

C. Bradyarrhythmias

    Bradyarrhythmias occur when impulse formation in the sinus node or impulse conduction in AV node or His-Purkinje system is impaired. Low cardiac output may ensue because of the slow rate and occasionally because of nonsynchronous atrioventricular contraction (as in complete heart block).

    The initial therapy in the management of symptomatic bradycardia is directed toward increasing the ventricular rate. The increase may be accomplished by:

    1. Increasing the sinus rate when AV transmission is intact.

    2. Accelerating AV conduction when AV transmission is impaired.

    3. Stimulating AV junctional automaticity.

    4. Stimulating ventricular automaticity.

1. Pharmacologic Management of the Bradyarrhythmias. Drugs capable of increasing the ventricular rate by one or more of those mechanisms are (1) the parasympathetic (vagal) blocking drugs (e.g., atropine sulfate) and (2) beta-adrenergic stimulators (e.g., isoproterenol).

   a) Atropine Sulfate. Atropine sulfate, a vagolytic drug, allows sympathetic effects on the heart to dominate. Atropine sulfate thus increases the sinus rate and accelerates AV conduction. It is a rapidly acting drug, easily administered IV as a bolus, and is thus frequently the drug of choice in treating symptomatic bradycardia. Small IV increments of atropine sulfate (0.4 to 0.6 mg) allow for more judicious management of the heart rate and less occasion for excessive rate response. Undesirable effects of atropine relate to its parasympathetic-blocking effect: urinary retention, dry mouth, facial flushing, and dilation of the pupils. Atropine is primarily excreted through the kidney and thus its effects may be accentuated in the presence of renal insufficiency.

   (1) What Nurses Should Know/Do About Atropine Sulfate Therapy

      (a) Continuous ECG monitoring for rate and rhythm is needed to prevent excessive acceleration of the heart rate.

      (b) Observe the patient for urinary retention due to atropine.

      (c) Note: Atropine is contraindicated in glaucoma because it increases intraoptic pressure (but in an emergency, the effects of atropine may be counteracted by pilocarpine-type eye drops).

      (d) With prolonged atropine therapy, observe the patient for changes in sensorium. (A mnemonic for the side effects of atropine: Red as a beet, dry as a bone, and mad as a hen.)

      (e) Note: Children are more susceptible to the effects of atropine than are adults.

      (f) Atropine is most effective in those settings in which the bradycardia (particularly sinus bradycardia) is due to enhanced vagal tone (i.e., vasovagal reactions, acute diaphragmatic myocardial infarction, and digitalis intoxication).

   b) Isoproterenol (Isuprel). Isoproterenol selectively stimulates beta-receptors of the sympathetic nervous system. Beta-receptors are found primarily in the heart and lungs. Isoproterenol may increase the heart rate by increasing automaticity in the sinus, AV junctional or ventricular tissue, and by accelerating AV conduction.

   Isoproterenol also stimulates myocardial contractility and causes bronchodilatation and peripheral vascular dilatation. It is administered as an IV drip with an infusion pump so that dosages can be carefully regulated. The patient must be carefully observed for therapeutic effects and for signs of overdose, such as atrial or ventricular premature beats and tachyarrhythmias. Isoproterenol is indicated as an emergency measure to temporarily increase the heart rate when atropine is ineffective, such as in block below the AV junctional tissue (Mobitz type II AV block) or in symptomatic AV nodal block during an acute diaphragmatic myocardial infarction. Isoproterenol increases oxygen consumption. But when the drug improves AV conduction and the heart rate, the increase in oxygen consumption is usually more than balanced by the benefits of the improved heart rate and rhythm.

2. Artificial Pacemaker Therapy for Bradyarrhythmias. Anticipating the need for an artificial pacemaker before an emergency occurs may be lifesaving. The capable nurse is skilled in diagnosing hemiblocks and bundle branch blocks from the ECG and knows the morbidity and mortality rate in bradyarrhythmias. The nurse must be familiar with the operation of pacing units so that they can be made to function smoothly in an emergency. (Artificial pacing is discussed in detail in Chapter 14.)

   a) What Nurses Should Know/Do About Bradyarrhythmias
      (1) Evaluate for signs of a critical decrease in cardiac output (changes in sensorium, cool or clammy skin, hypotension, and heart failure).
      (2) *Note:* Raising the patient's legs to augment the venous return and stroke volume may eliminate symptoms during a transient bradycardia. It may be used while the patient is awaiting drug or electrical management.
      (3) Watch for bradycardia-related ventricular arrhythmias.
      (4) Have atropine, isoproterenol, and an external pacemaker available.
      (5) Consider the possible etiologies of bradyarrhythmias:
         (a) Drugs (digitalis, beta-blockers).
         (b) Enhanced vagal tone (e.g., vasovagal reactions).
         (c) Acute myocardial infarction.
         (d) Sick sinus syndrome (Chapter 11).

III. CARDIAC EMERGENCIES DUE TO MECHANICAL DYSFUNCTION

Four main factors affect the pumping function of the heart:
   1. The peripheral vascular resistance (affects afterload).
   2. The venous return (affects preload).
   3. The inotropic or contractile state of the myocardium.
   4. The cardiac rhythm.

Disturbances in any one of those four factors can result in heart failure.

Congestive heart failure causes symptoms related to:
1. Failure to deliver sufficient blood to the tissue.
2. Congestion—the damming of blood in the vessels leading to the heart.

A. Pulmonary Edema (See also Chapter 2)

The clinical manifestation of acute left ventricular failure is pulmonary edema. When the left ventricle fails, left ventricular filling pressure and volume increase. The rise in pressure and volume is transmitted retrogradely to the left atrium and in turn to the pulmonary veins and capillaries. Elevated pulmonary capillary pressure results in interstitial and alveolar edema. Increased permeability of the pulmonary capillary membrane, a fall in plasma oncotic pressure, or alteration in interstitial lymphatic flow contributes to the development of pulmonary edema.

Pulmonary congestion may be manifested by the following symptoms: (1) dyspnea, (2) cough, (3) orthopnea, (4) wheezing, and (5) frothy sputum (often blood tinged). The heart rate increases in compensation for the falling stroke volume. Other compensatory symptoms of a falling cardiac output are cool or clammy skin, changes in sensorium, and decreased urinary output.

Therapy for pulmonary edema is directed at decreasing congestion and improving cardiac output.

1. Pharmacologic Management of Pulmonary Edema. Four classes of drugs are generally used in the management of acute pulmonary edema: morphine, diuretics, aminophylline, and vasodilators.

   a) Morphine Sulfate. The drug of choice in the management of pulmonary edema is morphine sulfate. Morphine has four important effects in pulmonary edema: (1) venodilatation, resulting in a reduction of the preload, (2) a decrease in anxiety, (3) a decrease in the rate of respiration, alleviating the severe dyspnea, and (4) a decrease in pulmonary venous pressure.

   b) Diuretics. Rapidly acting diuretics, such as furosemide (Lasix) and ethacrynic acid (Edecrin), are given IV. The immediate response to IV furosemide is peripheral venous dilatation, resulting in a decrease in the preload, which occurs prior to its diuretic effects.

   c) Aminophylline. Aminophylline is a pulmonary vasodilator and bronchodilator. It also stimulates myocardial contractility and has a mild diuretic effect.

   d) Vasodilators. Intravenous vasodilators, nitroglycerin and nitroprusside can provide rapid benefit in acute pulmonary edema. Nitroglycerin acts primarily by reducing preload because of its venodilating effects. Nitroprusside dilates both arteries and veins thereby affecting both afterload and preload significantly.

e) Digitalis. Digitalis is *not* a primary drug for the treatment of acute pulmonary edema but is effective in chronic therapy of congestive heart failure.

2. Additional Measures Used in Managing Acute Left Ventricular Failure.

a) Rotating Tourniquets. Decreasing venous return in pulmonary edema may be affected by the application of tourniquets. The principles of tourniquet application are: (1) apply the tourniquet high in the groin and axilla and reduce only the venous flow, (2) occlude only two limbs at a time, (3) rotate the tourniquets every 10 to 15 min, (4) discontinue using the tourniquets one at a time to prevent sudden increases in the venous return, and (5) do not apply the tourniquets if the patient is hypotensive, and discontinue the use of the tourniquets if hypotension occurs during their use.

b) Oxygen. Oxygen is administered to the patient who has pulmonary edema to increase arterial oxygen saturation and to reduce cardiac workload. Intermittent positive pressure breathing (IPPB) may be used to decrease venous return and to enhance ventilation. Oxygen should be administered by mask to patients who are mouth breathers.

c) Parameters to be Evaluated Frequently. Evaluation of the lungs and respiratory status is continuously made by: (1) observation of the rate and character of respiration, (2) auscultation of the lungs, and (3) analysis of blood gases.

d) Avoid Suction. Suctioning should be avoided in pulmonary edema, because it may produce bronchospasm and further decrease oxygen transport.

3. Evaluation of the Efficacy of Treatment. The efficacy of the treatment should be evaluated constantly, and the results should be documented.

a) What Nurses Should Know/Do About Pulmonary Edema

(1) Place the patient in the high Fowler's position (chair rest is ideal).

(2) Administer oxygen.

(3) Start an IV infusion to maintain venous access.

(4) Have tourniquets at bedside. Apply them as indicated, but do not apply them if the patient is hypotensive.

(5) Anticipate the need for morphine, diuretics, aminophylline, and vasodilators.

(a) With the IV administration of morphine, watch for hypotension and respiratory depression.

(b) With the administration of diuretic drugs, record the diuretic response; watch for electrolyte depletion.

        (c) With the administration of aminophylline, watch for nausea and vomiting, tachycardia, and ventricular premature contractions.

        (d) With IV vasodilators (nitroglycerin or nitroprusside) watch for untoward hypotension.

    (6) Have resuscitation equipment at the patient's bedside.

    (7) Explain any procedures that might frighten the patient (e.g., tourniquets, IPPB, and phlebotomy) and stay with him to decrease his anxiety.

    (8) Examine the patient's lungs and heart every 2 to 5 min until his condition stabilizes.

    (9) Monitor the patient's blood pressure, level of consciousness, skin color, and temperature for signs of decreased cardiac output.

   (10) If central venous pressure lines or a Swan-Ganz catheter is in place, monitor pressure changes to determine the effectiveness of drug therapy.

   (11) Avoid tracheal suctioning; it may induce bronchospasm.

B. Shock (See also Chapter 3)

    Shock is a hypotensive state accompanied by clinical signs of poor peripheral perfusion; that is, cold or clammy skin, poor mentation, and reduced urinary output.

    Hypovolemia, the most frequent cause of shock, is due to a reduction in circulatory volume per se or to a decrease in the effective circulating volume. A decrease in the effective circulating volume can result from (1) sequestration of fluid in one or more of the vascular compartments in which venous, capillary, or arterial tone has been altered, or (2) shifting of fluid into interstitial tissues.

    Marked tachyarrhythmias or bradyarrhythmias that result in a significant reduction in cardiac output may produce shock. Cardiogenic shock is usually due to extensive myocardial damage which produces serious impairment in contractility, and consequently, low cardiac output. During shock, the reduced peripheral perfusion creates tissue hypoxia and forces anaerobic metabolism and lactic acidosis.

    Constant monitoring of circulatory volume and fluid balance is important in all forms of shock so that an adequate fluid volume is maintained in the vascular space. Shifts of volume occur within the vascular space as a result of the compensatory responses to hypoxia and hypotension. Blood flow is distributed in such a way that nonvital areas receive less blood than do the vital organs—the heart, the brain, and the kidneys.

   1. Management. Therapy is primarily directed to the cause of shock:

     1. In hypovolemic shock, replace the circulatory volume.

     2. In arrhythmic shock, change the rate or rhythm to

improve cardiac output and to provide an adequate minute volume.

3. In cardiogenic shock, improve the relationship between oxygen supply and demand to ischemic and injured myocardium by (1) reducing cardiac work, and (2) improving coronary perfusion by augmenting diastolic volume and pressure (the time when the coronaries are perfused), using vasoactive drugs or mechanical cardiac support.

The selection of the appropriate IV fluid for volume challenge is based on the hemoglobin level, the oncotic pressure, the state of the myocardium, and the pulmonary artery wedge pressures. The nurse's job in fluid challenge management is the careful hemodynamic monitoring of the patient with regard to those parameters. Before manipulating fluid administration, it is important to find out from the attending physician what the target pressure is.

Therapy is directed toward (1) minimizing the demands for myocardial oxygen consumption, (2) improving coronary blood supply, and (3) optimizing left ventricular pump function.

The demands for myocardial oxygen consumption are minimized by:

1. Controlling the heart rate and rhythm.
2. Decreasing the preload (ventricular filling pressure).
3. Decreasing the afterload by the use of vasodilators.
4. Taking general ambient measures to lower tissue demands and thus reduce cardiac work; that is, making the patient comfortable and creating a calm, reassuring surrounding.

Myocardial oxygen demands may be decreased by vasodilator therapy, which decreases the preload and afterload. Coronary blood supply may be improved by vasoconstrictor drugs and by surgical revascularization. The intra-aortic balloon pump decreases demands, increases cardiac output, and improves coronary blood supply.

a) Sodium Nitroprusside (Nipride). Sodium nitroprusside is commonly used to reduce myocardial oxygen demands and to improve cardiac output. The drug acts directly on the blood vessels to produce vasodilatation. It affects both arteries and veins and thus is able to reduce both the preload and afterload. The drug should be administered by an infusion pump, with meticulous monitoring of the left atrial and systemic arterial pressures. Nitroprusside has a rapid onset and elimination that allows for ease of titration to therapeutic effect in hemodynamic emergencies. It is particularly useful in preshock states with low cardiac output and pulmonary vascular congestion. It is generally contraindicated, however, in cases of frank cardiogenic shock because of the danger of worsening hypotension.

(1) What Nurses Should Know/Do About Sodium Nitroprusside Therapy

(a) For initiating therapy with sodium nitroprusside, an arterial line and a Swan-Ganz catheter should be in place.

(b) Wrap the bottle and tubing in foil to protect the solution from light (which inactivates the drug) and indicate the time the solution was prepared; the unused portion must be discarded in 4 hours. Administer the drug with an infusion pump; do not add other medications to the IV solution containing sodium nitroprusside.

(c) Before starting therapy, find out from the physician what the target pulmonary capillary wedge and systemic arterial pressures are.

(d) Titrate the IV infusion and achieve a therapeutic response. A nurse should be in constant attendance to maintain the target pressures.

(e) If the wedge or arterial pressure falls below the determined critical levels, immediately slow down or discontinue the sodium nitroprusside infusion.

(f) Serum levels of the metabolite thiocyanate should be determined if the patient has been taking sodium nitroprusside for more than 24 hours. If levels exceed 12 mg/100 ml, sodium nitroprusside should be discontinued to avoid intoxication, which is manifested by deterioration of the patient's condition (acidosis and hypoxia), psychosis, and confusion. Cyanide poisoning antidote kits should be readily available.

b) Dopamine (Intropin). Dopamine is a sympathomimetic drug that has alpha-, beta-, and gamma-adrenergic properties. At low doses (< 10 μg/kg/min), beta-adrenergic effects predominate (increased myocardial contractility and vasodilation of renal and mesenteric vascular beds). At higher doses (> 20 μg/kg/min), alpha-adrenergic effects predominate resulting in peripheral vasoconstriction.

(1) What Nurses Should Know/Do About Dopamine Therapy

(a) Find out from the physician the target blood and wedge pressures.

(b) Find out from the physician the dosage in μg/min. Therapeutic effects are most evident at low to moderate dosages.

(c) Administer dopamine through an infusion pump; do not mix it with other medications.

(d) Monitor the patient's blood pressure and urinary output during infusion; watch for provocation of tachyarrhythmias.

c) Dobutamine (Dobutrex). Dobutamine is a beta-adrenergic stimulator that increases myocardial contractility directly. It is primarily used for cardiogenic shock.

(1) What Nurses Should Know/Do About Dobutamine Therapy

(a) Monitor rhythm, blood and wedge pressures, and urinary output as described with dopamine.

(b) Blood pressure may decline because of peripheral vasodilating effects.

(c) Dobutamine does *not* stimulate dopamine-specific receptors of renal and mesenteric arteries.

d) Norepinephrine (Levophed). Norepinephrine may be used to support arterial pressure and thus improve coronary blood flow. Norepinephrine causes arterial vasoconstriction (alpha-adrenergic effect) and produces a slight positive inotropic (beta-adrenergic effect). By enhancing afterload and stimulating contractility, norepinephrine may increase oxygen consumption. If, however, normal blood pressure can be restored, the benefits derived from improved coronary perfusion may outweigh the increase in oxygen consumption.

(1) What Nurses Should Know/Do About Norepinephrine Therapy

(a) Find out from the physician the end point of therapy.

(b) Administer norepinephrine with an infusion pump, through an Intracath.

(c) Monitor the patient's blood pressure and cardiac status.

(d) Avoid infiltration into subcutaneous tissue; norepinephrine can cause severe tissue sloughing. *Note:* The antidote for norepinephrine that infiltrates the tissue is phentolamine (Regitine) injected into the tissues involved.

(e) Patients receiving norepinephrine often have cold or clammy skin because of the drug's vasoconstriction effects.

(2) What Nurses Should Know/Do About Shock

(a) Place the patient flat or in Trendelenburg position (to maximize the blood flow to the cerebrum).

(b) Maintain oxygen therapy.

(c) Have resuscitation equipment at the bedside.

(d) Swan-Ganz catheters and arterial lines are

needed for sodium nitroprusside and dopamine therapy.

(e) Evaluate and treat the underlying causes:

i) Correct cardiac arrhythmias.

ii) Fluid replacement for hypovolemia.

iii) Elevate the patient's legs to increase venous return, and observe the patient's response.

iv) Check the central venous, pulmonary artery, and wedge pressures to determine whether they are low or low normal.

v) Rule out vasoactive mechanisms as the cause of shock; determine whether the shock is drug related (morphine, nitroglycerin, meperidine hydrochloride), is a vasovagal reaction or is caused by infection (sepsis).

(f) Evaluate the patient's lung status:

i) Examine the patient for rales.

ii) Investigate whether shock is due to depressed oxygen and carbon dioxide transport at lung level.

(g) Evaluate the patient's tissue metabolism:

i) Evaluate the rate and character of respirations. Are Kussmaul's respirations present?

ii) Watch for signs of deterioration in tissue perfusion.

iii) Analyze the blood gases. Is metabolic acidosis present, or is there a respiratory component?

iv) Evaluate the effectiveness of drugs.

(h) Evaluate the patient's renal perfusion status:

i) Is the patient uremic or oliguric?

ii) Is the urine concentrated in appearance?

iii) Observe the urine output closely (every hour) and correlate it with the IV therapy and pharmacologic interventions.

(i) If shock is determined to be cardiogenic:

i) Reduce the myocardial oxygen demand.

ii) Treat fever if present.

iii) Maintain the patient's heart in optimal contractile state by correcting acid-base electrolyte imbalances and by checking the central venous, pulmonary artery, and wedge pressures and the cardiac output.

iv) Support the patient with drugs as ordered.

(j) Monitor the cardiac and vascular effects of drug therapy. Observe the patient closely and correlate his signs and symptoms with his:

i) Cardiac rate and rhythm.

ii) Arterial pressure.

iii) Wedge pressure.

    iv) Central venous pressure.
    v) Rate and work of respiration.
    vi) Fluid intake and urinary output.

IV. CARDIAC TAMPONADE (See also Chapter 16)

Cardiac tamponade results when an increase in intrapericardial pressure due to fluid accumulation results in an impairment of the diastolic filling of the heart. The ability of the pericardium to accommodate or comply with the increase in fluid volume depends on the length of time over which the fluid accumulates. The pericardium, if stretched over a period of weeks, may accommodate a liter or more. If, however, an increase in contents occurs suddenly, as little as 100 to 200 ml may cause significant hemodynamic compromise. Tamponade can be readily recognized and even prevented if the possibility of its occurrence is considered in certain clinical states. Infection, inflammation, trauma, acute myocardial infarction, or neoplasm of the heart are common predisposing conditions of tamponade.

A. Signs and Symptoms

Cardiac tamponade is characterized by the following signs and symptoms: (1) a rising venous pressure, (2) a falling blood pressure and cardiac output—narrowing pulse pressure, (3) pulsus paradoxus, (4) distant heart sounds, (5) dyspnea, (6) electrical alternans or diminished voltage of the QRS complexes on the ECG, and (7) tachycardia. These manifestations correlate with the pathophysiologic aspects of tamponade. Elevation of the venous pressure and distention of the neck veins result from impedance to right ventricular diastolic filling. The fall in arterial pressure and cardiac output is a manifestation of decreasing left ventricular stroke volume and is usually associated with compensatory tachycardia. Pulsus paradoxus is defined as a greater than normal inspiratory decline in systolic arterial pressure (8 to 10 mm Hg are considered the upper limits of normal). That definition was first used by Kussmaul (in 1873) to describe the marked diminution of the peripheral pulse volume on inspiration in patients who have tamponade. The exaggerated fall in arterial pressure on inspiration can be measured by an arterial pressure monitor, or it can be detected by palpating or auscultating the peripheral pulse using a brachial sphygmomanometer.

B. Management

Therapy for cardiac tamponade is directed toward decreasing the intrapericardial pressure. Pericardiocentesis and surgical drainage are the usual modes of therapy. Pericardiocentesis is performed with a large-bore needle or catheter so that pus or blood can be readily evacuated. Preparation by skin anesthesia is desirable if time permits. The needle should be connected by an alligator clamp to the chest lead of an ECG apparatus to permit monitoring of the course of the needle. S-T segment elevation (seen in subepicardial injury) appears if the needle comes in contact with the ventricle. Emergency equipment should be at the patient's bedside during the procedure, and an IV line should be kept running. If no fluid is aspirated during attempted pericardiocentesis, a pericardiotomy is indicated.

1. What Nurses Should Know/Do About Cardiac Tamponade
    a) Be aware of the settings in which tamponade could occur, that is, chest trauma, pericarditis, postcardiac surgery, and acute myocardial infarction.
    b) Note the heart rate and rhythm change.
    c) Examine the patient for pulsus paradoxus:
        (1) Palpate the peripheral pulse and note if there is a diminution on inspiration.
        (2) Obtain the systolic brachial blood pressure reading with a sphygmomanometer. Deflate the cuff on expiration; after noting the peak systolic pressure, slowly deflate the cuff during inspiration and note the difference in systolic peak pressure between expiration and inspiration. A fall greater than 15 mm Hg is a sign of possible tamponade.
        (3) If the patient has an arterial line in place, note from the pulse wave patterns whether there is marked fall on inspiration.
        (4) Examine for narrowing of the pulse pressure (seen with low-stroke volume).
    d) Look for signs of decreased cardiac output: cool or clammy skin, sensorium changes, decreased urinary output, acceleration of the heart rate, and hypotension.
    e) Monitor the venous pressure of the patient suspected of having tamponade:
        (1) Check the central venous pressure.
        (2) Check for neck vein distention (occasionally exaggerated during inspiration).
        (3) Rule out other causes of an increasing venous pressure.
    f) Note the character of respiration—look for dyspnea, orthopnea, and a changing respiratory rate.
    g) Auscultate the chest frequently for heart sounds:
        (1) Establish a baseline for the patient's normal heart sounds.
        (2) Note if the heart sounds become distant.
        (3) Listen for pericardial friction rubs.
    h) Look for low voltage and electrical alternans on the ECG.
    i) Make sure an IV route is available.
    j) Have emergency equipment available.
    k) Anticipate supportive measures (volume expansion, isoproterenol).
2. What Nurses Should Know/Do About Pericardiocentesis
    a) Explain the procedure to the patient and stay with the

patient during the procedure; elevate the head of the bed to 30°.

b) Have a crashcart and defibrillator at the patient's bedside.

c) Start a slow IV infusion.

d) Connect the patient to a monitor (a dual-channel monitor or a monitor and an ECG machine should be used).

e) Have a pericardiocentesis tray available (if one is not available, a large bore needle or an Intracath may be used). Lidocaine and a syringe for local skin infiltration should also be available.

f) Connect the alligator clamp to the chest lead of the electrode cable and to the needle.

g) Monitor simultaneously for cardiac rhythm and needle position.

h) Have culture bottles available.

V. HYPERTENSIVE CRISIS (See also Chapter 17)

Acute hypertensive crisis is a life-threatening emergency characterized by a marked elevation in arterial pressure (generally diastolic levels are about 140 mm Hg). Clinical manifestations include acute encephalopathy, left ventricular failure, and renal impairment. Most hypertensive crises develop in patients who are known to be hypertensive, many of whom have neglected or discontinued treatment for hypertension. Hypertensive crises can often be avoided by educating patients about the need to adhere to long-term dietary and drug management.

Acute hypertensive encephalopathy is accompanied by a severe headache, a decreasing level of consciousness, blurred vision, or other visual disturbances. Nausea, vomiting, or focal neurologic sensory or motor disturbances may be the presenting signs. Funduscopic examinations frequently reveal exudates, papilledema, and hemorrhage. Those findings are manifestations of cerebral edema and increased intracranial pressure. The treatment of pulmonary edema in such a setting is similar to the usual drug regimen for pulmonary edema plus antihypertensive drugs.

The primary therapy for an acute hypertensive crisis is directed toward decreasing the arterial pressure with acute antihypertensive drugs and decreasing the cerebral edema with diuretics. Care must be taken to avoid precipitous drops in blood pressure, which may compromise the cerebral, coronary, and renal blood flows.

A. Pharmacologic Management

The primary nursing responsibility is the monitoring of the patient's response to therapy. The monitoring is done by:

1. Checking the blood pressure every 5 to 15 min (as drug therapy indicates).

2. Monitoring the heart rate and rhythm.

3. Monitoring the neurologic states—level of consciousness, pupil responsiveness, general movement, and focal neurologic signs.

    4. Monitoring the renal status, measuring the intake and output and the BUN and creatinine levels.

1. Direct Vasodilators.

    a) Diazoxide (Hyperstat). Diazoxide, a potent antihypertensive drug, is given rapidly by IV bolus to dilate the arterioles. It is given as a rapid bolus because it binds with serum proteins, which inactivate the drug. Renal blood flow remains stable, and the heart rate and cardiac output increase reflexively. Sodium retention may occur with continued therapy with diazoxide and necessitates the use of diuretics. Hyperglycemia may also occur with diazoxide, just as it does with other thiazide drugs.

    b) Sodium Nitroprusside. Sodium nitroprusside causes direct vasodilatation. It is administered in an IV infusion and titrated to achieve the decreased pressure. The drug may be especially helpful in acute left ventricular failure because of its effects on reducing both preload and afterload.

    c) Hydralazine (Apresoline). Hydralazine is a direct vasodilator, and, like diazoxide, it increases the heart rate and cardiac output. Hydralazine is usually given IV slowly over a 5-min period. A continuous IV infusion may be given subsequently. The drug usually begins to act in 15 to 20 min. Hydralazine has been reported to have unpredictable effects on encephalopathy in some patients.

2. The Ganglionic Blockers (Sympathetic Blockers). The ganglionic-blocking drugs produce their effects by interrupting transmission of impulses at autonomic ganglia. By that mechanism, they block the effects of both sympathetic and parasympathetic nerves. The inhibition of sympathetic signals produces vasodilatation and thereby decreases blood pressure. Trimethaphan (Arfonad) is the most commonly used ganglionic blocker. To enhance the therapeutic effects, it is recommended that the head of the patient's bed be elevated on shock blocks 10 to 12 in—so that the patient maintains a more upright posture.

    Because the ganglionic blockers produce parasympathetic as well as sympathetic blockage, complications, such as urinary retention, paralytic ileus, and pupillary dilatation, occur if therapy is continued. Inactivation of pupillary reflexes interferes with the evaluation of the patient's neurologic status. Reduction in the glomerular filtration rate may also be seen with the ganglionic blockers.

3. Antiadrenergic Agents

    a) Reserpine (Serpasil). Reserpine acts by depleting catecholamine stores at nerve terminals in the central nervous system. Reserpine is rarely used in hypertensive crisis because of its relatively slow onset of action and major adverse effects.

b) Methyldopa (Aldomet). Methyldopa achieves its antiadrenergic effect by acting as a false transmitter in both the peripheral and central nervous systems. Like reserpine, methyldopa has a gradual onset of action (4 to 6 hours), and it may cause somnolence secondary to central nervous system depression. Therefore, it is generally not used in crisis therapy as the initial drug.

c) Phentolamine (Regitine). Phentolamine is used specifically to manage hypertensive crisis associated with increased levels of catecholamines. The drug blocks the alpha receptors of the sympathetic nervous system, which are found primarily in the blood vessels, and thus produces vasodilatation. Phentolamine is used for patients who have pheochromocytoma and hypertensive crisis associated with monoamine oxidase (MAO) inhibitors (Chapter 17).

4. Diuretics. Furosemide and ethacrynic acid, rapidly acting diuretics, are administered IV in a hypertensive crisis. They may be useful as adjunctive therapy when combined with other agents already discussed.

a) What Nurses Should Know/Do About Hypertensive Crisis

(1) Administer oxygen.

(2) Place the patient in the reverse Trendelenburg position, if possible, to minimize cerebral pressure and to maximize the effects of drugs, especially the ganglionic blockers.

(3) Intravenous infusion and infusion pump—have an arterial line available.

(4) Have the crashcart and other emergency equipment at the patient's bedside.

(5) Anticipate the need for rapidly acting antihypertensive drugs:

(a) Diazoxide and hydralazine—for patients without primary cardiac involvement.

(b) Sodium nitroprusside and trimethaphan—for patients who have left ventricular failure or other types of compromised cardiac function.

(c) Phentolamine and sodium nitroprusside—for patients who have pheochromocytoma or a crisis associated with MAO inhibition.

(6) Know the physician's criteria for a therapeutic response:

(a) The target systolic and diastolic pressures.

(b) The amount of time allotted to reach the goal. (*Note:* Precipitous drops in blood pressure may compromise the coronary, cerebral, and renal blood flows.)

(c) The maximum infusion rate to titrate.

(7) Establish and document baseline data about the patient's:
  (a) Neurologic status.
  (b) Blood pressure.
  (c) Wedge pressure.
  (d) Renal status.
  (e) Urinary output.
  (f) BUN and creatinine levels.
(8) Anticipate the need for rapidly acting diuretics—furosemide and ethacrynic acid:
  (a) Monitor the fluid intake and urine output.
  (b) Monitor the serum electrolytes.
(9) Keep the peripheral vascular demands for oxygen down by:
  (a) Sedating the patient.
  (b) Maintaining a calm environment to decrease the patient's anxiety
  (c) Explaining all frightening procedures.
  (d) Controlling the traffic into the room.
(10) With diazoxide therapy, watch especially for tachycardia, fluid retention, and hyperglycemia.
(11) Diazoxide and hydralazine frequently cause reflex increase in heart rate and cardiac output and should be avoided in patients who have ischemic heart disease and dissecting aortic aneurysms.
(12) With sodium nitroprusside, protect the drug from light, change the bottle every 4 hours, and monitor the thiocyanide levels after 24 hours of therapy.
(13) With the ganglionic blocker trimethaphan, watch for urinary retention, paralytic ileus, and inactivation of pupillary reflexes.
(14) With reserpine and methyldopa, watch for increasing somnolence.
(15) During IV therapy with antihypertensive drugs, be in constant attendance and have norepinephrine (Levarterenol) and metaraminol available in case of hypotension.

VI. PULMONARY EMBOLISM AND INFARCTION (See also Chapter 4)
  Pulmonary embolism and infarction are apt to occur in people who are bedfast. In most cases, the source of pulmonary embolism is the deep veins of the legs, but there may be no clinical evidence of deep vein thrombosis. The clinical manifestations of pulmonary embolism depend on the size of the occluded pulmonary circulation and the previous state of the cardiovascular system.
  Clinical features of pulmonary embolism or infarction include:
  1. Dyspnea and tachypnea (and possibly cyanosis).
  2. Chest pain (typically pleuritic with infarction).
  3. Cough and hemoptysis (with infarction).
  4. Diaphoresis and apprehension.

5. Tachycardia.
6. Hypotension (with massive embolism).
7. Wide splitting of the second heart sound with a loud pulmonic component.
8. Right heart S_3 and S_4 gallop.
9. Distended neck veins.
10. Fever and leukocytosis (with infarction).
11. ECG manifestations of acute cor pulmonale (e.g., right axis deviation, P pulmonale, S_1, Q_3 pattern, inverted T waves in leads II, III, and aVF, and/or inverted T waves in leads V_{1-3}, acute right bundle branch block, and atrial tachyarrhythmias).

When pulmonary embolism occurs, blood flow to the area distal to the occlusion is obstructed. If a large area of lung is not perfused, the oxygen tension in the arterial blood falls significantly. The patient develops dyspnea and then tachypnea in an effort to compensate for the underperfusion. Infarction of lung tissue produces the classic complaint of pleuritic chest pain which may be associated with a pleural friction rub. Hemoptysis results from hemorrhagic necrosis of the lung tissue distal to the obstruction. Distention of the neck veins reflects increased pressure in the right heart which is due to acute pulmonary hypertension. Syncope may occur if the embolic obstruction is significant enough to reduce left atrial and left ventricular filling and the reflex tachycardia and peripheral vascular constriction cannot support cardiac output. The pulmonary component of the second heart sound is loud and delayed because right ventricular ejection time is prolonged against a high pulmonary artery pressure.

Therapy for pulmonary embolism is primarily medical. The main therapeutic intervention is the administration of anticoagulants (heparin and warfarin). Thrombolytic drugs, such as urokinase and streptokinase, may also be used.

    a) What Nurses Should Know/Do About Pulmonary Embolism and Infarction

        (1) Anticipate and look for signs of pulmonary emboli in patients at high risk:

            (a) Patients after surgery
            (b) Patients with leg injuries
            (c) Patients who are postpartum
            (d) Patients taking contraceptive drugs
            (e) Patients who have chronic peripheral vascular disease
            (f) Patients who have chronic congestive heart failure
            (g) Patients who have cardiovascular disease
            (h) Patients who have a history of thromboembolic phenomena
            (i) Patients who are obese.

        (2) Use anti-embolic stockings and foot and leg exercise for patients at risk; consider low-dose heparin (5,000

units subcutaneously every 12 hours) prophylactically.

(3) Administer oxygen when pulmonary embolism is
suspected.

(4) Place the patient in Fowler position when embolization is suspected.

(5) Anticipate the use of heparin. Investigate the
patient's clotting times (the prothrombin time and
partial thromboplastin time), explain the need for the
tests to the patient.

(6) Perform serial blood gases analyses to monitor therapeutic response.

(7) Monitor the patient's vital signs closely.

(8) Ease the patient's anxiety.

(9) Explain the diagnostic procedures to the patient (e.g.,
lung scan, angiography).

VII. CARDIOPULMONARY RESUSCITATION (See also Chapter 15)
What Nurses Should Know/Do About Cardiopulmonary Resuscitation (CPR)

The nurse has a primary role in CPR. Her ability to perform CPR
according to the established guidelines gives the patient the best
chance for survival. *Immediate* initiation of effective and uninterrupted cardiac compression and assisted ventilation is crucial to
successful resuscitation. The American Heart Association has
established CPR certification programs at both the basic and the
instructor levels. It is recommended that all nurses be certified at
one of those levels to establish the highest standard of care.

Other nursing responsibilities in cardiac arrest are related to the
preparation and administration of drugs. The nurse who under-
stands the mechanism of action and potential hazards of drugs
commonly used in cardiac arrest can act appropriately when a crisis
occurs.

A. Drug Therapy

The five most commonly used drugs in a cardiac arrest are
(1) epinephrine, (2) sodium bicarbonate, (3) calcium, (4) atropine, and (5) lidocaine. The nursing aspects of atropine and
lidocaine were discussed in the section on arrhythmias. Sodium
bicarbonate, epinephrine, and calcium are discussed in the following paragraphs.

1. Sodium Bicarbonate. Sodium bicarbonate, a naturally occurring buffer in the body, is used to correct metabolic acidosis
in cardiac emergencies. A normal pH improves the response
of the myocardium to resuscitative measures. Analyses of
arterial blood gases should be made periodically in order to
assess acid-base status (if not rapidly available, an additional
ampule of bicarbonate should be administered at 10 min
intervals).

2. Epinephrine. Epinephrine (adrenalin) is an endogenous catecholamine with both alpha- and beta-adrenergic effects.

Epinephrine stimulates electrical and mechanical activity in the heart and causes peripheral vasoconstriction. Its use during cardiac arrest can: (1) elevate coronary perfusion pressure during resuscitation, (2) improve myocardial contractility, (3) stimulate electrical activity in ventricular standstill, and (4) convert fine, low-amplitude fibrillation to faster, coarse fibrillation which is more responsive to electrical defibrillation.

The usual dose of epinephrine is 0.5 ml of a 1:1000 solution or 5 ml of a 1:10,000 solution by the IV route; repeat doses may be given at 5 to 10 min intervals if necessary because of its short duration of action. It may also be given as an intracardiac injection by trained personnel. Because epinephrine is rapidly absorbed in the lungs, it can be given into an endotracheal tube as an alternative route in an emergency.

3. Calcium. Calcium stabilizes the permeability of the cell to sodium and potassium and thus affects electrical activity. It is also a direct mediator of myocardial contractility. Calcium is used in electromechanical dissociation (absence of any pulse despite an electrical rhythm) and in restoring electrical activity during asystole. Calcium preparations are administered IV slowly and may produce sloughing of tissues if IV fluid infiltrates. Calcium precipitates if it is mixed with sodium bicarbonate. It is important to remember that calcium should be used cautiously in digitalized patients because it potentiates digitalis activity and toxicity.

VIII. SUMMARY

1. The role of the nurse in cardiac emergencies has become a vital one with the advent of intensive care units. Because cardiac emergencies may take place anywhere in the hospital, all nursing personnel should be required to have a working knowledge of cardiac emergencies.

2. In this chapter, cardiac emergencies have been discussed with emphasis on pathophysiology and pharmacology in order to provide a better understanding of diagnosis and management.

3. Cardiac emergencies may result from primary electrical dysfunction or primary mechanical dysfunction.

4. Arrhythmias result from disturbances in automaticity or conduction. The possible causes must be reviewed when a patient presents with an arrhythmia.

5. Ventricular arrhythmias generally have greater clinical significance because they may precipitate a symptomatic fall in cardiac output and may lead to fatal ventricular fibrillation.

6. The symptoms and the pathophysiologic aspects of pulmonary edema as a manifestation of acute left ventricular failure have been discussed. Therapy is directed toward acutely decreasing the preload and cardiac work and improving the cardiac output. Thus the acute management of pulmonary edema includes the

use of morphine, diuretics, vasodilators, and in certain instances aminophylline.

7. Shock is a hypotensive state accompanied by signs of poor peripheral perfusion. Hypovolemic, arrhythmogenic, and cardiogenic shock have been discussed with emphasis on the collaboration of the nurse and physician in monitoring the patient's hemodynamic status and fluid balance, minimizing the myocardial oxygen demands, and carrying out vasoactive drug therapy.

8. The presence of cardiac tamponade has to be considered whenever there is infarction, inflammation, trauma, acute myocardial infarction, or neoplasm of the heart. Nursing considerations for the early detection of tamponade are emphasized.

9. Hypertensive crisis is characterized by an acute and marked elevation in the arterial pressure with manifestations of acute encephalopathy or acute left ventricular failure. The primary therapy is directed toward decreasing the arterial pressure with antihypertensive drugs and decreasing the cerebral edema with diuretics.

10. The key to successful resuscitation from cardiac arrest is the immediate initiation of effective cardiac compression and assisted ventilation. Nursing expertise in basic CPR technique and emergency drug administration is vital.

11. Full cooperation must exist between nursing staff and physicians when dealing with any cardiac emergency. Any nurse working in the cardiac emergency setting should be ready to assist cardiologists and cardiac surgeons whenever necessary for the best therapeutic results.

12. In recent years, cocaine is found to be one of the most important predisposing factors in the development of various cardiac arrhythmias, myocarditis, angina pectoris, coronary artery spasm, acute MI, and even sudden cardiac death. This is particularly true among young adult males.

SUGGESTED READINGS

American Heart Association. Textbook of Advanced Cardiac Life Support. Dallas, American Heart Association, 1981.

AMA Committee of Hypertension: The treatment of malignant hypertension and hypertensive emergencies. JAMA 228:1673, 1974.

Anderson, J.L.: Clinical implications of new studies in the treatment of benign, potentially malignant and malignant ventricular arrhythmias. Am. J. Cardiol. 65:36B, 1990.

Antman, E.M. and Braunwald, E.: Acute MI: Management in the 1990s. Hosp. Pract. 7:65, 1990.

Bell, W.R., and Simon, T.L.: Current status of pulmonary thromboembolic disease: pathophysiology, diagnosis, prevention, and treatment. Am. Heart J. 103:239, 1982.

Benhorin, J., Moss, A.J., Oakes, D., et al.: The prognostic significance of first myocardial infarction type (Q wave versus non-Q wave) and Q wave location. J. Am. Coll. Cardiol. 15:1201, 1990.

Berns, E. and Naccarelli, G.V.: Management of tachyarrhythmias after MI. Hosp. Prac. 4:33, 1990.

Blankehorn, D.H., Johnson, R.L., Mack, W.J., et al.: The influence of diet on the appearance of new lesions in human coronary arteries. JAMA 263:1646, 1990.

Braunwald, E.: Heart Disease, 3rd Ed. Philadelphia, W.B. Saunders, 1988.

Burrel, Z.L., and Burrel, L.O.: Critical Care. St. Louis, C.V. Mosby Co., 1982.

Chung, E.K.: Principles of Cardiac Arrhythmias, 4th Ed. Baltimore, Williams & Wilkins Co., 1989.

Cohn, J.N., and Burke, L.P.: Nitroprusside. Ann. Int. Med. 91:752, 1979.

DeSilva, R.A., Graboys, T.B., Podrid, P.J., and Lown, B.: Cardioversion and defibrillation. Am. Heart J. 100:881, 1980.

Dhar, S.K., and Freeman, P.: Clinical management of hypertensive emergencies. Heart Lung 5:571, 1976.

Falk, R.H.: Impact of prospective peer review on pacemaker implantation rates in Massachusetts. J. Am. Coll. Cardiol. 15:1087, 1990.

Gemson, D.H., Sloan, R.P., Messeri, P., and Goldberg, I.J.: A public health model for cardiovascular risk reduction. Arch. Intern. Med. 150:985, 1990.

Gettes, L.S.: Physiology and pharmacology of antiarrhythmic drugs. Hosp. Pract. 10:89, 1981.

Goldberg, R.J., Brady, P., Muller, J.E., et al.: Time of onset of symptoms of acute myocardial infarction. Am. J. Cardiol. 66:140, 1990.

Goodman, L.S., and Gilman, A.: The Pharmacologic Basis of Therapeutics. New York, Macmillian Publishing, 1980.

Gulhoed, G.W.: Blunt and penetrating chest trauma. Fam. Physicians 17:100, 1978.

Hale, S.L., Alker, K.J., Rezkalla, S., et al.: Adverse effects of cocaine on cardiovascular dynamics, myocardial blood flow, and coronary artery diameter in an experimental model. Am. Heart J. 118:927, 1989.

Hancock, E.W.: Cardiac tamponade. Med. Clin. North Am. 63:223, 1979.

Harken, D.W.: Postoperative care following heart-valve surgery. Heart Lung 3:893, 1974.

Huss, P., Miller, J., Unverferth, D.V. and Leier, C.V.: The new inotropic drug, dobutamine. Heart Lung 10:121, 1981.

Igarashi, Y., Yamazoe, M., Suzuki, K., et al.: Possible role of coronary artery spasm in unexplained syncope. Am. J. Cardiol. 65:713, 1990.

James, T.N. and Riddick, L.: Sudden death due to isolated acute infarction of the His bundle. J. Am. Coll. Cardiol. 15:1183, 1990.

Kannel, W.B.: CHD risk factors: A Framingham study update. Hosp. Pract. 7:119, 1990.

Kao, W., Khaja, F., Goldstein, S. and Gheorghiade, M.: Cardiac event rate after non-Q-wave acute myocardial infarction and the significance of its anterior location. Am. J. Cardiol. 64:1236, 1989.

Kaye, W.: Invasive therapeutic techniques. Heart Lung 12:300, 1983.

Kinney, M.R., Dear, C.B., Packa, D.R., and Voorman, D.M.N.: AACN Clinical Reference for Critical-Care Nursing. New York, McGraw Hill Publishing, 1981.

Kugler, J.D. and Danford, D.A.: Pacemakers in children: An update. Am. Heart J. 117:665, 1989.

Kuhn, L., Scheidt, S. and Smith, D.A.: The cholesterol debate. Primary Cardiol. 16:38, 1990.

Lavie, C.J. and Gersh, B.J.: Mechanical and electrical complications of acute myocardial infarction. Mayo Clin. Proc. 65:709, 1990.

Maseri, A., Davies, G., Hackett, D. and Kaski, J.C.: Coronary artery spasm and vasoconstriction. Circulation 81:1983, 1990.

McGoon, M.D., Vlietstra, R.E., Holmes, D.R. and Osborn, J.E.: The clinical use of verapamil. Mayo Clin. Proc. 57:495, 1982.

Ram, C.V.S.: Hypertensive emergencies: recognition and management. Curr. Probl. Cardiol. 7:1, 1982.

Scroder, J. and Daily, E.: Techniques in Bedside Hemodynamic Monitoring. St. Louis, C.V. Mosby Publishing, 1976.

Sempos, C., Fulwood, R., Haines, C., et al.: The prevalence of high blood cholesterol levels among adults in the United States. JAMA 262:45, 1989.

Shabetai, R., Fowler, N.O. and Guntheroth, W.G.: The hemodynamics of cardiac tamponade and constrictive pericarditis. Am. J. Cardiol. 26:480, 1970.

Singer, I. and Kupersmith, J.: AICD therapy: Patient selection. Primary Cardiol. 16:27, 1990.

Sodeman, W.A., Jr. and Sodeman, W.A.: Pathologic Physiology: Mechanisms of Disease. Philadelphia, W.B. Saunders Publishing, 1979.

Spodick, D.H.: Medical history of the pericardium. The hairy heart of hoary heroes. Am. J. Cardiol. 26:447, 1970.

Squires, R.W., Gau, G.T., Miller, T.D., et al.: Cardiovascular rehabilitation: Status, 1990. Mayo Clin. Proc. 65:731, 1990.

Vinsant, M., Spence, M. and Hagen, D.: A Commonsense Approach to Coronary Care, 2nd ed. St. Louis, C.V. Mosby Publishing, 1975.

Wagner, H.R.: Parodoxical pulse: 100 years later. Am. J. Cardiol. 32:91, 1973.

Wajngarten, M., Grupi, C., Bellotti, G.M., et al.: Frequency and significance of cardiac rhythm disturbances in healthy elderly individuals. J. Electrocardiol. 23:171, 1990.

c h a p t e r

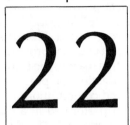

CARDIAC ELECTROPHYSIOLOGIC STUDIES

Soo G. Kim and Chung Whee Choue

Cardiac electrophysiologic studies involve recording of electrical activity of the heart using electrode catheters introduced percutaneously. Programmed electric stimulation is also given at various parts of the heart using catheters for diagnostic and therapeutic purposes. The uses and indications for cardiac electrophysiologic studies are expanding and evolving continuously. The technique was initially used mainly for diagnostic purposes. Subsequently, therapeutic applications such as drug therapy guided by electrophysiologic study, endocardial mapping for surgical therapy of ventricular tachycardia or WPW syndrome were added. Electrophysiologic studies are also used for risk stratifications of patients with various cardiac conditions such as conduction disturbances, nonsustained VT, WPW syndrome and others. Percutaneous transcatheter ablation of the AV junction for refractory SVT or WPW syndrome and ablation of VT are also performed by invasive cardiac electrophysiologists.

I. TECHNIQUES OF ELECTROPHYSIOLOGIC STUDIES

Cardiac electrophysiologic studies are performed in a cardiac catheterization laboratory. Multipolar electrode catheters are introduced percutaneously using femoral, subclavian, internal jugular, and antecubital veins. The catheters are advanced under fluoroscopic guidance to various sites of the heart, such as the high right atrium, the His bundle region, the right ventricular apex, and the

405

coronary sinus. Bipolar intracardiac electrocardiograms are recorded at these sites. The intracardiac electrocardiograms are usually filtered at 30 to 500 Hz. Multiple surface electrocardiograms (leads I, II, aVF and V_1) are simultaneously recorded. Electric stimulation is performed at various sites using an external programmed stimulator connected to the catheters. For this reason, the technique is also called programmed electrical stimulation or programmed stimulation (PES) of the heart. The risks and complications of electrophysiologic studies are very low when performed at a cardiac catheterization laboratory by experienced personnel. The reported mortality rates for electrophysiologic studies are lower than those for diagnostic coronary angiography.

A. Sinus Node Function Tests

Sinus function tests, such as the sinus node recovery time (SRT) or the sinoatrial conduction time (SACT), could be performed during electrophysiologic studies. In some cases, the intrinsic heart rate could be measured following autonomic blockade with atropine and propranolol to determine the mechanism of the bradycardia. However, the role of electrophysiologic studies is limited to clinical management of patients with abnormal or suspected abnormal sinus node function caused by a lack of sensitivity of the sinus function tests.

B. The His Bundle Electrocardiogram

The His bundle electrocardiogram allows evaluation of the conduction of various cardiac tissue (Fig. 22–1). The PR interval of the surface electrocardiogram could be divided into three segments, the PA, AH, and HV intervals. The PA interval is the interval from the onset of the p-wave to the atrial depolarization at the His bundle region, and represents the conduction time in the right atrium from the sinus node to the AV node. The AH interval, from the atrial depolarization near the His bundle region to the His bundle deflection, represents the conduction time in the AV node. The HV interval, from the onset of the His bundle deflection to the onset of the ventricular deflection, represents the conduction time in the His-Purkinje system. Measurement of the intervals, therefore, can elucidate and localize disturbances in the AV conduction.

The AH interval is prolonged by drugs, such as digoxin, beta blockers, calcium channel blockers, and adenosine, and by conditions such as an inferior myocardial infarction, myocarditis, or congenital heart block. The AH interval is shortened by atropine and isoproterenol. Class 1A antiarrhythmic agents such as procainamide mostly affect the HV interval. Heart blocks associated with an acute anterior wall myocardial infarction and bundle branch block are mostly caused by conduction disturbances in the His-Purkinje system and the block occurs at or below the His bundle (the infra-His block).

In patients with asymptomatic second-degree AV block not associated with myocardial infarction, the site of block is a

Normal Sequence

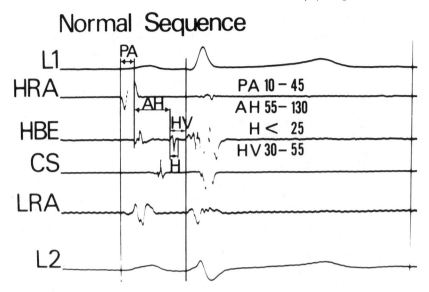

FIG. 22–1. The His bundle electrocardiogram during sinus rhythm. Normal values of PA, H and HV intervals are shown in msec. CS = coronary sinus electrocardiogram; HBE = His bundle electrocardiogram; L1 = lead I; L2 = lead II; LRA = Low right atrial electrocardiogram; HRA = High right atrial electrocardiogram.

determinant of long-term prognosis. Patients with a block at the AV node level (the supra-His block) have benign outcomes while patients with a block at or below the His bundle may develop sudden complete heart block with very slow ventricular escape rhythm. In patients with symptomatic second or third degree AV block, the level of the block is not important and a permanent pacemaker is indicated regardless of the level of the block. In patients with bundle branch block and symptoms suggestive of intermittent AV block, the measurement of the HV interval may be useful. A development of block at the HV level (atrial depolarizations followed by His bundle depolarizations but not by ventricular depolarizations—infra-His block) during atrial pacing is a sign of significant disease in the contralateral bundle branch and generally considered as an indication for a permanent pacemaker. Infra-His block during atrial single extrastimulus testing is not an indication for a pacemaker. The development of second or third degree AV block after intravenous infusion of procainamide is also generally considered an indication for a permanent pacemaker. Many investigators consider marked prolongation of the HV interval (e.g., greater than 100 msec) in patients with bundle branch block and intermittent symptoms an indication for a permanent pacemaker.

In asymptomatic patients with chronic bifascicular or trifascicular block without documented second degree or advanced AV blocks the His bundle electrogram is not indicated.

In patients with AV block associated with acute myocardial infarction, the presence of previously not documented bundle branch block is prognostically significant. Patients with transient second or third degree AV block associated with a new bundle branch block are treated with a permanent pacemaker.

C. Recording of the His Bundle ECG During Tachycardia

When a patient has a wide QRS complex tachycardia and the rhythm diagnosis is uncertain by the surface ECG, the recording of the His bundle ECG will clarify the diagnosis. During supraventricular tachycardia with aberrancy, the impulse is conducted via the His bundle to the ventricle. Therefore, the His bundle ECG always precedes the ventricular electrogram (the QRS complex). During ventricular tachycardia, the His bundle depolarization does not precede the ventricle depolarizations. Therefore, the His bundle deflections are not visible before the ventricular electrocardiograms.

D. Incremental Atrial Pacing and Ramp Atrial Pacing

Incremental atrial pacing (a stepwise increase of the pacing rate) or ramp pacing (a continuous and progressive increase of the pacing rate) is performed to evaluate the AV nodal conduction. As the rate of atrial pacing is increased incrementally, conduction via the AV node becomes slower due to decremental conduction property of the AV node, resulting in a gradual prolongation of the AH interval and the PR interval. At higher pacing rates, the conduction in the AV node is further slowed with an eventual development of Wenckebach phenomenon from a block at the AV node (the supra-His block or AH block).

The rate of atrial pacing at which the Wenckebach phenomenon is observed varies greatly. However, most adult patients develop Wenckebach phenomenon during atrial pacing at rates lower than 200/min. Patients with enhanced AV nodal conduction or patients with increased sympathetic tone such as in thyrotoxicosis or bronchial asthma, may exhibit 1:1 conduction at higher rates. The development of the Wenckebach phenomenon during atrial pacing at rates lower than 100/min indicates significant AV nodal dysfunction.

Decremental conduction (slower conduction at higher rates) noted in AV nodal tissue is usually not seen in other conduction tissues such as the His-Purkinje system or accessory pathways (Kent bundle). Therefore, the absence of decremental conduction during incremental atrial pacing suggests the presence of an accessory pathway.

E. Extrastimulus Testing

Extrastimulus testing is also used to evaluate conduction and refractory periods of cardiac tissues. By this technique, the right atrium is paced at a constant rate for 8 beats (the basic drive pacing) and a premature atrial extrastimulus is given at the end of the drive pacing. The coupling interval of the premature beat (the interval between the last drive pacing and the premature beat) is shortened progressively. The AH and HV intervals (the PR interval) and the configuration of the QRS complex following the premature atrial beat are observed.

Evaluation of the prolongation of the AH interval during progressively premature atrial stimuli can provide important diagnostic data. In patients with SVT caused by a dual AV node, there is a sudden increase in the AH interval when the premature extrastimulus reaches the refractory period of the fast pathway and the AV nodal conduction is exclusively via the slow pathway. The block at the fast pathway and the slower conduction via the slow pathway may initiate SVT due to AV node re-entry (see Induction of Tachycardia). In patients with WPW syndrome, when the premature extrastimulus is given, the conduction via the AV node becomes slow while the conduction via the Kent bundle is unchanged. While the impulse via the AV node is delayed, the impulse via the Kent bundle propagates to the ventricle without any delays causing preexcitation of a larger portion of the ventricle near the Kent bundle insertion (Fig. 22–2). As the extrastimulus becomes progressively premature, the delay in the AV node becomes progressively longer and a progressively larger portion of the ventricle is preexcited by the impulse propagating from the Kent bundle. The QRS complex, therefore, becomes progressively wider. When the extrastimulus reaches the refractory period of Kent bundle, suddenly AV conduction is exclusively via the normal pathway. The PR interval is abruptly prolonged with a normal narrow QRS complex without ventricular preexcitation. The development of a block at the Kent bundle accompanied by the slow conduction via the AV node may initiate an orthodromic tachycardia (see Induction of Tachycardia).

F. Evaluation of Retrograde Conduction

Retrograde conduction from the ventricle to the atrium is also evaluated during electrophysiologic studies. Extrastimulus testing and incremental or ramp pacing techniques described earlier are used for this purpose. The retrograde conduction should also exhibit the decremental conduction noted during antegrade conduction and the VA interval should prolong gradually with extrastimulus testing. Some patients with a normal AV conduction, however, may have no retrograde conduction at all. Others may exhibit only minimal decrement during the extrastimulus testing or ramp pacing in the absence of the Kent bundle. Administration of AV node blocking agents, such as adenosine, may unmask the decremental conduction. No decremental conduction is noted in the presence of the Kent bundle. Concealed WPW syndrome, in which the Kent bundle can conduct only retrogradely from the ventricle to atrium and not antegradely, could be easily diagnosed by this technique.

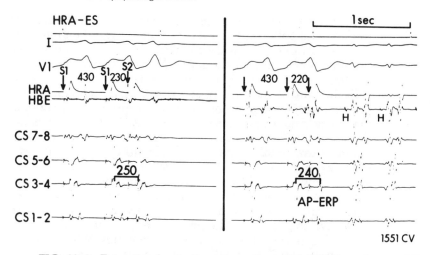

FIG. 22–2. Extrastimulus testing of a patient with WPW syndrome. AP-ERP = effective refractory period of accessory pathway; CS = coronary sinus electrocardiogram (recordings of left atrial and ventricular electrogram by a multipolar catheter placed in the coronary sinus). CS 1–2, 3–4, 5–6, and 7–8 indicate electrogram recorded at different sites in the coronary sinus; HBE = His bundle ECG; HRA = high right atrial ECG; HRA-ES = high right atrial extrastimulus. In the left panel, the high right atrium is paced at 140/min (S_1S_1 interval of 430 msec) and a single extrastimulus (S_2) is given after 230 msec. Because of the delay in the AV node, the ventricle is depolarized almost exclusively via the Kent bundle, with a resultant wide and bizzare QRS complex (the third QRS in V_1). In the right panel, the S_1S_2 coupling interval is shortened by 10 msec (from 230 to 220 msec). The Kent bundle becomes refractory (effective refractory of accessory pathway) and the atrial extrastimulus (S_2) is conducted exclusively via the AV node with a long delay in the AV node. Note the long AH interval in HBE and normal and narrow QRS complexes in leads I and V_1. This initiates a retrograde conduction via the Kent bundle as evidenced by the earliest atrial depolarization at CS 3–4 and AV re-entrant tachycardia. Numbers in CS 3–4 (250 and 240 msec) indicate coupling intervals of extrastimulus at the area.

The evaluation of the retrograde conduction is also important in the management of pacemaker-mediated tachycardia (PMT).

G. Induction of Tachycardia

Tachycardias from re-entry could be induced easily during programmed extrastimulus testing. The requirement for re-entry includes a potential circuit, unidirectional block, and slow conduction. One clear example of arrhythmias due to re-entry in the human is the AV re-entrant tachycardia (reciprocating tachycardia) in the WPW syndrome (Fig. 22–2). In this condition, the potential circuit is comprised of the AV node, the His-Purkinje system, the ventricular myocardium, the Kent bundle and the atrium. An APC blocked at the Kent bundle

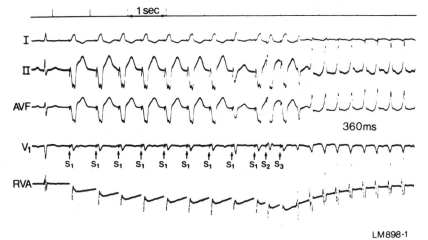

FIG. 22–3. Induction of ventricular tachycardia by programmed stimulation. RVA = right ventricular apex electrocardiogram; S_1 = pacer artifact for basic drive pacing at 100/min; S_2 = the first extrastimulus; S_3 = the second extrastimulus. Double extrastimuli (S_2S_3) induced a ventricular tachycardia of 170/min (tachycardia cycle length = 360 ms).

caused by refractoriness of the Kent bundle may be able to conduct slowly via the AV node. When the impulse finally reaches the ventricular insertion site of the Kent bundle, the Kent bundle may no longer be refractory. The impulse will, therefore, propagate retrogradely to the atrium from the ventricle via the Kent bundle. The re-entry initiated by unidirectional block (the antegrade block from the atrium to the ventricle with preserved retrograde conduction from the ventricle to the atrium) and slow conduction perpetuates to maintain the AV re-entrant tachycardia. During electrophysiologic studies, the re-entry can be reproduced. A critically timed premature extrastimulus will create the unidirectional block in the Kent bundle and the slow conduction in the AV node and will initiate a re-entry tachycardia (see Extrastimulus Testing). Other tachycardias from re-entry, such as the AV nodal re-entry or certain ventricular tachycardias, can also be induced by the extrastimulus testing by creating the unidirectional block and slow conduction. Sometimes 2 or 3 extrastimuli (doubles or triples) are necessary to create the critical conduction delay and unidirectional block necessary for the initiation of the re-entry (Fig. 22–3). Rapid burst or ramp pacing could also be used to initiate tachycardias. Sometimes drugs, such as isoproterenol or atropine, could be used to facilitate the induction.

The induction of these common clinical arrhythmias enables us to investigate further their anatomic origin, responses to

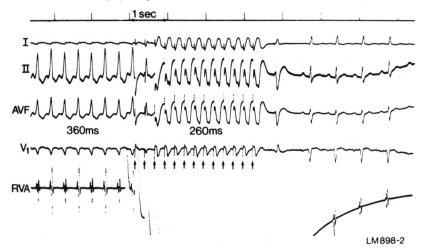

FIG. 22–4. Termination of ventricular tachycardia by rapid ventricular pacing. The ventricular tachycardia induced by PES (Fig. 22–3) was terminated by rapid ventricular pacing at 230/min (pacing interval = 260 ms). Arrows indicate pacing artifacts.

pharmacologic or nonpharmacologic interventions, and mechanisms and characteristics.

H. Termination of Tachycardia

Tachycardias induced by programmed stimulation or spontaneous tachycardias can often be terminated during electrophysiologic studies. A single extrastimulus could terminate slower tachycardias due to re-entry by altering the refractory period and the conduction velocity of tissues involved in the re-entry. However, multiple extrastimuli or burst pacing are often necessary to terminate rapid tachycardia (Fig. 22–4). Atrial flutter, SVT due to AV node re-entry, AV re-entrant tachycardias in WPW syndrome and ventricular tachycardia can often be terminated by rapid pacing, thus avoiding DC cardioversion.

II. MECHANISMS OF TACHYCARDIA AND PROGRAMMED STIMULATION

There are three potential mechanisms of tachycardias, i.e., automaticity, triggered activity and re-entry.

Automaticity is the result of spontaneous phase 4 depolarization and could be categorized into two groups, normal and abnormal, according to the resting membrane potential. Inappropriate sinus tachycardia is a clinical example of arrhythmia due to *normal automaticity. Abnormal automaticity* may be the mechanism of accelerated ventricular rhythms after myocardial infarction. Automatic rhythms cannot be reliably initiated or terminated by programmed stimulation.

Triggered activity results from after-depolarization. This is divided into two types: early and late after-depolarization. *Early after-depolarizations* occur before complete repolarization and have been noted in hypokalemia, acidosis, and during antiarrhythmic drug therapy. Arrhythmias associated with early after-depolarizations are bradycardia-dependent. Torsades de pointes from the congenital long QT syndrome, or drug-induced long QT may be caused by early after-depolarizations. This arrhythmia cannot be initiated or terminated by programmed stimulation. *Delayed after-depolarizations* occur after complete repolarization. Some digoxin-induced arrythmias may be due to this mechanism. Triggered rhythm from this mechanism is less reliably initiated and terminated by programmed stimulation: rapid pacing is a more reliable method to induce this arrhythmia.

Re-entry results from unidirectional block and slow conduction in anatomic or functional circuits (see Induction of Tachycardia). Arrhythmias from re-entry are reliably induced and terminated by programmed stimulation. Examples are AV re-entrant tachycardias in WPW syndrome, AV nodal re-entrant tachycardias, some ventricular tachycardias especially in patients with chronic coronary artery disease, and atrial flutter.

III. CLINICAL APPLICATIONS OF ELECTROPHYSIOLOGIC STUDIES

A. Evaluation of Effects of Antiarrhythmic Drugs

Evaluation of antiarrhythmic drug effect is one of the most important clinical applications of cardiac electrophysiologic studies. The reproducible induction and termination of many clinical arrhythmias prompted the use of this technique in evaluating the efficacy of antiarrhythmic agents. If a tachycardia is still inducible by programmed stimulation during drug therapy, the drug is considered ineffective. If the tachycardia is no longer inducible by programmed stimulation during a therapy, the therapy is considered effective. This technique has been used extensively in patients with sustained ventricular tachycardia and other arrhythmias. Electrophysiologic studies are also used to evaluate the effects of drugs on the various conduction systems in the heart.

B. Endocardial Mapping

By recording intracardiac electrocardiograms at multiple sites simultaneously during a tachycardia, the sequence of depolarization of various sites in the ventricle or atrium can be determined and the site of origin of the arrhythmia can be localized. This is essential for successful surgical therapy or ablation therapy of conditions such as WPW syndrome or ventricular tachycardia.

C. Evaluation of Patients for Antitachycardia Devices

Certain tachycardias could be reliably terminated by rapid antitachycardia pacing. If a patient does not want to take medications for an indefinite period of time, or if medications are ineffective or not tolerated, supraventricular tachycardias caused by the AV node re-entry often can be treated with rapid atrial pacing using a permanent pacemaker. Electrophysiologic studies are mandatory to determine the efficacy of this technique before implanting pacemakers.

Implantable automatic defibrillators are widely used for treatment of ventricular tachycardias or ventricular fibrillation. Electrophysiologic studies are necessary for proper selection of patients, selection of an appropriate device, intraoperative testings including the measurement of DFT (defibrillation threshold), and postoperative testing and management.

D. Evaluation of Conduction Disease

Electrophysiologic studies are used in the assessment of conduction disease to determine the need for a permanent pacemaker (see the His-bundle Electrocardiogram).

E. Percutaneous Transcatheter Ablation

The precise origin of an arrhythmia is essential for nonsurgical percutaneous transcatheter ablation. Ablation could be achieved by DC shocks or radiofrequency (RF) energy. Ablation therapy is used in SVT due to AV nodal re-entry, AF with rapid ventricular response refractory to drug therapy, and WPW syndrome. Ablation of VT focus, although less effective, could also be performed.

F. Diagnosis of Arrhythmias

Electrophysiologic studies are useful in patients with wide QRS complex tachycardias for determining the mechanism of the tachycardia. In patients with a narrow QRS tachycardia, the precise mechanism of the tachycardia could be determined by electrophysiologic studies for better management of the arrhythmia. In patients with syncope of unknown origin, when other causes are excluded, electrophysiologic studies could reveal cardiac arrhythmias.

G. Risk Stratification of Certain Clinical Conditions

The measurement of Kent bundle refractory periods is important in predicting the risk of malignant arrhythmias. Electrophysiologic studies are also used by some investigators for risk stratification of patients in clinical conditions such as post-myocardial infarction, nonsustained ventricular tachycardia, congestive cardiomyopathy, and hypertrophic cardiomyopathy.

IV. ELECTROPHYSIOLOGIC STUDIES IN SPECIFIC ARRHYTHMIAS

A. Sinus Dysrhythmia

Electrophysiologic studies are not very sensitive in detecting intermittent severe bradycardia from sinus node dysfunction. Although sinus re-entry tachycardia may be reproduced by programmed stimulation, electrophysiologic studies are usually not indicated in this condition.

B. Atrial Fibrillation and Flutter

Rapid atrial pacing can often be used to terminate atrial flutter. Epicardial temporary pacing wires left after an open heart surgery are used for rapid atrial pacing in postoperative atrial flutter. For patients with atrial flutter in whom a DC cardioversion is undesirable for various reasons, a transvenous temporary pacing catheter placed in the right atrium could be used. The role of PES-guided drug therapy for prevention of atrial fibrillation and flutter is not established. Electrophysiologic studies are necessary when electric ablation of the AV node to control ventricular response is attempted.

C. Supraventricular Tachycardias

Electrophysiologic studies of normal QRS complex tachycardia can define the mechanism, like junctional re-entry or concealed accessory pathway, and are helpful in selecting the appropriate therapy such as drugs, antitachycardia pacing, or ablation (see Extrastimulus Testing and Induction of Tachycardia). PES-guided drug therapy may be desirable but is optional in many patients with these non-lifethreatening arrhythmias. In addition, the PES-guided therapy may not be reliable because the arrhythmia substrate in SVT is easily modulated by automatic influences. However, when curative surgical or ablation therapy is considered or when antitachycardia therapy is considered, electrophysiologic studies must be performed. Paroxysmal atrial tachycardias, non-paroxysmal junctional tachycardia, and multifocal atrial tachycardias are not reproducibly induced by programmed stimulation.

D. WPW Syndrome

In patients with symptomatic WPW syndrome, electrophysiologic studies are indicated to document the mechanism of the arrhythmia and to estimate the risk of sudden death from ventricular fibrillation. Atrial fibrillation is induced during electrophysiologic studies to determine the shortest preexcited R-R interval. Patients with an R-R interval of less than 250 msec may be at risk of sudden death from ventricular fibrillation in the event of atrial fibrillation. Orthodromic or antidromic AV re-entrant tachycardia is easily induced by programmed stimulation (see Extrastimulus Testing and Induction of Tachycardia). The diagnosis of concealed WPW syndrome could only be made by electrophysiologic studies. The effects of antiarrhythmic agents on the refractory periods of the Kent bundle could be determined by electrophysiologic studies. Endocardial mapping study could localize the precise location of the accessory pathway and guide curative catheter ablation therapy or surgical resection. PES-guided drug therapy is useful but of limited value because the re-entry circuit of the AV re-entrant tachycardia is easily modulated by autonomic influences and effects of drugs on spontaneous atrial fibrillation cannot be reliably predicted by PES. The role of electrophysiologic studies in asymptomatic patients with ventricular preexcitation on a routine ECG has not been established.

E. Bundle Branch Block and AV Block

See the His bundle ECG.

F. Wide QRS Complex Tachycardia

Electrophysiologic studies are useful to determine the mechanism of wide complex tachycardias. Supraventricular tachycardia with aberrancy could be easily distinguished by electrophysiologic studies. A diagnosis of antidromic AV re-entrant tachycardia of WPW syndrome could be established by electrophysiologic studies. Most wide complex tachycardias are, however, ventricular in origin.

G. Sustained Ventricular Tachycardia in Coronary Disease

Electrophysiologic studies are most commonly used in this condition. Ventricular tachycardias not associated with an acute myocardial infarction in chronic coronary disease are easily induced by programmed stimulation. The reproducible induction of VT by programmed stimulation makes it possible to evaluate the effects of drug therapy on the inducibility of arrhythmias by programmed stimulation. When VT becomes no longer inducible during a drug therapy, the therapy is very effective in preventing recurrences of the arrhythmia. A failure to suppress the inducibility during a therapy, however, does not indicate good long-term outcomes especially in patients taking amiodarone.

The nonspecificity of the induced VT by PES during a therapy led to alternative efficacy criteria by PES. If VT remains inducible by PES but the patient tolerates the induced arrhythmia well because the rate of VT is slower during the drug therapy, the patient may survive spontaneous recurrence of VT. Changes in the mode of induction of VT (for example, requiring more extrastimuli to induce VT during a therapy as compared to the baseline) are not useful in predicting drug efficacy.

An alternative approach to the PES-guided drug therapy is drug therapy guided by Holter monitoring and exercise testing. The limitation of the noninvasive approach is poor sensitivity. A suppression of VPCs during drug therapy does not preclude poor outcomes. Therefore, invasive and noninvasive methods (PES and Holter and exercise testing) have values as well as limitations and are complementary. Both methods together may be more useful than either alone in identifying optimal antiarrhythmic drug regimens.

Endocardial catheter mapping studies are important for surgical treatment of VT in chronic ischemic heart disease and crucial in catheter ablation of VT.

H. Sustained VT in Congestive Cardiomyopathy

Re-entry may be the predominant mechanism of sustained VT in congestive cardiomyopathy. VT from bundle branch re-entry is not rare. VT could be reliably induced by PES in 60 to 70% of patients as compared to 90 to 95% in patients with chronic coronary disease and VT. PES-guided therapy is commonly used, although the technique is somewhat less reliable than in patients with chronic ischemic heart disease.

I. VT in Apparently Normal Heart

Repetitive monomorphic VT occurs in the young and middle aged, and often is associated with exercise or emotional stress. The morphology of VT is left bundle branch block and normal or right axis configuration. A burst of nonsustained VT and intervening sinus rhythm are typical. The VT is not reproduced by PES but is provoked by exercise or catecholamines, suggesting a mechanism of abnormal automaticity. *Paroxysmal sustained monomorphic VT* is similar to repetitive monomorphic VT but longer in duration and may be induced by PES. It may be a triggered rhythm from delayed after-depolarizations. *Idiopathic left ventricular tachycardia* is also noted in young patients with apparently normal hearts. This VT is of right bundle branch block and left axis configuration, may be caused by fascicular re-entry, and is inducible by PES. VT is responsive to verapamil therapy. Beta blockers are usually not effective.

J. Arrhythmogenic Right Ventricular Dysplasia (ARVD)

This condition is characterized by fatty infiltration and fibrosis of the right ventricle. It is typically noted in males and causes recurrent VT, syncope, and cardiac arrest. The morphology of VT is left bundle branch block pattern. VT may be induced by PES in some patients.

K. Hypertrophic Cardiomyopathy

The mechanism of sudden death in this condition may be multifactorial including but not limited to supraventricular tachyarrhythmia and ventricular arrhythmias. Although polymorphic VT is more often induced in patients with a history of cardiac arrest, the role of PES in risk stratification and the role of PES-guided therapy have not been established.

L. Mitral Valve Prolapse

The mechanism of VT or cardiac arrest in this condition is not well known. VT is not reproducibly induced by PES.

M. Cardiac Arrests

Many patients with poor ventricular function due to ischemic heart disease or dilated cardiomyopathy die suddenly. Cardiac arrests and sudden deaths are usually caused by rapid ventricular tachycardia, ventricular tachycardia degenerating into ventricular fibrillation, or ventricular fibrillation. Bradyarrhythmias may be the mechanism in some 10 to 20% of cases. Preventing a recurrence of cardiac arrest in patients who survived an out-of-hospital sudden death remains a challenge in modern cardiology. The recurrence rate of cardiac arrests not associated with an acute myocardial infarction or reversible causes such as drugs, electrolyte imbalances or myocarditis may be approximately 35% in 2 years. Electrophysiologic studies are used for the management of survivors of out-of-hospital cardiac arrest. VT induced by PES in this condition is usually very fast and poorly tolerated. Polymorphic VT or ventricular fibrillation may be the only arrhythmia inducible by PES. Drug therapy is guided by PES if VT is induced by PES. Drug therapy guided by PES in patients with inducible VF or polymorphic VT may not be as reliable as in patients with inducible monomorphic VT by PES. Implantable defibrillators, amiodarone and Holter-guided therapy are alternative methods used by some investigators.

Some patients with a history of a cardiac arrest do not have any PES-inducible tachyarrhythmias. These patients tend to have a better prognosis if the left ventricular function is preserved or if the initial event was associated with reversible causes, such as acute ischemia, and the cause is corrected. The optimal therapy of this condition is controversial. Holter-guided therapy, amiodarone or implantable defibrillators are used in this situation. No PES-induced VT in patients with a poor ventricle, especially in patients with dilated cardiomyopathy, is associated with a poor outcome. Amiodarone or implantable automatic defibrillators should be used in this situation.

N. Syncope of Unknown Origin

Electrophysiologic studies are indicated in patients with syncope if the cause cannot be identified after careful screening. Electrophysiologic studies may uncover cardiac arrhythmias such as VT, SVT, or bradycardia. The diagnostic yield is higher in patients with a known cardiac disease and relatively low in patients with apparently normal hearts. Treatment of arrhythmia uncovered by electrophysiologic study often improves the symptoms. Negative electrophysiologic studies do not preclude cardiac syncope, especially syncopes associated with the long QT syndrome, intermittent bradycardia due to sinus dysfunction, vagotonia, or other autonomic dysfunction. Carotid sinus massage or a tilt table test may uncover abnormalities.

O. Nonsustained VT

Nonsustained VT in patients with poor ventricular function is associated with increased cardiac mortality from sudden and nonsudden death. The degree of ventricular dysfunction is the most powerful prognostic indicator. Programmed stimulation has been used for risk stratifications. If a sustained VT is inducible by PES, the risk of sudden death is higher. If no VT is inducible, the risk of sudden death may be lower especially in patients with coronary disease. However, the role of PES for risk stratification and selection of therapy in this clinical setting has not been firmly established.

P. Post-myocardial Infarction Patients

The presence of VPCs, late potentials in the signal averaged ECG and decreased left ventricular ejection fraction are predictors of late sudden deaths after acute myocardial infarction.

The role of PES in predicting late sudden deaths after myocardial infarction is controversial.

Q. Proarrhythmia

Proarrhythmia is a worsening of arrhythmias caused by antiarrhythmic agents. Proarrhythmia is caused by the effect of drugs like prolongation of the QT interval, slowing of conduction velocity, or changes in the refractory periods of cardiac tissues. These effects are considered antiarrhythmic effects and in some situations may facilitate arrhythmogenesis, cause a new arrhythmia, or aggravate existing arrhythmias.

Proarrhythmia from class 1A antiarrhythmic agents (quinidine, procainamide or disopyramide) manifests as torsades de pointes, associated with a prolongation of the QT interval. Bradycardias, hypokalemia, or hypomagnesemia often precipitate this arrhythmia. This arrhythmia may be due to early afterdepolarizations and cannot be induced by programmed stimulation. Therefore, PES cannot be used to predict this proarrhythmia. Torsades de pointes due to antiarrhythmic drugs could be treated by magnesium, isoproterenol infusion, or by preventing bradycardia using a temporary overdrive pacing.

Proarrhythmia from class 1C agents, such as flecainide and encainide, manifests as intractable sustained monomorphic VT not easily terminated by DC shocks, or as a development of a new sustained VT that the patient has never experienced. The mechanism of the proarrhythmia may be in part related to slowed conduction in re-entry circuits without significant prolongation of refractory periods. Ischemia may play an important role in the genesis of proarrhythmia. Risk factors for proarrhythmia from class 1C agents include ventricular dysfunction, a history of sustained VT or a higher dose or too rapid upward titration of the dosage of these agents. The development of sustained VT is often preceded by a marked suppression of spontaneous VPCs. Therefore, Holter monitoring is not useful in predicting this type of proarrhythmia. The role of PES in predicting this type of proarrhythmia is unknown. Exercise testing may unmask proarrhythmic effects of class 1C agents and induce malignant arrhythmias.

By Holter monitoring, a marked increase (for example a seven-fold increase) in VPCs or asymptomatic nonsustained VT after initiation of an antiarrhythmic agent is considered proarrhythmia. However, the clinical significance and long-term effects of this type of proarrhythmia are unclear.

By PES, a conversion from an induction of nonsustained VT to an induction of sustained VT and an induction of VT in previously noninducible patients after drug therapy may be considered proarrhythmia. The clinical significance of these is unknown. An easier induction of VT during therapy is not considered proarrhythmia. For example, if VT is inducible by double extrastimuli during therapy as compared to triple extrastimuli before the therapy, the therapy is not considered proar-rhythmic.

R. Congenital Long QT Syndromes

Torsades de pointes in patients with idopathic congenital long QT syndromes may be caused by early after-depolariza-tions. This arrhythmia is not induced by PES: therefore therapy cannot be guided by PES. Sympathetic imbalance and left stel-late ganglion stimulation may be related to this arrhythmia. Beta blockers and left stellate ganglionectomy are effective in preventing this arrhythmia and sudden death.

S. Acquired Drug-Induced Long QT Syndrome

Torsades de pointes from drugs such as quinidine may also be caused by early after-depolarizations. Unlike the congenital long QT syndrome, beta blockers are not used for the treatment of the arrhythmia. Beta blockers may precipitate torsades de pointes by inducing bradycardia (see Proarrhythmia). This arrhythmia is not induced by PES.

T. Surgical Therapy of Arrhythmias

Surgery for the WPW syndrome involves resection of the Kent bundle. Preoperative and intraoperative electrophysio-logic studies and mapping are essential. The cure rate is greater than 95% and the surgical mortality is less than 1% when per-formed by experienced surgeons and electrophysiologists. AV node re-entry tachycardia could also be treated surgically by modifying the AV nodal conduction without producing com-plete AV block, thus avoiding a permanent pacemaker.

Surgery for ventricular tachycardia is performed when recur-rent ventricular tachycardia cannot be controlled by medical therapy. In patients with VT and previous myocardial infarc-tion, the VT often originates from surviving endocardium near the scar tissue. Endocardial resection guided by preoperative and intraoperative mapping studies often eliminates the sub-strate of the tachycardia. A blind resection of scarred endocar-ium without guidance of mapping study is also used. In patients with VT from noncoronary disease, the focus of the arrhythmia may not be in the endocardium. Cyrosurgery guided by endocardial and epicardial mapping studies is often used. Surgical therapy for VT is used in fewer and more selected patients nowadays because of the relatively high surgical mor-tality of 10 to 15% and the advent of implantable defibrillators.

Coronary bypass surgery is usually ineffective in preventing recurrent VT. However, the outcome of patients with ventric-ular fibrillation may improve after bypass surgery especially when the event may be related to ischemia.

U. Antiarrhythmic Devices

Implantable automatic defibrillator is very effective in pre-venting sudden death due to malignant ventricular tachyar-rhythmias. Upon detecting rapid rhythm, the device will deliver an electric shock of up to 30 joules to terminate the arrhythmia. For sensing, bipolar epicardial or endocardial electrodes are used. For defibrillation, two large epicardial patch electrodes are usually used. Some models have rapid pacing capability for termination of VT in addition to the high energy defibrillation. Electrophysiologic studies are necessary for proper selection of patients, selection of appropriate devices, and testing of efficacy of the device.

The use and indication of implantable defibrillators are evolving as the technology and surgical technique improve. Currently, most defibrillators require a thoracotomy. The surgical mortality ranges between 2% and 5%. Future devices will be implanted by a nonthoracotomy approach and will have multiple programmable functions. Surgical mortality and morbidity will be decreased in the future and the use of the device therapy will expand rapidly. Using currently available defibrillators, sudden death rates are reduced to 2 to 6% per year. The sudden death rate, however, overestimates benefits of the defibrillator therapy. The true benefit of the defibrillator therapy is represented by the total arrhythmia-related death including sudden death, surgical mortality (caused by the therapy), and arrhythmia-related nonsudden deaths. When total arrhythmia-related deaths are considered, the benefits of defibrillator therapy become less dramatic.

Pacemakers capable of automatic or manually triggered rapid pacing are used to terminate recurrent SVT or VT in patients carefully selected by electrophysiologic studies. Automatic antitachycardia pacers for VT without a back-up defibrillation capability are not advised, because of potential acceleration of the VT.

V. Percutaneous Transcatheter Ablation

Refractory supraventricular tachyarrhythmias such as atrial flutter or fibrillation with rapid ventricular response or recurrent SVT due to the AV node re-entry could be treated by transcatheter ablation therapy. The His bundle and AV node are destroyed or modified by a high energy DC shock delivered by the catheter electrode. Radiofrequency energy is also used for this purpose. After the ablation, a permanent pacemaker is implanted. Late sudden deaths have been reported by some investigators in 2% of patients treated by this technique. The ablation therapy is also used for WPW syndrome due to posterior septal pathways. Ablation of left freewall pathways using radiofrequency energy may be used in many patients in the future, avoiding open heart surgery. Ablation of ventricular tachycardia is less successful and appears to be of limited value especially in patients with chronic ischemic heart disease. Ablation of the right bundle branch can abolish ventricular tachycardia caused by bundle branch re-entry often in dilated cardiomyopathy.

ACKNOWLEDGMENTS

We express our appreciation to Ms. Sandra Lenofsky for her secretarial assistance in the manuscript preparation.

SUGGESTED READINGS

Cooper, M.J., Anderson, K.P., and Mason, J.W.: Invasive electrophysiological studies. *In* D.P. Zipes and J. Jalife (eds): Cardiac Electrophysiology from Cell to Bedside. Philadelphia, W.B. Saunders Co., 1990.

Fisher, J.D., Furman, S., Kim, S.G., et al.: Tachycardia management by devices. *In* S.S. Barold and J. Mugica (eds): New Perspectives in Cardiac Pacing. Mount Kisco, N.Y., Futura Publishing Co., Inc., 1991.

Gallagher, J.J., Selle, J.G., Sealy, W.C., et al. Variants of pre-excitation: Update 1989. *In* D.P. Zipes and J. Jalife (eds): Cardiac Electrophysiology from Cell to Bedside. Philadelphia, W.B. Saunders Co., 1990.

Kim, S.G. Values and limitations of programmed stimulation and ambulatory monitoring in the management of ventricular tachycardia. Am. J. Cardiol. 62:71–121, 1988.

Kim. S.G. Management of survivors of cardiac arrest: Is electrophysiologic testing obsolete in the era of implantable defibrillators? J. Am. Coll. Cardiol. 16:756–762, 1990.

Kim, S.G., Fisher, J.D., Furman, S., et al. Benefits of implantable defibrillators are overestimated by sudden death rates and better represented by the total arrhythmic death rate. J. Am. Coll. Cardiol. (In press).

Martins, J.B., Constantin, L., Kienzle, S.L., et al. Mechanism of ventricular tachycardia unassociated with coronary artery disease. *In* D.P. Zipes and J. Jalife (eds): Cardiac Electrophysiology from Cell to Bedside. Philadelphia, W.B. Saunders Co., 1990.

Sung, R.J., Huycke, E.C., Keung, E.C., et al. Atrioventricular node reentry: Evidence of reentry and functional properties of fast and slow pathways. *In* D.P. Zipes and J. Jalife (eds): Cardiac Electrophysiology from Cell to Bedside. Philadelphia, W.B. Saunders Co., 1990.

Zipes, D.P. Cardiac electrophysiology: Promise and contributions. J. Am. Coll. Cardiol. 13:1329–1352, 1989.

INDEX

Page numbers with **bold letters** indicate the major discussion; "f" indicates illustrations.